The Bedside Torah

The Bedside Torah

wisdom, visions, and dreams

Rabbi Bradley Shavit Artson

Edited by Miriyam Glazer, Ph.D.

Contemporary Books

Chicago New York San Francisco Lisbon London Madrid Mexico City
Milan New Delhi San Juan Seoul Singapore Sydney Toronto

Library of Congress Cataloging-in-Publication Data

Artson, Bradley Shavit.
    The bedside torah / by Bradley Shavit Artson.
      p.   cm.
    Includes index.
    ISBN 0-7373-0587-8 (alk. paper)
    1. Boble. O.T. Pentateuch—Meditations.   I. Title.

BS1225.4 A73   2001
222'.107—dc21   2001028745

Contemporary Books

A Division of The McGraw·Hill Companies

4 5 6 7 8 9 0 DOC/DOC 0 9 8 7 6 5 4 3

ISBN 0-7373-0587-8

This book was designed and set in Garamond MT by Lovedog Studios
Printed and bound by R. R. Donnelley—Crawfordsville

Cover design by Laurie Young
Cover illustrations by Kristina Swarner

McGraw-Hill books are available at special quantity discounts to use as premiums and sales promotions, or for use in corporate training programs. For more information, please write to the Director of Special Sales, Professional Publishing, McGraw-Hill, Two Penn Plaza, New York, NY 10121-2298. Or contact your local bookstore.

This book is printed on acid-free paper.

For

ELANA,

I have nothing more precious than you.

Pesikta de-Rav Kahana 22:2:4

For

JACOB and SHIRA,

My child, more than a calf wants to drink,

the cow wants to suckle.

Pesashim 112a

And for

My *haverim* in the study of Torah

JEREMY BENSTEIN, LEE BEARSON,

DANIEL ORNSTEIN, ELIE SPITZ, ZALMAN MARCUS,

No matter what other doubts we may entertain,

we cannot question the reality of friendship.

And in a world where so little is certain, that is a great deal.

Rabbi Milton Steinberg, *As a Driven Leaf*

Contents

Leviticus

Numbers

Deuteronomy

Foreword

"Is my word not like . . . a hammer that shatters rock?" God once asked his prophet Jeremiah (Jer. 23:29). Jeremiah's reply on that occasion is not recorded, but we may be sure that, having spoken on other occasions as if he himself were the rock whom God's hammer was shattering, the prophet agreed. In later Jewish tradition, this vivid image underwent a remarkable inversion. God's word, once the hammer, now became the rock, and interpretation became the hammer. To borrow a pair of rabbinic terms that recur frequently in this book, the *pshat* or plain meaning of God's word became the rock, while *drash* or inventive commentary became the hammer.

Inventive commentary? Once commentary starts to invent, how can it remain mere commentary? The honest answer is that it cannot remain *mere* commentary, but traditional Jewish commentary has always gloried in its freedom to be more than *mere*. The Talmud itself gives the commentator his work permit: "As the hammer splits the rock into many splinters, so will a scriptural verse yield many meanings" (Sanhedrin 34a).

The hammer of traditional commentary begins by breaking the rock of Torah into fifty pieces, fifty portions or *parashiyot*, one for each of the fifty weeks of the lunar year. But this is no more than the beginning. Past this point, some strong hand must seize the hammer each week and strike anew. This is where Rabbi Bradley Shavit Artson comes in, making his own the venerable but still daring principle that it is "incumbent every moment to labor in the study of Torah and *to innovate to the full extent of one's abilities*."

Torah has its agenda, and its attitude. Artson arrives with an American agenda, and plenty of American attitude. The result? Sparks fly, rock splits, and veins of gold sparkle in the sudden light. Artson's hammer strikes three times upon each of the fifty *parashiyot*. As the year rolls by, the reader comes to know Torah better, but he or she also comes to know an American Jewish mind rather as the reader of an op-ed page comes to know the regular columnists. Something happens in Washington, and you know just what that opinionated so-and-so will have to say about it. You find yourself framing his thoughts for him, just to have the satisfaction of rebutting them. In other words, you take up your own hammer, you strike your own sparks, you mine yourself a little gold of your own.

But there is something else, something much gentler, to be said about this "bedside Torah." Different Jews go (or don't) to different synagogues, and few Gentiles ever enter to a synagogue at all, but at the end of the day everyone, Jew or Gentile, crawls into his own bed. Artson, who sees Torah as a treasure that no longer belongs exclusively to Israel, offers his work without discrimination to each man and each woman, believer or unbeliever. As a Gentile, I must admit that I hear this Jewish conversation as, from my bed, I might overhear a conversation from the other side of a hotel room wall. But have you never, perhaps as a child on the verge of adult awareness, overheard a conversation from your bed and discovered not the shameful secrets of the speakers, perhaps your parents, but their earnest aspirations, their touching admissions, their struggles?

This is what a Gentile reading this book may discover about American Judaism in the 5761st year since the creation of the world. And God's question to Jeremiah, to fill in the ellipsis above, was "Is my Word not *like a fire that burns* and like a hammer that shatters rock?" To play with Torah, make no mistake, is to play with fire, but a fire that burns is also a fire that, on a cold night, can warm, and who, Jew or Gentile, will not welcome a little extra warmth in bed?

—Jack Miles,
author of *God: A Biography*

Acknowledgments

Earlier versions of these meditations have already been published as a weekly Torah column in the *Orange County Heritage,* and I would like to thank that paper's editor, Dan Brin. It was my friend and mentor, Sam Smotrich, who insisted that I write these columns. Like so many of my rabbinic involvements, this one would not have happened but for his loving insistence. I owe him a great deal and miss him often.

Some of these essays also appeared in my weekly on-line Torah list, "Today's Torah," capably established and administered by Cheryl Peretz. I thank her and the many readers of "Today's Torah" who took the time to respond so thoughtfully to these reflections. I also gratefully acknowledge my debt to the Jewish Publication Society; its translation of the Hebrew Bible (*TANAKH: A New Translation of the Holy Scriptures According to the Traditional Hebrew Text,* Philadelphia, 1985) is the finest available. It forms the basis of all of the biblical quotations in these reflections. Additionally, many of these columns were reprinted in the Homiletics Service of the Rabbinical Assembly, the international association of Conservative rabbis. I consider it a great privilege to be able to share Torah with my colleagues, and their encouragement has led me to seek publication, so that these reflections might find a broader audience.

If you would like to receive "Today's Torah," at no charge,
please send a message to listserv@uj.edu with the following in the body
of the message: "SUBSCRIBE torah."

I am deeply grateful to the University of Judaism and its Ziegler School of Rabbinic Studies, which has provided me home, community, and fellowship beyond my greatest desires. The faculty, students, administrators, and lay leadership form a passionate and caring partnership in pursuit of Torah, and I am thrilled to be with them. It is a privilege to work with the university's president, Rabbi Robert Wexler, who is mentor, friend, colleague, and more. I learn from him daily, and am forever grateful for his leadership, his vision, and his steady friendship.

The editor of this volume is a remarkable scholar and friend. Professor Miriyam Glazer brings passion, zest, and depth to any project she pursues. Thank you, Miriyam, for the unanticipated joy of working together on this book. Your talents, energy, and warmth pervade every page.

I would also like to thank Rena J. Copperman, of McGraw-Hill Companies. Rena was the consummate professional, who took an unruly manuscript and nurtured it into a real book. Throughout this process, her ability to attend to minute details while holding on to the big picture was a source of inspiration and comfort. She has become both friend and colleague and I thank her.

My thanks also to the Jewish Theological Seminary, where I was ordained as a rabbi and where I still cherish my friendships and many close ties with faculty, administration, and students.

My deepest thanks to Maria Lara for all her care and assistance to me and to my family.

This collection is dedicated to my partners in Torah study *lishma* (Torah for its own sake) over the years, Jeremy Bernstein, Lee Bearson, Rabbi Daniel Ornstein, Rabbi Elie Spitz, and Rabbi Zalman Marcus; to my wife, Elana Shavit Artson; and to our children, Shira and Jacob.

For Jeremy, Lee, Daniel, Elie, and Zalman: Each one of these dear friends helped me to form my Jewish soul and to find my Jewish voice. All gave me a precious gift—their insights into our heritage, their love of Judaism and the Jewish people, and the chance to study in their presence. Each continues to work on behalf of our God, Torah, and Israel in ways that reflect his unique gifts of love, mind, and spirit.

Elana has been, in so many ways, the point of origin for many of the ideas found here. Her life is itself a commentary on the Torah and its values. Her deeds, her kindness, her love and compassion, and her passion for justice all embody in action what these words hope to express.

Being with her is a pleasant way to learn what Torah can mean for human living. I love her now even more than the day I married her, and consider our marriage God's greatest gift to me.

Shira and Jacob are the song in my heart. Their vitality, curiosity, challenges, and love fill my life. They constitute the most concrete demonstration of God's love in our lives. Their love of Judaism in general, and of Torah in particular, is a matter of great delight to their Ema and to me. I pray that the light of Torah will always make sure their step, and joyous their way.

And, *aharon, aharon haviv,* I am grateful beyond words to the Holy Blessing One, whose Torah I have been allowed to study, to teach, and to observe. *Modeh ani lefanekha, Adonai elohai, sheh-samta chelki mi-yoshvei beit ha-midrash.*

Introduction:
Reading Torah and
Hearing God's Voice

The Torah: it keeps a person from all evil in youth, and it offers
a future and a hope in old age.

—*Mishnah Kiddushin* 4:12

The public chanting of Torah marks the apex of Jewish worship. After
warming up with the recitation of psalms and entering God's presence
with the *Amidah,* the standing silent prayer, the congregation is ready as
individuals—now joined together in sacred community—to receive
God's teaching anew. For the revelation of Sinai, the moment of the
giving of the Torah, is renewed every time Jews take the Torah out of
the Ark, carry it among the congregation, and sing its words. Holding it
aloft, Jews point to our Torah in precisely the same way the Roman
masses would point to their conquering general or emperor at a tri-
umphal march. But the Latin words "*Ho Imperator*" have been replaced
with "*Ve-zot ha-Torah!* This is the Torah!" With that change, the arrogance of human might recedes before the infusion of divine energy,
light, and life of the Torah. Our simple ritual of removing the Torah
from the Ark, marching it around the sanctuary, reading from it, and
raising it recurs so often that we rarely pause to reflect on how odd this
Jewish practice is. While other religions *do* something at the core of their
services—transfigure the communion wafer, arrange an offering—we
Jews *read about* doing something. Thus, there is a strange passivity at the
pinnacle of our worship, and worse, there is often boredom: With
Hebrew a foreign language to many Jews, the Humash (the five books
of Moses) remains a closed book both literally and figuratively.
Torah-reading time during religious services is often treated as
"recess"—a time to attend to personal needs or to schmooze with a
friend. Yet, when Torah-reading intersects with a key life cycle juncture,

such as a Bar or Bat Mitzvah, hearing those ancient words read by the young man or woman can become the most powerful and inexpressible Jewish moment for exactly those same Jews who were, just the week before, schmoozing away.

This apparent contradiction—being moved to tears by a ritual that one otherwise often finds dull—is but the beginning. At a deeper level, the paradox of the Jewish People and our Torah is the contradiction of revering a book that remains largely unread and often ignored. No Jew alive implements every word of the Torah as its *p'shat,* its contextual meaning, would dictate. From the strictest literalist to the freest allegorist, we read the words of Torah through the filter of our choosing (a filter often selected along denominational lines). Consequently, none of us even attempts to enact every *mitzvah,* every commandment, in its biblical form. We don't ask *kohanim,* priests, to make legal rulings for us; we don't each write a Torah scroll manually; we don't practice polygamy, to name just a few biblical practices that are generally forgone. Most Jews, indeed, have changed the Torah from text into symbol. Strangely enough, however, though its content may be no longer embodied or even studied, Jews still grow weepy when they hear the words of Torah they don't understand and when they point to elevated words they cannot read. What's going on here? What accounts for the perplexing power of the ritual of holding the Torah aloft? Of hearing it chanted by a young person we love?

Why is this unread book capable of summoning such profound responses?

For some Jews, the power of Torah-reading is like the power of a photo album from childhood, or an old high school yearbook. Even without opening its covers, the sight of the album inspires love, along with a sense of nostalgia, a feeling of belonging, and a bittersweet joy at memories enshrined in the heart. Seeing the yearbook reminds us of where we've been, who we are, how far we've journeyed. The photos may not win any prizes, but for their owners, they are irreplaceable gateways to a crucial part of identity and to values.

For other Jews, Torah-reading is more like an empty ceremony, much like looking into someone else's wedding album. The key, as with other areas of Jewish passion, is to realize that it is not someone else's at all: It is *our* album, *our* betrothal, and *our* wedding. When we are emotionally receptive, when the Torah-reading reflects identification and involvement, its songs become our own. Seeing the scrolls just as they looked when we sat with our grandparents for a holiday, hearing the same singsong we first learned in Hebrew school, ignite a mix of nostalgia, identity, and reverence largely independent of the Torah's actual content or its "objective" value. In that sense, our passivity is a mask, our boredom a pose. Face to face with the connection to our past, the symbol of our essence, the sounds of our destiny, Jews respond with deep feeling. Just as we flip mindlessly through the pages of our photo albums, stopping when a particular photo grabs our attention, so we drift during the Torah-reading, reconnecting periodically for a passage we notice, for a child we love, for an *aliyah* that speaks to our hearts. And that rootedness of heart is all right, for, after all, "God wants the heart" (*Sanhedrin* 106b). The mind is a wonderful thing, but it follows the heart, amplifying the music the soul sings, reflecting the light of our shining spirit. Torah can ignite our hearts, and the heart is the true home of the *"pintele Yid,"* the spark of the Jew within us.

Rabbis and teachers of rabbis, trained in the intricacies of mind, celebrating a spirituality of intellect, often mistake the sanctuary for the classroom, confusing wisdom with knowledge, cutting the text with the scalpel of critical thought when what is called for is the softening touch of identification and intuition—an inner listening. The *kriyat ha-Torah,* the public chanting of the Torah, is an opportunity to ignite the flame of Sinai in each Jewish heart, enhanced with useful facts and grounded in knowledge, to be sure. But the goal is inspiration, not information, dedication, not mastery. *Drashot,* commentaries on the Torah, should build on the often-dormant emotional link between Jew and Torah, awakening the slumbering soul to a sense of wonder in the words that live again. The commentaries which follow seek to do just that. They do convey information: The *parashah* summaries detail the names and explain events that fill the Torah portions. But these commentaries aim for more than just a learned brain—they seek to address the heart.

Sinai is more than a mountain, and Torah is more than a text. As text, it is deep and worthy of serious study; for example, in Bible study fellowships, *Hevra Torah,* that meet before services or during the week, and offer rich, thought-provoking encounters with the text. Yet Torah is also a brush with holiness that comes straight from the heart and, as the Talmud reminds us, "What comes from the heart goes to the heart." Just as we need to study Torah, so, too, we need to hear the Torah sung. When coupled with the depths of emotion that a sense of belonging can evoke, when linked to the life passages of our loved ones or our community, when contemplating our own lives in the light of our spiritual journey, experiencing the chanting of Torah can become a renewed encounter with the mystery of the sacred, a second Sinai. We need to learn the language of the heart, and then to sing its song.

On the Value of Regular Torah Learning

Most of us could use some support to refrain from doing what we know is wrong. And when life seems overwhelming, a steady stream of encouragement, community, and faith can restore joy and wonder, invigorating us for the tasks ahead. A feeling of hope and a sense of purpose, as well as moral restraint: These, say the ancient sages of the *Mishnah,* are precisely the role that the first five books of the Bible, known as the Torah, can play in our lives. Perhaps that is why Jewish tradition sees the Torah as a gift from God.

Rabbinic law exhorts Jews to read the weekly Bible portion—what we will call throughout *The Bedside Torah* by the Hebrew word *parashah*—at least three times each week. To accommodate that expectation, it has become a custom to call worshipers to thank God for the gift of the Torah and to publicly chant from the scroll during the morning minyan, or prayer service on Monday, Thursday, and Saturday mornings. This commonsense approach ensures regular exposure to Israel's most sacred writings, permitting no more than a two-day interval between each new encounter with the Holy Scripture. The reflections in this collection take advantage of that same schedule, offering three different commentaries on each *parashah* for the entire year of Torah-readings. Having three commentaries, three different "takes," frees us to see the *parashah* from different perspectives, to ask different questions and to seek different answers, all of which enrich and enliven our daily living and nourish our desire for spiritual growth. The commentaries seek to reveal a contemporary application of each weekly *parashah,* utilizing the insights of ancient rabbis and sages, medieval commentators and philosophers, and modern scholars and religious leaders.

My writing was guided by the conviction that, in the words of my teacher, Rabbi Alan Miller, the Torah is a "high-voltage book" still giving off sparks, still enlightening those who make themselves channels for its power. Entering the electric world of Torah and its commentaries, the common inheritance of Jews, Christians, and all humanity, can only strengthen a sense of God's presence and an experience of comfort with one's own religious traditions. "Takes" in *The Bedside Torah* frequently draw upon classical Talmudic and medieval commentaries, viewed through the lenses of contemporary issues and perspectives. Those readers educated in the Israel of biblical antiquity alone will thus discover a window into the religious roots of Judaism's "daughter" faiths, Christianity and Islam, as they also become aware of the continuing vitality of a venerable people. For all, these meditations provide a forum for wrestling with questions of ultimate worth and perennial concern. I pray that these thoughts will inspire and enrich the religious lives of all who read them. I pray that these meditations are worthy of that awesome responsibility, and that in some small way they provide a peek underneath the sacred canopy, where Israel and the Holy One first consecrated a love relationship still retaining its ability to startle, to excite, to soothe, and to sanctify.

When Reading Torah Isn't Easy

In a famous passage, the Book of Proverbs lauds the "Woman of Valor" because she opens her mouth with wisdom, and on her tongue is *Torat hesed,* a Torah of love. The description poses a curious dilemma: Doesn't the mention of a Torah of *hesed,* of steadfast love or loving kindness, imply that there is a Torah that is not of love? Can there be a Torah where loving kindness does not rule?

If we understand God's revelation of Torah as a finite text given on a specific day, it is hard to avoid the conclusion that there are passages in it that cause serious religious and ethical problems for sensitive and enlightened readers. Yet it is precisely the most troubling parts of Torah from which we can learn most deeply. First of all, the passages that provoke us to thought challenge us to seek spiritual and ethical value even where it is not easily evident. Second and crucial, precisely because a passage is challenging for us, we are driven to engage in the process of *drash,* of interpretation. We begin to experience how, while the Book is the vehicle for God's voice, God's voice is to be located in how we read the entire Torah, not with the content of particular passages within it. Identifying God's voice with specific verses, moreover, assumes a single, intrinsic meaning inherent in the text. Yet the ancient rabbis—as well as many of our most sophisticated contemporary critics—understand that Torah is what emerges from the interaction among reader, written word, and interpretive community: "When two people meet and exchange words of Torah, the *Shekhinah* [the Divine Spirit] hovers over them" (*Avot* 3:3). It is not the passage, but how we read it, that creates a Torah of love.

Here is a vivid example of what I mean. There is a Biblical verse that may shock us on first reading: It condemns a *ben sorer u-moreh*, a stubborn and rebellious son, to death. The rabbis of the Talmud went out of their way to assert the value of continuing to study that passage even as they rendered the verse legally unenforceable. Why? Because they understood that that law is a poignant reminder of the value of honoring parents. If we simply eliminate passages like that of the rebellious son from our Torah, we deprive ourselves of a moving opportunity to contemplate why the commandment to honor our parents may be so powerful. We would be precluded from a chance to stretch ourselves spiritually.

The Bedside Torah is an expression of my belief that the voice of God can emerge from every passage of the Torah, provided we read that passage in a way that allows that voice to become audible. Such reading takes honesty, effort, and spiritual imagination, which is precisely what God would have us bring to an encounter with Torah. As the *Turei Zahav* notes, "One is perpetually commanded to derive new teachings from the Torah, for it is incumbent every moment to labor in the study of Torah and to innovate to the full extent of one's abilities."

How Do We Articulate God's Voice in Torah?

Reading the Torah to hear God's voice through its words, as with any strategy of reading, begins with certain assumptions. The first premise is that God is loving, wise, just, and compassionate. The second assumption is that the Torah, when read with reverence, will reflect those divine values.

Hence, when we read Torah and it appears to be hateful, unjust, or callous, we must read it differently. Even when the *p'shat* supports a harsh explication, our religious premise precludes identifying that *p'shat* with the voice of God. And it is God's voice of love, not the *p'shat*, that is commanding.

In *Parashat BeHar*, for instance, we read of the laws of slavery, both for an *eved Ivri*, a Hebrew slave, and an *eved K'nani*, a Canaanite slave. The

Hebrew slave is an indentured servant, limited in the duress he must endure and limited also to a finite term of service. But the *eved K'nani* enjoys none of those prerogatives. The Torah allows the master to impose onerous burdens on his slave, and prohibits the master from ever liberating the slave or the slave's children. If God's revelation is the *p'shat,* this part of the book forces us to ask what kind of a God would allow slavery as part of an eternal revelation.

What kind of a God would mandate the ownership, and would permit the degradation, of another human being?

There are many Jews who have a literal notion of Torah *min ha-Shamayim,* Torah from the Heavens, as if God indeed dropped the book down from the sky to earth. They grapple with such a text and try to interpret it in as humane a way as possible, adding that the Jewish slave laws weren't actually as harsh as those in other cultures. For many other Jews, however, such a reading seems forced and untenable. Worse, it puts God in the obscene position of mandating slavery, of permitting the ownership of another human being. Are we forced to simply concede that this passage is cruel and edit it out? What, then, of Torah and its holiness? What, then, of God and our Covenant?

Rejecting the voice of this passage renders the entire Torah suspect, and encourages us to simply bypass it when seeking spiritual or moral growth.

The solution to this dilemma is to be found in another traditional understanding of the idea of Torah *min ha-Shamayim*: the idea that Torah is best conceived as a process of interpretation through which God interacts with the Jewish people and all humankind. First initiated at Sinai, that process of the *midrash* continues with full force in the interpretations of biblical Prophets, the rabbis, and the medieval and even contemporary sages. God's voice cannot be contained between the covers of any book or even any collection of books; it is the interaction among the book, the reading community, and the inherited tradition, that is electric.

In that dynamic, a Torah of love emerges. Each new interpretation marks another refraction of the limitless light of God's Torah. In this sense, Torah *min ha-Shamayim* is eternally and vividly alive.

How would this approach perceive the traces of a loving and just God amidst the painful presence of slavery in the Torah? To begin with, we would define the issue not in terms only of what was present in Leviticus, but in terms of how Jewish tradition insists on reading God's voice in that presence.

Our question would concern how the process of Torah deals with the existence of slavery in Leviticus. For it is the process—the *drash*—that is authoritative. It is in the *drash,* the mode of reading, in which God's voice is to be found. As the mystical Book of Splendor, the *Zohar,* recognizes, "Just as wine must be in a jar to be preserved, so the Torah must be contained in an outer garment." The "garment" is made up of tales and stories, but we are bound to penetrate beyond it. Let us penetrate beyond the outer garment, the Book of Leviticus, to uncover the process of Torah within.

The great medieval rabbi, Moses ben Maimon, known as the Rambam, offered one such authoritative *drash.* He wrote, "Though the law makes its permissible to work an *eved K'nani* with rigor, both piety and the way of wisdom are that a man be merciful and pursue justice and not make his yoke heavy upon his slave or distress him, but give him to eat and to drink of all foods and drinks. The sages of old let the slave eat of every dish that they themselves ate and they fed the slaves before they themselves sat down to eat. Thus, also the master should not disgrace them by hand or by word, because Scripture has delivered them only to slavery and not to disgrace. Nor should he heap upon the slave oral abuse and anger, but should rather speak to him softly and listen to his claims."

Here, the Rambam accepts the fact of the *p'shat*: Slavery was technically permissible and one could ruthlessly oppress one's slave. Yet he also understands the values of Torah as moving us beyond the *p'shat,* creating a religious obligation to be merciful and just toward slaves. In fact, he insists that one ought to share the same foods, and allow the slaves to eat first, as a demonstration of compassion. A good master is one who speaks softly and listens to what the slave has to say. In short, for the Rambam, a Jewish master is one who affirms that the slave, too, is made in God's image. Ultimately, our understanding that all people are made in God's image precludes the very possibility of slavery at all.

Verses in the Torah that are morally problematic call on us to have the religious courage to read against the grain, so that we can hear God's loving voice in the process of reading. As one commentary says, "Those who constantly create new interpretations of Torah are harvesting [Torah]" (*Or ha-Hammah* on *Zohar* 3:106a). In that process, we make God's gift of Torah our own, and affirm our status as *b'nei rahamim,* the merciful children of a merciful God.

As you move through *The Bedside Torah,* I hope you will be moved to reread the Torah portion of the week and discover interpretations of your own as, three nights a week, you contemplate mine. Like any classic, the Torah appears in different guises with each rereading. Its infinite layers of meaning offer the opportunity to harvest anew, without any fear of exhausting its supply of wisdom, counsel, and *kedushah,* holiness, for to encounter Torah is to encounter God.

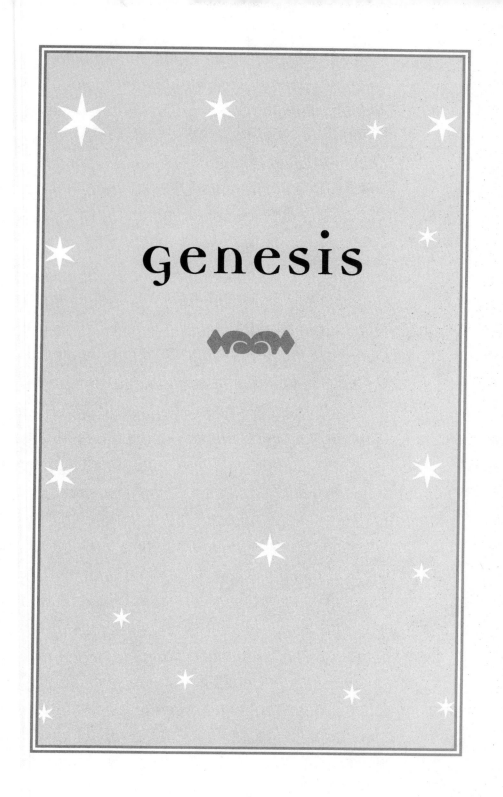

genesis

B'RAISHEET/In the Beginning
Genesis 1:1–6:8

B'raisheet *means beginnings and that is the concern of this opening Torah portion, as it is of the book that bears its name, known in English as Genesis. Like many ancient religious narratives, the Bible begins with the creation of all that is, culminating in the creation of life on earth. Distinct to this telling, however, are two significant variations. Instead of creation as the result of a cosmic battle requiring great effort, the God of the Torah creates easily simply by issuing a brief, effortless verbal command, "Let there be." The incomparable ease by which God summons the sun, moon, stars, water, sky, earth, and life into existence and that God does so without the aid or counsel of any other being marks this God as truly incomparable and unique.*

The second distinctive feature of the Torah's creation account is that it culminates not with the creation of humanity as the servants of the deity and the building of a temple in which the deity can dwell but with the cessation of all labor, hence, the creation of a Day of Rest—the Sabbath, Shabbat. That God's efforts should culminate in the gift of rest to the Jewish nation establishes a radical new reality. Made in God's image, human beings are free. And the fullest expression of their humanity is to be found in their freedom, demonstrated by leaving aside their chores and turning back to their God, to Torah, and to community.

At the end of the process of creation, God declares the cosmos, the world, and living things to be very good. In the Garden, humanity is given one solitary commandment—to not eat from the fruit of the tree of knowledge of good and evil. Enticed by the snake, first Eve and later Adam ate of the fruit, resulting in their moral responsibility, their expulsion from paradise, and their mortality. That mortality is immediately apparent as one of their sons, Cain, murders Abel and is doomed to wander. The parashah closes with the record of Adam's genealogy to Noah and the foreboding recognition that Adonai saw how great was man's wickedness on earth and how every plan devised by his mind was nothing but evil all the time.

Parashat B'raisheet/Genesis

Take 1

Genesis Is More Than Chronology

In our own age, and for the last several hundred years, learned men and women have argued about the meaning of the Creation story. Are these tales of a seven-day unfolding of the cosmos meant as the Biblical rendition of history, the record of how Creation actually happened? Or are the opening chapters of *B'raisheet* (Genesis) intended to convey a different lesson?

The question is of more than merely academic relevance. Several court cases around the United States seek to gain equal time in the classroom to teach "Creationism," the biblical account of the origin of life and the cosmos.

Proponents of Creationism maintain that the narrative in the Bible is divinely inspired in a literal way. They therefore read of the marvels in the Torah in a fundamentalist light—insisting that to accept the divinity of the Torah means to accept it as a historical record that is literally true. Their approach offers the comfort of certainty, the clarity of simplicity. It also, however, reduces Judaism's most sacred book to the status of an ancient newspaper—relating all the news that's fit to print.

There is another, equally religious way of understanding the Torah and of perceiving its sanctity. Rather than reading the Torah simply as a chronicle of ancient events, a listing of facts (what was created on which day), we can understand the Torah as Judaism's founding statement about the *meaning* of human, and specifically Jewish, life and community. While perhaps less successful in compelling acceptance of biblical "facts," the strength of this view is that it does recognize the concerns and priorities of the Torah as primarily religious and spiritual.

The Torah doesn't focus on lists of events so much as on what life and history reveal about the Creator of the universe and our *brit* (covenant) with God. The Torah tells us how to live, not merely how others have lived.

No less an authority than Rashi, the preeminent medieval commentator on the Bible and the Talmud, took such a stand on the story of Creation.

Rashi thought a literal approach to the biblical tale "astonishing." Instead, he insisted, the only way to understand biblical Creation is according to the *midrash* (rabbinic interpretation). A superficial, historical reading of Creation would miss the point of the story.

What captures the Torah's attention is not facts, but the meaning of those facts. We need to see the significance of the biblical tale for our own lives and our communities. And in seeking that significance, imagination, as Einstein suggested, is more important than knowledge.

For imagination is the ability to connect facts into meaningful patterns, the willingness to transform an "is" into an "ought." Such use of imagination has characterized our traditions at their best.

Jewish traditions, starting with the Creation story, provide a way of reading the world not simply as a random collection of phenomena, but as a coherent message of morality, holiness, and hope.

Out of that vision of meaning and coherence, a society committed to establishing God's sovereignty, one that can implement God's love, becomes possible.

The task awaits; the reading is possible.

Parashat B'raisheet/Genesis
Take 2

The Equal Rights Amendment in Eden

It is a fact of history that all of the rabbis of the Talmudic age were men. Actually, every rabbi in history was a man until 1972, when the first woman rabbi was ordained. Through the ages, in other religious and secular traditions as well, the male perspective dominated—to the extent that the word *man* itself was until recently used to mean *humanity* and the pronoun *he* was considered gender neutral.

Throughout history, then, the male perspective was considered the "normal" one, while the female viewpoint was disregarded, downplayed, or regarded as true *only* for women.

Occasionally, however, recognition of the harm caused by this suppression of women peeks out from under the smothering blanket of male domination. Such a moment of insight emerges from the story of Adam and Eve in the Garden of Eden.

The rabbis of the Talmudic age, sensitive and honest readers of the Torah, noticed a discrepancy between the command of God to Adam and the way Adam paraphrases that command to Eve.

God instructs Adam, "You must not eat of the tree of knowledge of good and bad; for as soon as you eat of it, you shall die." Dutifully, Adam informs Eve of God's command. But he apparently also adds one small phrase. When Eve relates her husband's words to the snake, she paraphrases God's instruction as, "You shall not eat of it, nor touch it, lest you die"—the version she most likely received from her husband.

Just as in the children's game Telephone, the more people who transmit a message, the more distorted and garbled that message becomes. God-to-Adam-to-Eve-to-the-snake seems to have been one layer too many.

The *Midrash B'raisheet Rabbah* tells us that the snake "took her and thrust her against [the tree]." The snake's action forced Eve to see that, in fact, *touching* the tree did not cause her death. And so, she reasoned, if *touching* the tree was actually perfectly safe, why would eating of it be any different? We still live with the tragic outcome.

According to *Avot de-Rebbi Natan,* an ancient *midrash* to *Pirkei Avot* (The Teachings of the Sages), Eve logically concluded that Adam had lied to her. Yet, Eve is not the villain in this story. While she *is* responsible for choosing to eat the fruit, she is also a victim of patriarchal exclusion. Adam had not clearly communicated God's will to Eve, and thus is equally responsible. God, too, is partly responsible, having spoken only to Adam while intending to obligate Eve as well.

The lesson of the *midrash* is quite clear: The disproportionate centrality of men and male dominance breeds disaster. Invidious hierarchy among people, assigning a greater worth to one human being over another, is misguided and dangerous. The *midrash* says that in those days, "Eve addressed Adam only as 'my master.'" But mastery of another person corrodes both individuals—master and underling—while simultaneously muting God's word. After the expulsion from Eden, Eve stopped viewing Adam as master, moving humanity down the long and still unfinished journey toward true equality.

For only as equals can men and women be a source of insight, support, love, and guidance to each other. Only as equals can we guide each other on the road ahead.

Parashat B'raisheet/Genesis
Take 3

For Every Thing, a Purpose

One of the great debates within the environmental community is the proper human posture toward the preservation of diverse species.

On the one hand, there are those who argue that extinction is the normal method through which nature keeps itself trim. Throughout the eons, a great many species, unable to compete successfully for a habitable niche in a difficult world, have gone the way of the dodo bird and the stegosaurus. This constant cycle of evolution and extinction may be unfortunate from the perspective of the individual dodo, but it represents a real strength through natural adaptation to changing conditions.

Through extinction, life remains vital.

In recent ages, human beings have become a significant factor in deciding which species survive. The High Holy Day prayer repeating the phrase "who shall live and who shall die" emits an eerie pall in the light of our own excessive impact on other species. In the past, extinction embodied the slow reconciliation among living things and their environments. Today it is the rapid—sometimes in only a few decades—intrusion of human thoughtlessness on the natural order. Many species that would be fully capable of surviving in the world cannot cope with what people are doing to our planet.

As we overfish our seas, deplete our forests and tropical jungles, pollute our air and water, destroy the ozone layer, and pile up mountains of nondegradable garbage, we need to refocus our attention, to stop and inquire about the worth of all living things—are animals and plants simply tools for humans to use as we choose, or is there a purpose to all things under the heavens?

In the Creation story, the Torah relates a magisterial unfolding of order over chaos, of life over death, as God's word becomes tangible. Creation moves from simplicity to complexity, from homogeneity to diversity, and, paradoxically, from chaos to order.

The rabbis of *Midrash B'raisheet Rabbah* express their viewpoint unambiguously: "Even those things which you may regard as completely superfluous to the creation of the world, such as fleas, gnats, and flies, even they too are included in the creation of the world, and the Holy Blessing One carries out the divine purpose through every [living] thing, even through a snake, a scorpion, a gnat, or a frog."

It is no coincidence that the rabbis choose animals that repel most human beings. We don't hang up pictures of fleas or gnats on our refrigerator doors or draw their images on greeting cards. What poet rhapsodizes about the beauty and grace of a frog?

Too often, we presume to judge the worth of Creation by its appeal to our human perspective.

The *midrash* insists that this criterion is insufficient. The world does not exist merely to please us. While human beings may be the pinnacle of God's creation, the world and the cosmos remain *God*'s creation, not our own. The standards of value therefore come not from us, but from God.

Stories in the *midrash* reveal the prescient ability of the sages to recognize scorpions and snakes, frogs and leaves, as "intended to perform God's commission." They, too, have a role to play and a purpose. We all need to refocus our vision to discover our divine "commission," the proper role for *us* to play.

The complex interdependence of living creatures—of the myriad plants and animals that populate our globe—is essential to the continuation of life, just as the remarkable range of cells and structures in the human body all contribute to the body's vitality. We diminish that variety at our own peril.

But the danger is more than simply one of physical survival. A second danger, more subtle but no less real, emerges when we coddle our egocentric insistence that the world should answer to human standards and human utility. In the words of the psalmist, "How vast Your works, O Lord. Your designs are beyond our grasp." The glory of the world of which we are a part is directed beyond us, reflecting the grandeur and transcendence of its sacred Source.

Noah/Noah
Genesis 6:9–11:32

God turns to the one righteous person on earth, Noah, and instructs him to build an ark of gopher wood in which to save his family and representatives of every species of every land-dwelling animal. God also tells Noah to store away enough vegetables to feed him and the animals in the ark. Foretelling the institution of Temple sacrifice and kashrut, *the Jewish dietary laws*, Noah takes seven of each tahor *(ritually permissible)* species, and only two each from the tamei, *the ritually impermissible*. He gathers this menagerie into the ark. Then for forty days and forty nights, it rains without letup, submerging even the highest mountains under the deluge. The waters cover the earth for 150 days, and then begin to recede as the ark settles on the summit of Mount Ararat. For three more months, the waters continue to diminish; at the end of forty days, Noah opens the window, sends out a raven, then a dove that is unable to find enough dry land to rest. After another seven days, Noah sends the dove out again. This time, it returns clutching an olive branch. After yet another seven days, the dove flies out and never returns. God instructs Noah and his family to replenish life on land. As his first act after the flood, Noah builds an altar and sacrifices every kind of tahor animal. God is pleased with the offering, pledging, "Never again will I doom the earth because of humanity, since the devisings of the human mind are evil from their youth." As a sign of that covenantal promise, God sets the rainbow in the sky. In recognition of human nature God makes animals fear humans, and permits eating meat, provided that the blood is separated from the meat (as is still performed during kosher meat preparation). Noah's three sons, Ham, Shem, and Japheth, emerge with him from the ark. Noah becomes a vintner and gets drunk. His son, Ham, sees his father's nakedness, which his other sons cover without looking. As a result of this incident, Ham (Canaan) is cursed; Shem, ancestor of the Semites, is blessed; and Japheth is made large.

Amidst tracing the record of the descendants of Noah through his three sons, the Torah recounts how a uniform humanity attempts to build a tower to make a name for itself. God responds to this arrogant *overreaching by dividing and multiplying the languages of humanity and by scattering humanity over the face of the whole earth. The parashah ends by tracing Shem's descendants through Terah to Avram and Sarai.*

☙❦❧

Parashat Noah/Noah
Take 1

Choosing Noah and Noah Choosing

Among other puzzles, the story of the Flood provides us with an enigmatic figure struggling through a difficult experience. Noah is a man who is called to build an ark to save himself, his family, and representatives of different species. Provoked to outrage by human misconduct, God has resolved to wipe out most of humanity and to start over.

It's difficult to know what to make of this story. How could a loving Creator deliberately cause such devastation? And why was Noah the one selected to continue the line of human existence? What merit did *he* possess to warrant that distinction?

"Noah was a righteous man; he was blameless in his age," says the Torah. The description is puzzling, for the two parts of the verse elicit contradictory understandings of who this man Noah really was.

Midrash Tanhuma, an early medieval compilation, asks, "What is meant by 'in his age'? . . . It means righteous in *his* age, but not in others. To what may this be compared? If someone places a silver coin among copper coins, the silver appears attractive. So Noah appeared righteous in the age of the flood."

According to this interpretation, Noah's distinction was merely contextual. Had he lived in an age of *real* righteousness, he would not have been noteworthy at all. It was only because of the total corruption around him that Noah appeared special.

But the same *midrash* also offers a very different way of understanding Noah's distinctiveness. "Others interpret the verse to Noah's credit. How so? It may be compared to a jar of balsam placed in a grave, and giving off a goodly fragrance. Had it been inside a home, how much the more so!"

Here the *midrash* argues that Noah was able to be decent *even though* he lived in a barbaric age. Had he been alive when truly compassionate people predominated, he would have been able to be even more outstanding.

Those two ways of looking at humanity apply in our own day as well.

Is human character a product of environment, or does it result from something innate and internal?

Are we who we are because of the way we were raised, or because of our own genetic composition?

As usual, reality is more complex than any single response. People are very much products of their backgrounds. Parents, grandparents, relatives, friends, income, education, and myriad other factors influence our personalities and our interests in powerful ways. Righteousness has a context.

Yet not everything is contextual. Two children raised in the same home and the same circumstances will grow up to be very different people. Our internal makeup also has a significant role in determining who we become.

And, finally, whether the parameters of our personalities are established by our upbringing or by our biology, we are still responsible for the choices we make in our lives.

Our tradition transmits the teaching that "all is in the hands of heaven, except the fear of heaven." Human beings can choose, within limits, how they will live their lives. We can choose to reflect the best of our environment and our nature. Just as Noah could rise above the conventions of his age, so, too, can we.

✦✦✦

*Parashat Noah/*Noah
Take 2

Evil Cannot Be Contained

Every schoolchild is familiar with the story of Noah and the Flood: God tired of the cruelty and immorality of humans and vowed to destroy the entire species through a spectacular deluge. But God selected one righteous family, that of Noah, and saved them by instructing them to build an ark. Noah did so and saved himself, his family, and representatives of all the different types of animals and birds.

When the floodwaters receded, Noah, his family, and his passengers began the long, gradual task of repopulating the planet.

Conventionally, the tale of the Flood is explained as reflecting God's intolerance of evil. Humanity became so corrupt and so violent that we ultimately disgusted God. Humanity exhausted God's limitless patience.

But there is still something disquieting about the whole episode. Even if every single human soul was wicked and cruel, why did God have to kill all those innocent animals? Why did fish survive the deluge just because they knew how to swim? Couldn't some of the people have been given a good scare and then told to do better? Why did there have to be so much death?

No matter how we read it, the Flood seems unfair.

And maybe that is precisely the point. Even when it comes from the God who is "slow to anger and abounding in kindness," destruction bursts beyond manageable or fair limitations. Even punishments originally intended to be measured and reasonable provoke unanticipated suffering and hardship.

Rashi teaches us that "whenever you find immorality and idolatry, indiscriminate punishment comes upon the world and it kills good and bad alike."

Once violence is launched, Rashi suggests, there is no foretelling its sweep or its destruction. In the words of the *Mekhilta*: "However mighty the man, once the arrows leave his hand he cannot make them come back. . . . However mighty the man, once frenzy and power take hold, he strikes even his father, even his mother, and even his nearest kin as he moves in his wrath."

Perhaps the discomfort we feel with the Flood story—with its epic devastation and its universal horror—is precisely the response we are intended to have. By demonstrating that even in the best of hands violence soon escalates beyond all control or direction or justice, the Torah's story urges us to work toward a day when disputes are not resolved through force, when children are not taught through blows, when lovers don't express their rage through beatings, when nations do not wage bloody conflicts.

We live in a world wedded to violence and war. It need not be that way forever. At the end of the Flood, God offers humanity a rainbow—a multicolored symbol of peace, a sacred pledge to refrain from destruction.

The rainbow is a reminder of the need to build coalitions with others. The rainbow is a call to confirm God's pledge "not to doom the earth because of humanity . . . not [to] ever again destroy every living thing."

Out of the horror of the Flood can emerge a new commitment to life and to peace. God has already spoken. Have you?

Parashat Noah/Noah
Take 3

God of the Jews, God of Humanity

Is Judaism a particularistic religion, concerned with the well-being and sanctity of the Jewish People only, or is it also one of the universalistic faiths, expressing a concern for all humanity in every region of the globe?

Enemies of our people have portrayed Judaism as a narrow, legalistic, and particularistic religion. *The Chosen People* has been defined as referring to the Jews alone. Moreover, by its own admission, Judaism doesn't actively seek converts; those who are attracted to our ways are welcome, but there is no burning drive to "get the word out." The God of the Bible is one who liberates the *Jews* from slavery, who gives them a path of life, who provides them with a Promised Land. Doesn't that focus make everyone else peripheral, even perhaps negligible?

On the other hand, the God of the Bible is also the Creator of the Universe, of the planet Earth, and all that it contains. The Bible explicitly speaks of God's covenants with other people as well—the Assyrians and the Egyptians, to name just two. So if God were the God of the whole world, then wouldn't God have the same relationship with everyone?

The Torah presents that paradox to us: God is the God of the Jewish People, and also the God of all humanity. That dual set of concerns is mediated through the Laws of the *B'nai Noah,* the Children of Noah, a way that Judaism and *halakhah* (Jewish law) incorporate God's sovereignty and love for all people with God's unique mission for the Jews.

Noah is the direct ancestor of all people. Through one son, Shem, he is the father of the Jewish People, and through his two other sons, Ham and Japhet, he is the ancestor of Asians, Africans, and Europeans, as well as their modern descendants (scholars note that Native Americans descend originally from Asia). All humanity is related through Noah.

The rabbis of the *Tosefta,* a rabbinic compilation from around the time of the *Mishnah,* specify seven commandments binding on all the *B'nai Noah*:

1. establishing courts of justice and rule of law,
2. prohibiting idolatry,
3. prohibiting blasphemy,
4. prohibiting sexual immorality,
5. prohibiting bloodshed,
6. prohibiting theft,
7. prohibiting tearing a limb from a living animal.

These rules establish a fundamental base of moral interaction, justice, and compassion for other human beings and for the animal world, as the basic requirement of human society. All humanity is commanded by God, all people have *mitzvot* to observe. These Seven Laws of Noah are the fundamental expectation that God has for all.

According to Judaism, then, God judges humans not according to their particular creed, not according to which group or institution receives their support, but rather for the kind of people they make of themselves. God commands decency, morality, and goodness, from everyone—Jew or Gentile. Based on just how godly persons are, to that extent are they beloved of God. In the words of Rabbi Moses ben Nahman, the medieval sage called the Ramban: "Whoever accepts the seven commandments and carefully observes them, is among the pious ones of the nations of the world, and enjoys a share of the hereafter— provided that [he] accept and perform them because the Holy Blessing One ordained them."

A righteous Gentile is a full child of God, to be cherished by all who give God allegiance, regardless of their religious affiliation. What matters, according to traditional Judaism, is goodness. That same requirement binds Jews as well. After all, we too are "Children of Noah." What distinguishes Jews from other *B'nai Noah* is that the rest of the *mitzvot,* the entire web of sacred deeds that nurtures and gives expression to the specific *brit,* also privilege us with the covenant between God and our People. It is those additional standards that make our relationship specific and unique.

God demands goodness of the Jew no less than of the non-Jew, and loves the Gentile no less than the Jew. And so should we.

LEKH LEKHA/
Take Yourself, Go Forth
Genesis 12:1–17:27

God commands Abram, "Go forth from your native land and from your father's house to the land that I will show you." Promised that he will become a great nation, Abram leaves Haran with his wife, Sarai, his nephew, Lot, and their entourage, and they reach the city of Shechem in Canaan. God promises this land to Abram's descendants, and Abram builds an altar to God at Beth El. A famine forces Abram and Sarai down to Egypt, where Pharaoh lusts after Sarai, thinking she is Abram's sister. God prevents Pharaoh from touching her. Instead, Pharaoh gives Abram great wealth and expels the group to Canaan.

There the servants of Lot and Abram quarrel; the two agree to separate, with Lot choosing the cities of Sodom and Gomorrah in the well-watered plains of Jordan. God reiterates the promise that the land will belong to Abram's heirs who will number the dust of the earth. Four kings battle five kings, and in the process capture Lot. When Abram hears of this, he musters 318 fighters, routing them near Damascus and rescuing Lot and the residents and wealth of Sodom. In gratitude, King Melchizedek of Salem—later Jerusalem—blesses Abram in the name of God Most High.

God tells Hagar that her son, Ishmael, will become a great nation, and that she must, in the meantime, return to Abram and Sarai. God changes Abram's name to Abraham ("father of a multitude") and Sarai's name to Sarah ("princess"), ordaining the mitzvah of the brit milah, the ritual circumcision binding on all Jewish males throughout the generations. God promises that Sarah will bear a son—despite being ninety years old—and that the boy will be called Isaac. Abraham circumcises himself and all his followers. Responding to Abraham's complaint that he is still childless, God tells him to look toward heaven and count the skies: "So shall be your offspring." God tells Abraham to sacrifice a heifer, a goat, a ram, a turtle dove, and a bird. Abraham sleeps between *the split carcasses, and God tells him that his descendants will be enslaved for four hundred years but that God will liberate them with great wealth and Abraham will die in peace. Sarah takes matters into her own hands and has Abraham sleep with her servant, the Egyptian handmaid Hagar. Hagar conceives and thereafter disdains her barren mistress. In response, Sarah treats her harshly; Hagar runs away. An angel tells her to return.*

✦

Parashat Lekh Lekha/Take Yourself, Go Forth
Take 1

Arise, Walk About the Land . . .

For more than 2,500 years, the majority of the Jewish People has lived outside of the Land of Israel. Since 586 B.C.E., the first exile to Babylon after the destruction of King Solomon's Temple, we have seen the Land of Israel as more than mere territory. *Israel* is also a value, an embodiment of Jewish wholeness, of being sheltered, of being at home.

Parashat Lekh Lekha begins with God's call to Abraham: "Go forth from your native land and from your father's house to the land I will show you" (12:1).

From the outset, this *parashah* is one of transitions and new beginnings. God tells our ancestor Abraham to sever his connection to a past rooted in convention and idolatry, and seek a new orientation, go to a new place.

To go to Israel is not merely to change one's address. Israel represents a shift in consciousness, a place that can nurture deeper spiritual insight by virtue of the events and institutions that will emerge from its soil. The Land of Israel will become the home base of the people of Israel during their period of greatest freedom and their earliest religious creativity.

From this soil, the judges and the house of David will guide the Jewish People in the service of their God. In the center of Jerusalem, on Mount Zion, King Solomon will erect the Temple, where our ancestors fulfilled the sacrificial requirements of the Torah, with a few exceptions, for a thousand years.

That site was so important that it occasioned the rebellion of the Maccabees and the rededication of the Temple, an event we still celebrate annually with the lights of Hanukkah.

It was in the Land of Israel that the Torah was compiled, that the prophets spoke, that the psalms were composed and chanted. In that little land our people lived out the earliest phases of our history.

Years later, that same soil was the site of the creation of the *Mishnah,* the earliest work of rabbinic law, and of the *midrashim,* the creative rabbinic expansions of the Bible. Here the institution of the synagogue was nurtured and the schoolhouse, the *Beit Midrash,* was born. In Israel, the Jewish calendar was developed and maintained.

The Talmud teaches that the sanctity of the Land of Israel and of the people of Israel are one. Having blossomed as a people, having cultivated a covenantal love with God in Zion, the Land of Israel acquired holiness through our many experiences there.

Not the least of its miracles was its centrality in the process of Jewish renewal of the last two centuries. In the words of the Israeli anthem, *Hatikvah,* we prayed for two thousand years "to be a free nation in our land, the land of Zion and Jerusalem."

The Zionist movement transformed Hebrew, for centuries a language only of scholarship and piety, into a living tongue. Hebrew now lives in the mouths of Israelis and has enjoyed a resurgence in American synagogues as well. Along with our language, the existence and achievements of Israel also resurrected Jewish pride and a sense of mission.

What can we do for our land in response? God instructs Abraham, "Arise, walk about the land, through its length and breadth, for I give it to you" (13:17).

That instruction applies to us as well. The land has always been a source of resurgence and identity for us, but only to the extent that we make Israel a part of our being, an unveiling of our personalities and our souls.

As Rabbi Eliezer explains in *Midrash B'raisheet Rabbah,* "If one walks in a field, whether along its length or its breadth, one acquires it."

By renewing our connection to Israel, by traveling there, studying there, living there, we establish our claim to the land, and allow the land to exercise its claim on us.

Parashat Lekh Lekha/Take Yourself, Go Forth
Take 2

Righteousness and Faith

At a ripe old age, Abraham receives a message from God, telling him that he will produce an heir, and that the child will inherit both his father's property and his father's covenant with God.

Surely God's promise would strain the credulity of even the most devoted follower. Long barren, Abraham's wife, Sarah, is now ninety years old, way beyond her childbearing years. Abraham himself is no youngster. "Shall a child be born to a man one hundred years old?" he laughs. Yet, despite this biological reality, God insists that Abraham and Sarah will have a child, and that their descendants will outnumber the stars in the sky!

In response to God's astounding promise, the Torah states simply that Abraham "trusted the Lord and deemed it as righteous merit on his part" (15:6).

In that one ambiguous sentence, the Torah contrasts the rich complexity of biblical faith to the flimsy notion of faith today.

For most religious Americans, "faith" means belief in certain claims about the metaphysics of reality. Faith is perceived as the absence of doubt. In this view, true faith requires a willingness to avoid too much thought, to ignore the difficult questions which life inevitably raises.

As a result, when those questions do arise—as indeed they must—this faulty "faith" shatters easily.

The biblical-rabbinic understanding of faith is radically different.

Our *parashah* shows Abraham filled with tensions and doubt. He worries about his lack of heirs, the state of his covenant with God, his relations with his neighbors.

In the midst of these struggles, Abraham has a conversation with God. What emerges from that conversation is a radically different kind of faith experience. For Abraham comes to understand that faith is not the passive acquiescence to an idea, nor does faith require the obedient stifling of doubt. Rather, Abraham learns that faith is a willingness to trust *through* one's tensions and *despite* one's doubts.

Faith, then, is trust. The simplest reading of our biblical verse is that God valued Abraham's trust and rewarded him for his merit. Rashi comments that Abraham's trust was an expression of his *tzedakah,* his righteousness, for rather than ask God to prove he would have heirs, he "believed" and did not ask "for a sign."

A relatively recent work of biblical commentary, the *Torah Temimah* by Rabbi Barukh Epstein of early twentieth-century Russia, understands our ambiguous sentence differently. He interprets it to mean that Abraham trusted God and considered God's promise as evidence of *God*'s own righteousness.

We often take it for granted that we live in a habitable universe—the sun rises and sets with predictable regularity, the earth produces material, which in turn nourishes living things, and human beings are able to produce and raise children to adulthood. While the world may be far from perfect, it is nonetheless regular, reliable, and vital. Evidence of God's promise is not hard to find.

One way of understanding our verse, then, is to see in it God's willingness to trust Abraham. Another way to read the verse is to recognize Abraham's willingness to trust God. Both are far from predictable. Both represent little miracles.

There is insight in both readings. For both Abraham and God, faith is the willingness to trust, despite the reality of setbacks and suffering.

In this *parashah* and elsewhere, Judaism insists on a rich trust, demonstrated through deeds.

Parashat Lekh Lekha/Take Yourself, Go Forth
Take 3

To Call upon God by Name

One of the striking facts about religious faith around the world is the array of ways in which human beings conceive of, and worship, the Divine. The sacred claims a myriad of names—Ahura Mazda, Brahma, Nirvana, Wanka Takan, Osiris, Zeus, Jupiter, Wodan. Given how many names the Divine is called, it is particularly striking that the Jewish conception of God doesn't really have a name at all.

Or, at the very least, our God's name is suspiciously like no name at all. Our two daughter religions, Christianity and Islam, have inherited this quirk as well—a supreme God who lacks a name. Christianity calls the Divine "God the Father." But "God" isn't a name; it's a job description, a title. In Christianity, "God the Son" may have a name, but God the Father doesn't. Similarly, in Islam, the appellation "Allah" is comparable to the Hebrew name "El." El means "god," but it isn't a name; again, it's a title.

All of which springs from the interesting history of the God of the Torah.

Our portion mentions that Abraham "built an altar to the Lord and invoked the Lord by name" (12:8).

What does it mean to invoke a nameless God by name?

Building on the explanation found in the ancient *Midrash B'raisheet Rabbah,* the Ramban explains that this phrase means that Abraham established God's service in new lands and proclaimed the identity and oneness of God to people who had never encountered monotheism before.

To name something is to reveal something about its essence, to exert a kind of control, to assert a comprehension of its nature, its limits, and its potentials. Certainly, when the Torah says that Abraham called on God by name, it means to tell us that Abraham enjoyed an intimacy with God that others of his generation did not. It teaches that Abraham knew God with a thoroughness that no one before him could equal.

And yet, the name that Abraham knew sounds suspiciously like no name at all.

The name consists of four Hebrew letters: Y-H-V-H. Lacking vowels (or hard consonants, for that matter) the word "Y-H-V-H" is virtually impossible to articulate. It sounds like a breath, like air passing in and out of the lungs. Perhaps it tells us that God is the breath of the universe.

Grammatically, the name is a mixture of the verb "to be" in three different tenses: Y-H-Y-H (*was*); H-V-H (*is*); and E-H-Y-H (*will be*). The odd combination of all three in one asserts that God transcends time, categorization, and limit. God is eternal, and radically different from anyone (anything?) else to which we relate in life.

When Moses asks God to reveal the divine name, God refuses, asserting that no one can see God's face and live. But God also leaves Moses with the bizarre "WAS-IS-WILL BE" and tells Moses to transmit that "name" to the Jewish People.

And the history of that name reveals that the Jews understood that they should treat that awkward word with reverence, for it was unlike any other name in the world. Its articulation was restricted to the holiest day of the year, Yom Kippur, by the holiest person in biblical Judaism, the *Kohen Gadol,* the High Priest, in the holiest place in the world, the Holy of Holies in the Temple in Jerusalem.

Since the destruction of the Temple some two thousand years ago, no observant Jew has pronounced that "name," the ineffable sign of our unique God.

To say that God is ultimately unnamable is to suggest that the Divine is ultimately beyond the totality of our experience, beyond our comprehension. Without actually *being* God, we cannot fully *know* God.

What we can do, however, is *relate* to God: to seek to embody godly traits and, in all of our actions, to cultivate God's loving presence.

VA-YERA/He Saw
Genesis 18:1–22:24

As Abraham sits in the opening of his tent, he sees three men coming toward him. He offers them hospitality, they accept, and as the food is prepared they ask after Sarah. One of the guests tells Abraham that when he returns a year later, he will have a son. Overhearing this, Sarah, in one of the most famous moments of Genesis, laughs. "Is anything too wondrous for Adonai?" God—who is apparently one of the guests—responds. The focus of the scene abruptly changes, as God tells Abraham that he intends to destroy Sodom and Gomorrah. Rather than resign himself to God's announcement, Abraham argues with God against such collective punishment. God listens, and agrees not to destroy the cities if there are ten righteous people there. Two angels go to Sodom to warn Lot of the impending catastrophe; he invites them to stay, as the townspeople surround his house and demand that he surrender the guests to them for abuse and humiliation. Pleading with them not to violate his hospitality, Lot offers his daughters to the mob instead. But the angels pull Lot back inside, blinding the townspeople and protecting the daughters. Lot and his family flee as the cities are annihilated—and in one of the images that has come down through the ages, Lot's wife turns back, becoming, by doing so, a pillar of salt. The plains are destroyed. Convinced that they are the only humans to survive the destruction of the planet, Lot's daughters sleep with their intoxicated father in order that the human race should continue. One conceives Moab—ancestor of the Moabites (and later of Ruth)—and the other, Ben Ammi, ancestor of the Ammonites.

Once again, Abraham tries to pass his wife off as his sister, this time to King Abimelech of Gerar. Again God protects her, and Abraham and the king part amicably. As promised, Sarah conceives and bears Isaac. After an ambiguous incident, she insists that Abraham expel Hagar and Ishmael, a demand that God tells Abraham to meet. Hagar and her son move to the wilderness of Paran. Abraham and Abimelech sign a friendship pact.

Now comes one of the most overwhelmingly difficult moments in the whole of the Bible. God tests Abraham, telling him to sacrifice his son,

"Isaac, whom you love." The two proceed in silence for three days until they arrive at Mount Moriah. At the top of the mountain, Abraham builds an altar, straps his son onto it, and lifts the knife to slay his son. "Abraham, Abraham," calls an angel, interrupting him; "Hineni," responds the patriarch, "Here I am." The angel tells him not to harm the boy. Looking up, Abraham sees a ram caught in a nearby bush, and slaughters the ram in Isaac's stead. In response to Abraham's obedience to a commandment, God again promises to multiply Abraham's descendants and to give them Eretz Yisrael. "All the nations of the earth shall bless themselves by your descendants, because you have obeyed My commands," God tells him.

Parashat Va-Yera/He Saw
Take 1

Honesty as Idolatry

Idolatry is the practice of treating something that may be of relative importance as though it were of ultimate significance. In our idolatrous age, we often act as though money, career, sex appeal, or prestige are of ultimate importance, when in fact they are worthwhile only to the degree that they contribute to our becoming better, more compassionate, and more responsible people.

Today's Torah-reading highlights another source of idolatry. We are accustomed to regarding honesty as possessing the highest value possible. We justify an unkind remark with the observation that it is true; we make a virtue of "telling it like it is," regardless of the effects of what is really a self-centered "integrity."

The conversation between Sarah and God casts a very different light on that behavior. After God reveals that the aged Sarah will bear a son, Sarah laughs: "Now that I'm so old, and my husband is so old, am I to bear a son?" she responds, her tone in all likelihood expressing the pent-up disappointment of years, along with the hope.

God reports her words to her husband, Abraham, but makes a slight—and vital—modification. As if God understands that he would be hurt by Sarah's assertion that her husband was too old to father a child, God tells Abraham that Sarah said, "Shall I really bear a child, old as *I* am?"

In changing Sarah's words, God acts to preserve both Abraham's dignity and family harmony. As Rashi notes, "Scripture altered her statement for the sake of peace."

Mip'nei darkhei shalom—for the sake of peace, we are instructed by Jewish wisdom to modify our statements. While precious, honesty is of value only insofar as it helps human beings live together in peace. When scrupulous honesty can damage a relationship, Jewish wisdom teaches that the higher value is to protect a person's feelings of self-worth and love.

The *Mishnah*, for example, teaches that on her wedding day a bride is to be told that she is beautiful, regardless of how she really looks. Why? *Mip'nei darkhei shalom*, for the sake of peace.

If serving the Lord does not lead to caring for the dignity of other human beings, does not lead to a willingness to protect another's feelings even at the cost of being "honest," then there is something lacking in our notion of what God wants.

According to the Torah, and according to rabbinic tradition, God values most human caring.

Honesty in the service of compassion and growth is a *mitzvah*, even if the truth is painful. Honesty at the expense of another human's feelings, simply to air one's own viewpoint, is a betrayal of God.

Parashat Va-Yera/He Saw
Take 2

Freed from the Trap of Experience

Personality is molded by experience. How we live our lives and the events that we confront serve to shape our very beings. We respond to each new situation by referring to earlier ones—always seeking to avoid past mistakes, always looking to improve on earlier interactions.

In this light, our response almost always comes one event too late. We become trapped by our most recent experience.

The story of Hagar and Ishmael conveys that essential insight into human nature. Expelled from the security of the caravan, Hagar takes her young son, Ishmael, into the desert. Unwilling to watch him die, she sets him down under a plant and then wanders off to a distance, where she sits down and sobs.

God hears the wailing of the boy, and calls to Hagar, telling her not to despair, for her son will become the ancestor of a vast nation. "Then God opened her eyes and she saw a well of water" (21:19). She gives her son water to drink.

The Torah does not claim that God created a *new* well for her. The miracle of the well is that it was there all along; Hagar had not noticed it before, and now she is able to see it. Trapped by her own despair and her own past, she had been unable to recognize possibilities for her own survival. Her awareness of God and the resurgence of hope liberate her from the shackles of her own experience.

Modern scholars have applied this same insight in their own fields of expertise. Professor Ernest May of Harvard University, in his book *Uses of the Past,* argues that the errors committed in America's last several military conflicts all spring from the fact that our generals applied the lessons of the previous war to the next conflict, always operating one war too late. In Korea, we tried to rectify the errors of World War II, but those errors (and insights) didn't apply to such a different environment. Then we tried to correct the errors made during the Korean War in Vietnam, again with disastrous effects.

May argues that the dynamics of history itself lead people to seek to apply a model to each new situation, and that logic and memory dictate that the model they apply is the one they best remember, the most recent occurrence that seems relevant.

Sigmund Freud perceives a different motivation, arguing that each of us strives to correct deficiencies or painful encounters from our childhood. Thus we unconsciously construct similar situations as adults, over and over again, desperately trying to master the pain and frustration we felt in the past by engineering a new resolution today. Most often, however, we simply repeat past encounters, perpetuating a cycle of trauma and disappointment. We become trapped in "repetition compulsion."

To escape our enslavement to past experience requires a radical openness to the present, a willingness to see the world afresh each moment that we live.

As the *Midrash B'raisheet Rabbah* notes, "All may be presumed to be blind until the Holy Blessing One opens their eyes."

We smother ourselves in convention and expectation and experience, until we learn to open ourselves to the marvels undergirding existence. Then we can see the liberating vision of a humanity redeemed and of a God who cares. Like Hagar's, our eyes will be opened.

Parashat Va-Yera/He Saw
Take 3
The Mitzvah of Hospitality

Ours is an age of institutions.

Inured to depersonalization, we turn to computer services for dating and discreet professionals to worry about death. We expect our schools, not our families, to instill moral values and build character in our children, and our rabbis, cantors, and catering companies to fulfill the spiritual roles the community—our neighbors, our friends—used to perform.

In today's Torah portion, Abraham and Sarah receive three visitors—complete strangers—and drop everything they are doing to welcome these wanderers into their homes. *Hakh'nasat or'him,* hospitality, is a central value of Judaism, one of our distinctive *mitzvot.* Abraham rushes about, offering water for his guests' dusty feet, choosing a calf from his herd for their dinner. Sarah kneads dough for cakes.

How differently we respond to the hungry today. We delegate feeding the hungry to soup kitchens, house the homeless in shelters, and integrate newcomers with "welcome wagons."

While these groups may be essential, they lack the grounding of community and friendship, and thus the emotional sustenance that could provide a warmer context for the food, clothes, or shelter. We may adequately meet basic physical requirements, but those requirements are stripped of emotional or personal nurturance. What of the humanity of those in need?

Efficiency can never replace caring, concern, and personal involvement. A single hand can touch where a battalion cannot.

The mobility and instability of most American families erode a precious sense of community and belonging. We may not be able to stop the moving from place to place, but we can make ourselves into "booby traps" along the way—little explosions of caring and involvement that invite weary and desensitized people to join, to trust, and to share. We can expand our sense of community to include people we have never met before, or those we will only see once.

That inclusiveness is true *hakh'nasat or'him,* true hospitality. In the words of the Passover *Haggadah,* "let all who are hungry come and eat."

By opening our homes as places of respite from the frenzy of an economy and society moving at breakneck speed, by creating a haven where strangers are welcomed and shown that no one is really a stranger after all, we have the power to renew a sense of connection and belonging. By providing for the hungry and sheltering the homeless, we can offer tangible relief from the suffering of fellow human beings. By reaching out to newcomers and greeting visitors with warmth, we make the world a little more intimate, a little more like *mishpakhah.*

Ultimately, hospitality is a question of defining our community broadly enough so that no one is left out. Just as we feel a sense of responsibility to share our food and companionship, so we can cultivate a sense of family for the entire household of humanity. The *mitzvah* of *hakh'nasat or'him* offers us a compromise: Rather than abandoning contemporary society entirely—with its rush, its transience, and its outcasts—rather than surrendering to a faceless world of institutions and anonymity, this *mitzvah* reveals the human faces in our midst and restores the caring heart to its rightful place in our lives.

Hahk'nasat or'him is about welcoming people into our lives, into our living. It is about sustaining other people and deriving sustenance from the encounter. It is, through deed, affirmations of God's love that provide a habitable world and of our potential to emulate that love.

Hahk'nasat or'him, then, reclaims our humanity, and God's.

Got any plans for lunch this *Shabbat*?

Parashat Akedah/The Binding of Isaac
A Special Section

All of us have, on occasion, experienced a time in which time itself stands still, when the normal pulsing heartbeat of the world seems suspended and the rhythmic breath of life is hushed. At such moments our perception of the world is jolted, we see in a new way, as if for the first time.

If we are open to the opportunity, these are moments that offer insight, occasions when we might develop a new profundity and a deeper wisdom.

Today's Torah-reading presents a figure who could respond to that moment with such radical insight, a moment which forever altered his personality and his future. Traditionally, Isaac is known merely as a link—as the son of Abraham and the father of Jacob. He has few deeds to plead his cause as one of the founding ancestors of Israel.

The Torah tells us little about Isaac's childhood. We know that he was the beloved progeny of his parents' old age. We know also that his father, Abraham, was the leader of a powerful clan, forever conducting diplomacy and warfare with local rulers, with the Pharaoh of Egypt, and even with God directly. We don't see Abraham as a loving husband or an involved father.

Like other prominent leaders, he was preoccupied with important affairs on behalf of his group. Abraham's greatness lay in being the first patriarch and in spreading an awareness of the one Creator of the universe.

Isaac's mother, Sarah, also appears as an extraordinary woman—running an enormous household, managing the servants, chiding her husband, and herself conducting several conversations with God. Sarah's greatness lay in her being the first matriarch of the Jewish People.

Everything in Isaac's youth pointed to a future of public prominence and of communal leadership. We expect Isaac to be like his parents. But later generations of Jews, finding no evidence of his public greatness, regarded Isaac as the least of Israel's founding ancestors, as little more than a link.

In making that assessment, however, posterity failed to appreciate Isaac as an individual of deep insight and character. Later generations simply applied the wrong standards, external standards of prowess, wit, and oratory.

Isaac turned away from a life of public leadership because of one transforming event that we read about today, because of the *Akedah*.

God decided to test Abraham, the public leader, by ordering him to sacrifice his beloved son. Ever obedient to his God, Abraham responded immediately. With his son and two servants, Abraham gathered the necessary supplies and marched to a still-undesignated place to perform God's will. "He bound his son Isaac (22:9)." Then Abraham took up the knife to slay his son. Only at the last moment did an angel of God order Abraham to stop. A substitute for Isaac, a young ram caught in a bush, appeared and was sacrificed instead.

The Torah reports the *Akedah* primarily as an event in Abraham's life. The intention of the narrator is to show the important virtue of the fear of heaven, and, secondarily, to record God's disapproval of human sacrifice.

We are never told how Isaac responded. Indeed, once the ram appears in the thicket, the Torah's interest in Isaac seems to dissipate completely. Read superficially, the Torah implies that the *Akedah* did not affect Isaac at all—his life appears unchanged. We don't see Isaac again until his father has found a bride for the boy, yet another event recounted because of Abraham's involvement, rather than revealing any direct interest in Isaac himself.

What happened to Isaac during his ordeal on the altar? What did he see when he was under the knife? For a brief and agonizing moment, Isaac came face to face with the reality of his own mortality, with the certain knowledge that he would someday die. Such an insight must permanently affect the perspective of any human being, must forever change a person's priorities and conduct.

We see instances of deepened perception emerging from moments of crisis in the Torah and in daily life itself. Several summers ago, I was a chaplain at Memorial Sloan-Kettering Cancer Center in Manhattan. I functioned as rabbi and counselor for cancer and AIDS patients on three floors of the hospital. Daily, my job was to walk into the rooms of people I had never previously met; to introduce myself; and to talk with them about their fears, their concerns, and their pain. Mostly, my job was to listen and to empathize.

Like Isaac, the people in Sloan-Kettering were, in a sense, under the knife. They, too, were experiencing their own mortality—a reality which the rest of us deny for as long as we can. Some patients, like Isaac, got a reprieve. Some were not so fortunate. How does such a brush with death change someone? Can one even speak of insights gained in such a terrible moment?

The Torah helps us to understand that we can. The portrait painted of Isaac is so unique, so unlike that of any other biblical leader, that we are justified in assuming that only some unique and overpowering event could have molded his character in such a special way.

When next we see Isaac after the *Akedah,* the Torah reports "that he is walking in the fields (24:63)." The Midrash understood that Isaac was davvening *Minhah,* praying and meditating, in the words of the Psalmist (77:7), "communing with his heart and searching his soul." Walking quietly, lost in a world of thought and contemplation is something we have not seen in a biblical figure, nor something we shall see again. Isaac has become more attuned to an inner life than was his father or his mother.

Isaac also relates to others in an unprecedented way. He marries Rebekah and the Torah tells us "he loved her (24:67)." In itself, Isaac's ability to love is rare. Only one other husband-and-wife couple, Jacob and Rachel, are reported this way in the *Tanakh.* For a man in antiquity to care so deeply for a woman is striking and noteworthy. In fact, Isaac cares so deeply for his wife that he intervenes with God when his wife becomes barren. The Torah says, "Isaac pleaded with the Lord on behalf of his wife, because she was barren (25:21)." No other biblical figure is able to empathize to this degree. Isaac so identifies with his wife's suffering that he takes it on as his own as well.

And his care for Rebekah is the fullest expression of mature intimacy. Isaac is singular among biblical figures in his ability to integrate his love for his wife with his sexual attraction for her. Isaac and Rebekah share a sexuality that is both loving and playful. The Torah tells us that "Isaac fondled his wife Rebecca (26:8)."

Isaac is unique in the depth and seriousness of his relationship with Rebekah. This is no youthful passion, no lustful fling. Rebekah and Isaac share an adult love, the union of two souls who can be fully themselves in each other's presence. They share each other's sorrows and they learn to laugh with each other. Theirs is the Torah's truest romance.

But Isaac's insight extends beyond the realm of love. He is also a man of peace. Three times he digs wells of water, and three times those wells are contested by Philistine chieftains. Each time, Isaac cedes his wells rather than wage war.

An early rabbinic figure, Ben Zoma, asks: "Who is rich? One who is happy with his portion (Mishnah Avot 4:1)." Isaac did not measure wealth by the number of wells one possessed, or even how much money one has stockpiled. His life, his family, the safety of his own followers was worth more than a few wells of water. Having himself been offered on an altar, Isaac was not going to sacrifice young lives for material wealth. Isaac was a man who knew the profound value of peace, a commitment that was well-rewarded. Three times he permitted the Philistines to claim his wells. God blessed him and made him prosper. The Philistines were taught a lesson in human kindness and priorities by Isaac's behavior. Impressed by his grandeur and magnanimity, they sought Isaac and exchanged oaths of friendship.

Ben Zoma has wisdom to offer here too. "Who is mighty? One who conquers his evil impulse, as it is written, 'One who is slow to anger is better than he who conquers a city'" (Proverbs 16:32). *Avot De-Rebbe Natan,* a later commentary, adds that wisdom consists of transforming an enemy into a friend (38a). In converting the Philistines into allies and friends, Isaac demonstrated that special wisdom.

Isaac's steadfast faithfulness, his commitment to maintaining a relationship, extended even to the land of his birth. Alone of all the patriarchs, Isaac never left the Land of Israel. Even in time of famine, Isaac's attachment to *Eretz Yisrael* never wavered. He expressed his relation to the Land by never leaving it, and he cultivated that attachment by being the first patriarch to engage in agriculture. Both of those facts require a depth of commitment, a patience, and a level of maturity that is rare even in our day.

Isaac possessed that solidity, that fidelity and commitment. He was a loving partner with Rebekah, a man who went out of his way to keep peace with his neighbors, and one whose commitment to the Land of Israel and the God of Israel was total.

Where did he gain that perspective?

I suggest to you that Isaac learned the importance of love, of inner depth, of relationship, when he was bound on the altar on Mount

Moriah. Isaac looked at that glistening blade, and he saw in its reflection his own eventual death. Awareness that his life would one day end changed him forever. In an instant, Isaac could see that public fame, lofty speeches, the glitter of wealth or power were all meaningless in the face of death. The only possession of ultimate worth is the love of other people, a sense of connectedness with a community and with God, having lived life with meaning, sensitivity, and love.

Isaac saw, in that instant, that it was possible to go through a lengthy life without ever truly living. That one could forever pursue pomp and acclaim and be, in reality, alone and poor. But a person who knows love, a person who deepens his or her own insight and sensitivity and character possesses a richness eternal.

Isaac learned that lesson, and the Torah recounts it for our benefit in its own unique way. But Isaac is not alone in confronting his own death. Each week, countless people face the same glimpse of their own mortality, and struggle to learn the same lesson about life. This summer, I watched numerous people wrestle with their cancer, and I saw them develop a new insight about how they would live differently in whatever time was left to them. Over and over, people in the hospital told me that they had indeed learned from their cancer.

Few people, the saying goes, spend their last moments on their death beds wishing they had spent more time at work. Illness can teach that what matters most in life is the people we love.

Thank God, we are not at this moment facing death. The story of Isaac's binding, and indeed of Isaac's life, comes as an annual reminder that yet another year has passed, never to return. We are all one year closer. Are we also one year wiser?

Yet again the Torah presents, in the story of Isaac, an opportunity for us to grow in perspective without ourselves lying under the knife. Isaac offers us all a role model not often followed: a man who did not give great speeches, lead mighty armies, or create a popular movement. Quietly, and without pretensions to greatness, Isaac spent his time building relationships—with his wife, with his Heritage, with himself, and with his God. By insisting on living a meaningful life, Isaac makes it possible for each of us to do the same. Let us claim his insight while we can.

HAYEI SARAH/The Life of Sarah
Genesis 23:1–25:18

Despite the name of this parashah, it opens with the death of Sarah in Hebron, and Abraham's need to acquire a burial site for her remains. He purchases the Cave of Machpelah, marking the first time a Hebrew owns land in Eretz Yisrael. Recognizing the need to assure the transmission of the covenant, he then arranges for her servant to return to his homeland and find a wife for his son Isaac from among his extended family. The servant discovers Rebekah, of Abraham's family line, at the well in the oasis, fulfilling exactly the signs for which the servant had prayed. Returning to her home with her, he meets the rest of the family; both her brother, Laban, and her father, Bethuel, recognize the handiwork of God in this fortuitous connection, and ask Rebekah if she wants to return with the servant and marry Isaac. She does.

As the caravan of Rebekah approaches, Isaac is out walking — or meditating — in the fields. They see one another, and, in a powerfully moving moment, the Torah tells us that as she alights, Isaac brings her into the tent that had been his mother's, loves her, and is comforted for his mother's death.

Abraham marries again, this time to Keturah, and though he provides for all his progeny, only his son Isaac inherits his blessing, remaining wealth, and his land. By now 125 years old, Abraham dies, and, like Sarah, is buried in the Cave of Machpelah.

*Parashat Hayei Sarah/*The Life of Sarah
Take 1

Generosity, Meekness, Humility

One of the central features of this week's Torah portion is the attention it lavishes on Abraham's efforts to acquire property in the Land of Israel.

In the town of Hebron, in the middle of the West Bank of the River Jordan, Abraham faces the death of his wife and friend, Sarah. He speaks to the local residents, the Hittites, about purchasing a plot. "I am a resident alien among you," Abraham says. "Sell me a burial site among you, that I may remove my dead for burial."

Responding with equal dignity and graciousness, the Hittites reassure Abraham: "You are the elect of God among us. Bury your dead in the choicest of our burial places."

The elaborate ritual of purchasing a plot continues, as Abraham reveals which site he wants to buy and speaks to the owner. With finesse and a sense of great propriety, the two settle on an appropriate price for the Cave of Machpelah. Paying four hundred silver shekels, Abraham gains eternal title to the field of Ephron in the town of Hebron.

Nothing remarkable so far, right? Just the patriarch of the Jewish People buying some land to bury his dead, while establishing his people's legal claim on the Land of Israel at the same time. An ordinary transaction.

Yet something is strangely missing here; there is no reference in this description to the Divine gift of the land to Abraham and his descendants. Isn't one of the principal points of Genesis the proclaiming of God's conferral of ownership of *Eretz Yisrael* on Abraham and his heirs, the Jews, for all time? And since God gave the land to Abraham, why would the patriarch feel any need to negotiate its ownership with any human possessors? He already has God on his side.

Why indeed? Aren't there people today who claim an exclusive possession of the truth, who insist that their monopoly on morality, or compassion, or divine will, allows them to slander, to slight, to distort, or to oppress? From the liberal chic to the conservative smug, all over the world self-appointed spokespeople of the "correct" view trumpet their own infallibility and moral superiority.

If anyone ever had a right to take that position, Abraham was that person. And yet, despite his knowledge of God's gift of Israel to the Jews, Abraham still made a point of respecting the humanity of his pagan hosts, still insisted on taking seriously the perspective of the Hittites, their customs, and their proprieties.

We who claim to be the descendants of Abraham and Sarah would do well to hearken to the wisdom of the Talmudic volume, *Avot De-Rebbe Natan*:

One who possesses these three traits is one of the disciples of our father, Abraham: a generous eye, a meek spirit, and a humble soul.

Abraham didn't doubt God's word, or his accurate awareness of the divine will. But he also knew that no one possesses an exclusive hold on truth, that other well-meaning people also pursue the truth to the best of their ability. Without relinquishing his own convictions, Abraham never abandoned the religious humility that accepts the possibility of being wrong.

A generous eye, a meek spirit, and a humble soul. Who would have guessed that these traits would provide the strength for Abraham's people to thrive into eternity?

Parashat Hayei Sarah / The Life of Sarah
Take 2

The Service of the Heart

One of the universals of human culture is the need to commune with something larger, something that extends beyond ourselves. We all feel the desire to speak, to create, to perform. One aspect of the human urge to communicate is worship—awakening to the awe of existence, the staggering marvel of the world and its order. Awe moves us to a silent expression of gratitude and wonder. Awe moves us to worship.

For many Jews, worship has come to mean the formal ritual of reading the prayers of other, earlier Jews from the printed *Siddur* (prayer book); listening to the chanted words of the Torah and the *Haftarah*; and absorbing the insights of the rabbi's sermon. Worship is public, planned, and cyclical. How many of us, though, approach God with the simple outpouring of our own hearts? Isn't it true that the notion of just speaking with God in our intimate personal voices sounds strikingly un-Jewish?

Yet consider today's Torah portion. Abraham's nameless servant is assigned the task of traveling to a distant land to find a bride for the patriarch's son. Overwhelmed by the gravity and seriousness of his mission, unable to summon a special revelation through sacrificing an animal, the servant simply sits and speaks. "O, Lord, God of my master Abraham," he prays with neither formula nor poetry, "grant me good fortune this day, and deal graciously with master Abraham" (24:12).

The servant speaks to God with a directness borne of necessity. Filled with a sense of the uncertainty of his task, aware of his own limitations, he turns to the Source of Life and shares his fear.

Note also that the servant establishes criteria for judging the successful accomplishment of his mission, and then prays that his standard should be God's as well (13–14). Those standards are themselves an insight into the human heart—he asks for a woman who is generous, compassionate, and willing to act on behalf of others. Such a person is indeed a fitting mate.

We are no less in need of pouring out our hearts today than were our ancestors. We, too, are daily sent on missions which test our limits, which force us into territory we have not previously explored, and for which the stakes may be very high indeed. Sustaining a marriage, cultivating a friendship, raising children, or pursuing a career all test us every day.

With as great an emotional burden as that faced by Abraham's servant, with no less need to cry out and to absorb the comfort of having been heard, many of us have nonetheless cut ourselves off from God's listening ear.

Do we worry that speaking to God is superstitious? That God doesn't answer prayer? That God doesn't *hear* prayer? That there is no God?

Yet discomfort with spontaneous prayer does a disservice to our sacred tradition, to our deepest needs, and to our relationship with God.

Prayer is not philosophy; it need not justify itself at the bench of reason, consistency, or sophistication. Prayer is what the Talmud calls "the labor of the heart." It is answerable to the heart alone.

Our possible discomfort with spontaneous prayer can lead us to the very first prayer we need: "Help me, Lord, to pray." Or, in the words preceding the *Shabbat Amidah,* the silent standing prayer, "Open my mouth, Lord, and my lips will proclaim Your praise."

If you are uncomfortable praying with words, teach yourself to sit with silence. Let your awareness of your need become your prayer; let your awareness of God's love be your answer.

If you need to pray, if your sorrows or your joys move you to speak, from a simple "thank you" to an elaborate speech, then pray. If you rise from your prayers a more sensitive and aware person, your prayer was worthwhile.

Parashat Hayei Sarah/The Life of Sarah
Take 3

The Power of Love

God's love for humanity is revealed in the love two people feel for each other. Our tradition repeats the insight that human beings are fulfilled through their love for one another and in the loving deeds they can perform for each other.

Today's Torah-reading testifies to that power of love.

After burying his beloved wife, Sarah, and mourning her passing, Abraham turns to his servant Eliezer and instructs him to find a wife for his son Isaac. Eliezer returns from his mission with Rebekah, who gazes on Isaac as her caravan approaches the encampment. She descends from her camel, and then, in a way that illumines the power of love potentially within us all, the Torah tells us, "Isaac then brought her into the tent of his mother, Sarah, and he took Rebekah as his wife. Isaac loved her and thus found comfort after his mother's death." Rebekah, indeed, will become one of the great figures of the Hebrew Bible.

Parents, most often the mother, are our first source of love in life. The mother attends to her infant's needs even before the child is aware of having them. Food, comfort, clothing—all seem to be magically provided, along with smiles, kisses, and hugs. As the child grows, the mother is there—and the father too—to provide support, encouragement, and insight.

But at some point in the child's life, it becomes apparent that the parents can no longer meet every emotional need or resolve every fear. As the child begins to see glimmerings of the parents as limited human beings, they slowly "die" as parents. They emerge as people.

Through most of our adult lives, we may maintain some amalgam of both attitudes, our parents are *parents* and adults separate from us at the same time. But didn't something precious die within us when we lost that vision of parents as perfect sources of love, protection, and wisdom?

Do we lose intense closeness forever? The Torah suggests not, for in its description of Isaac's response to Rebekah, it hints to us that, in a loved spouse, we all have the opportunity to regain some of the security, affection, and intimacy first enjoyed by infants and their mothers. In a very real way, the love of our spouses comforts us for the "death," the loss, of the infant's image of Perfect Mother.

That comfort is as close a replica of the love of God as one can know in this world. In the care, trust, decency, and goodness of one's spouse, we have the chance to reaffirm the lesson learned in our mothers' arms—that in this sometimes difficult life there is a haven, and that our love for each other can serve as a witness to God's love for all human beings.

TOLDOT/Generations
Genesis 25:19–28:9

Toldot *tells the story of the second generation of patriarchs and matri-*
archs, and begins the dramatic story of the third. Scenes from this
parashah *are among the most famous in the Bible. The saga begins when*
Isaac is aged forty, and Rebekah is experiencing a difficult pregnancy.
Learning from God that she is pregnant with twins who will become
ancestors of different peoples, Rebekah is also told by the Divine that
the older of the twins will someday serve the younger. Esau and Jacob
are born—the first famously red and hairy, and thus named "Esau," the
second emerging clutching the heel of his brother, and hence named
"Jacob." In a poignant line, the Torah tells us that Isaac loved Esau
because he brought him food, but "Rebekah loved Jacob."

Impetuous from birth, Esau, a hunter, returns from a hunt so hungry
one day that he agrees to sell his birthright to his younger brother in
exchange for a bowl of the lentil stew that Jacob is preparing.

The scene changes, and what follows is a series of incidents that echo
nearly identical ones from the life of Abraham, again involving
Abimelech and the attempt to pretend his wife is his sister; once more the
Hebrew patriarch is protected by the king, and grows rich. Then forced
from place to place by avaricious Philistines, Isaac leads a nomadic life.
As God once blessed his father, Abraham, in Beersheva, so God blesses
Isaac there.

Next comes one of the most powerful incidents in all of Torah. Now
blind and frail, Isaac decides the time has come to bless his elder son,
and so he sends him out to hunt game and to prepare a dish for Isaac to
eat before he bestows the blessing. At Rebekah's behest and with her
help, Jacob masquerades as his brother, approaches his blind father,
offers him food, and asks for the blessing. In words that have resounded
through history, Isaac responds, "The voice is the voice of Jacob, but the
hands are the hands of Esau," and blesses his son.

Esau returns and discovers that his younger brother has stolen his
blessing; distraught, he begs his father for a blessing as well, and plans
to kill Jacob as soon as Isaac dies. Rebekah sends Jacob away to safety

with her brother Laban, telling her husband that Jacob needs to find a non-Canaanite bride. Isaac agrees, and now, in a blessing indeed intended for his younger son, says, "May God grant the blessing of Abraham to you and your offspring, that you may possess the land where you are sojourning, and which God bequeathed to Abraham."

⧈

Parashat Toldot/Generations
Take 1

Our Legacy: Can You Dig It?

Isaac is one of the least appreciated of the biblical patriarchs. While his father, Abraham, was the founder of ethical monotheism and a public leader, and his son Jacob will establish the Jewish People and wrestle with God, Isaac is remembered mostly for being the near-sacrifice during the *Akedah,* the binding on Mount Moriah. In this Torah portion we meet that same Isaac—unimpressive, merely going along and doing again what his more prominent father had done in the past.

The Torah tells us that Isaac's warlike neighbors were sniping at the Jewish community. "The Philistines stopped up all the wells, filling them with earth, which his father's servants had dug in the days of his father Abraham." Isaac's response shows persistence, if not sparkle: "So Isaac dug the wells again, which had been dug in the days of his father Abraham, and he gave them the same names that his father had given them."

Not very impressive, is it? The most Isaac can muster himself to do is to redig the same old wells. He can't even think up new names for them, relying on his father's creativity rather than his own. As the great thirteenth-century Spanish commentator, rabbi, and philosopher known as the Ramban remarked, "There would seem to be no benefit nor any great honor to Isaac, given that he and his father did the identical thing!"

But why should the Torah, normally so concise and laconic, waste words just to inform us that Isaac was unoriginal, that he went through life simply doing what his father had pioneered before him?

The *midrash* gives us a hint. "How many wells did our father Isaac dig in Beersheva?" asks *Bereishit Rabbah.* "The Rabbis said, 'Five,' which corresponds to the five books of Torah." In other words, the *midrash* implies, the act of redigging those same old wells was a way of expressing loyalty to the spiritual values and practices that Isaac had inherited. Isaac's was no mere act of repetition. Instead, by stubbornly holding on to his parents' tradition, Isaac was assuring that Judaism would thrive beyond his own lifetime.

In a similar reading, the thirteenth-century French rabbi Hizkuni remarked that giving the wells the same names that Abraham had given them was an act of merit, "for these names [show] that the wells were in his possession because of his father's legacy." These wells had significance to Isaac because they were part of the legacy of Abraham.

Ours is a culture that places great value on originality, on innovation. Creativity, openness, a willingness to change—all are considered the approach most likely to produce useful discoveries and helpful insights. And, certainly, the wondrous creativity of modern men and women has produced great works.

But the other side of focusing on the new may be a certain rootlessness, a restlessness. How can we feel settled in a world where everything is up for grabs, where every custom or value is subject to question, objection, analysis?

Isaac's example points to the need to balance creativity with loyalty, innovation with fidelity to tradition. Change is good, but change is not God. When change is rife, our lives can border on the chaotic. With no consistency or trust, human living and human relating become impossible. The example of Isaac teaches us to cling to the sublime and the vital from our own inheritance, to honor the spiritual path others have successfully trod before, to respect a tradition the light of which has illumined countless lives through the good times and the bad.

Parashat Toldot/Generations
Take 2

Schwartzenegger Meets Jacob

Esau is surely one of the most tragic figures of the Bible. He is a simple man, whose robust nature leads him to exult in his own health, strength, and energy. Esau loves to hunt, reveling in the outdoors and in surpassing all limits.

He is a man of impulse. Like Rambo or the heroes played by Arnold Schwartzenegger, Esau thrives on his tremendous power, his physical courage, and his own inner drives.

Modern America admires that. We distrust the intellectual—someone who thinks too much, is too sensitive to the feelings of others. We prefer a man who can impose his own will through a show of determination and strength, someone who doesn't need to plan in advance, who can relish the moment and trust his passions.

America accepts the romantic notion that the truest and best expression of who we are lies in the spontaneous release of our feelings. Our feelings should not be subject to control.

But the Torah asserts exactly the contrary. For the Torah, every aspect of being human—heart, mind, and soul—needs constant training, direction, and restraint. The story of Esau and Jacob is exactly the story of these two conflicting approaches to becoming human.

Esau comes home from a day of hunting. He is hungry. He wants to eat. Meanwhile, Jacob has been home; he's prepared a pot of lentil stew. The man of action meets the man of forethought. Acting on impulse, Esau demands to be fed. Responding with calculation, Jacob agrees to sell his brother the stew in exchange for Esau's birthright.

How easy it is to identify with Esau when he agrees to Jacob's deal. He *is* hungry, after all, and having a birthright doesn't satisfy his hunger; lentil stew does. That's what he feels, that's what he acts on—it is so easy for us to identify with him!

Jacob, on the other hand, lives with one foot in the future. Less physically powerful than his burly brother, Jacob compensates by using his mind and by weighing consequences. He prefers to skip a meal if that means he will acquire the birthright of the covenant.

And ultimately it is Jacob who is the Torah's model for us of the truly developed human. "Who is powerful?" asks the *Mishnah*. And it answers, "those able to conquer their own impulses." And even though Jacob's ability to control his own drives, to restrain himself now in order to thrive in the future, is profoundly out of touch with mainstream American values today, it is, ironically, precisely that trait that lifts a person above the moment and makes the future possible.

Immigrants: The Strangers in Our Midst

Most Jews in America were born here, so it's easy to forget the remarkable combination of courage, vision, and sacrifice that it takes to move to a new place, surrounded by a foreign culture, language, and expectations. It's easy for those of us whose ancestors showed such pluck to look with scorn upon today's immigrants—those brave souls who must resemble our grandparents and great-grandparents—and to see them as threatening "our" way of life or "our" jobs, just as earlier Americans viewed our families when they first arrived here.

Today's Torah portion portrays one of our earliest ancestors, the Patriarch Isaac, as an undesired alien, blamed for being industrious and prosperous, and expelled by the anti-immigrant bigots of his day. Isaac, during a time of famine, moved his family to Gerar, a region inhabited by the Philistines and their king, Avimelekh. In a new land, like so many other immigrants, Isaac turned to agricultural work to support himself and his loved ones. The Torah records that "Isaac sowed in that land and reaped a hundredfold the same year." His willingness to work so hard (perhaps at jobs that the Philistines considered beneath their dignity) earned him only the jealousy and animosity of the surrounding people: "The Philistines envied him."

The Philistines responded to Isaac's willingness to accept back-breaking labor, and his ensuing devotion to his family and his people, by trying to cut off his access to the bounty of the region: "The Philistines stopped up all the wells which his father's servants had dug . . . filling them with earth." Apparently, only the native-born Philistines were entitled to the basic necessities of life; the immigrant Isaac would have to do without.

Ultimately, the Philistines' attempt to deprive Isaac of all social support was but the first step in a campaign the ultimate goal of which was expulsion. After cutting off his water, the Philistines finally command Isaac, "Go away from us, for you have become far too big for us."

Feeling threatened by the new immigrant Isaac, the Philistines ultimately were content only with his banishment. Rather than respond to his industry by working harder themselves, rather than seeing his presence in their midst as another source of skill and community, rather than seeing the presence of another culture as a source of enrichment, the Philistines preferred to blame Isaac for his admirable drive and diligence, and to see him as a threat to their own existence.

The Philistines of antiquity are not alone in their willingness to blame their own problems on the newcomer and the immigrant. The renovated exhibits at Ellis Island, where most Jewish immigrants came to America's shores, testifies to the continuing appeal of xenophobia (the fear and hatred of foreigners) as a recurrent pattern in American political life, as unscrupulous politicians attempt to distract the voters from their own failings and ride to victory by appealing to the fears and bigotry of the electorate.

At the turn of the century, from 1880 to the mid-1920s, a wave of immigrants came to the United States. The largest group came from Italy, and the second largest were the Jews of Eastern Europe. In response to the swelling immigration, nativists launched a campaign to close America's borders to any newcomers who threatened to "dilute America's purity." Groups such as the Ku Klux Klan sponsored speakers and marches to protest that these new immigrants were taking America away from the true Americans, stealing jobs, contributing to the crime rate, benefiting from American largess, and degrading American culture. The primary targets of this inflammatory rhetoric were Jews, African Americans, Asians, and Catholics. While there were some brave leaders who stood up for the immigrants (notably Congressman James Curley of Boston), the United States Congress ultimately closed off immigration, dooming millions of our relatives to lives of poverty, fear, and suffering in the Soviet Union and Eastern Europe. Ultimately, those Jews and their children were murdered in the Nazi death camps.

Rather than face the real problems of American society and economic life, most politicians preferred to coddle their constituents and to distract them by blaming the immigrants who, after all, had no vote.

Yet the benefits that this wave of immigrants and their children brought to America—in the realms of culture, scholarship, science, government, and commerce—contributed to our greatness as a world power during the Second World War and beyond.

Philistines of all ages prey on fear and hatred, bigotry and greed. We, the children of immigrants, and the descendants of Isaac, need only recall that hatred of immigrants was directed against us earlier in this century. We need only recall that in the struggle between the hateful Philistines and the immigrant Isaac, God blesses Isaac and takes his side. Ultimately, the Philistines realize the riches that industrious immigrants can bring, telling Isaac, "We now see plainly that *Adonai* has been with you."

The Philistines of our age would do well to ponder the story of the immigrant Isaac, and to recall that the most frequently repeated verse in the Torah is "You shall have one law for yourself and the stranger who dwells in your midst."

VA-YETZE/He Went Out
Genesis 28:10–32:3

On his way to his uncle's house, in the middle of the wilderness between Paran and Beersheva, Jacob prepares to sleep, a stone for a pillow under his head. He dreams of a stairway reaching from the ground to the heavens, with angels at once ascending and descending, and of God standing by his sleeping form and repeating the promise he had made to his ancestors: "Your descendants shall be as the dust of the earth, and you shall spread out to the west and to the east, to the north and to the south; all the families of the earth shall bless themselves by you and your descendants."

When Jacob awakes, he recognizes that God had surely been present, and he had not known it. He vows that if God protects him along his way, Adonai will be his God. Jacob reaches his destination and, in the town center, sees Rachel and rolls the stone from off of the well where she has brought her flocks to be watered. Thus begins the story of their romance. Jacob works for her father, Laban, for seven years in order to marry her, but Laban substitutes his older daughter, Leah, in disguise for Rachel in the nuptial bed. Angered by the deception, Jacob nevertheless agrees to labor another seven years for Rachel.

Over the years, Leah and Rachel compete with one another for children. Leah bears many sons, and one daughter, for Jacob, hoping, with each birth, that her husband will love her. Desperate for a child, too, Rachel (like Sarah before her) arranges for Jacob to sleep with her handmaid Bilhah, who, in turn thus becomes the mother first of Dan and then of Naphtali. Leah responds by having Jacob sleep with her handmaid Zilpah, who bears Asher, and then, with Rachel's assent, sleeps with Jacob and bears him another two sons and a daughter. Finally, Rachel herself gives birth to Joseph. Later, she will bear the family's youngest son, Benjamin.

Having amassed significant wealth, Jacob wants to return home, despite Laban's protests. As Jacob and his family are leaving, however, Rachel steals her father's household gods. Discovering that his daughters and their family are missing and that his idols have been stolen as well, Laban pursues them, and accuses them of the theft of his gods. Having no idea at all that it is his beloved Rachel who has stolen the household gods, Jacob tells Laban that the one who has the idols, shall not live, thus tragically foreshadowing his wife's early death. Rachel, pretending to be menstruating, hides the idols underneath her and blames her inability to rise and greet her father on her "condition."

The parashah *ends with Jacob and Laban agreeing to separate permanently, and Jacob continues on the road home.*

❧❧❧

Parashat Va-Yetze/He Went Out
Take 1
The Power of the Imagination

Through the power of imagination each of us retains the ability to transform the world. Cultivating our creative powers—learning to imagine as a community and to channel our social inventiveness toward visions of justice and of holiness—is one of the central functions of Judaism.

Our religion trains us to visualize a better world, in which we are more passionate and observant, kinder, and more cooperative than we are now. Judaism nurtures that creativity as a source of inspiration and guides us, through *mitzvot,* toward translating that vision into a living reality.

Today's Torah-reading reveals the power of imagination in its full dimension. Jacob has just fled his parents' home. He is on his way to his uncle, Laban, and to a future shrouded in uncertainty and doubt. Exhausted by his journey, Jacob uses a stone as a pillow, and falls fast asleep under the heavens.

Jacob dreams.

In his sleep, he sees angels mounting a ladder to heaven, and other angels descending another ladder toward earth. God speaks to Jacob, renewing the covenant between God and Abraham, between God and Isaac. God clearly extends that covenant to the third patriarch, and through Jacob to the Jewish people as a whole.

"Surely the Lord is present in this place and I did not know it," Jacob says when he awakens.

The Torah never clarifies whether Jacob's dream was merely the product of his own vivid imagination, or whether his imagination provided him with a deep insight into reality. Nevertheless, Jacob acts on his dream as a new understanding of truth.

Jacob's dream was a turning point for him, a crucial step in recognizing the presence of God in his life.

The medieval French commentator Rashi approaches this paradox by explaining that when Jacob said, "I did not know it," he meant, "For had I known, I would not have slept in such a holy place." But had he not slept there, he would never have known that the place was holy at all!

To understand that the location was sacred, Jacob had to trust his ability to imagine, his own inner power to construe.

Every human being has this power. Each of us looks at the world as it is, but we then select which facts matter, and how they are to matter in our own understanding. We look at the world as it is, and we imagine it as it should be.

For Jews that process of imagination takes two principal forms. By reading the world through the perspective of the rich stories of the Torah and of rabbinic tradition, we see ourselves in the timeless world of Jewish values and ethics. We make ourselves contemporaries of Moses and Miriam, of Rabbi Meir and Rabbi Beruriah. It is as if each of us leaves Egypt personally.

And through *mitzvot*—deeds of holiness in time—we train our imaginations to view the world as a place where Jewish behavior, whether lighting *Shabbat* candles or caring for a widow, can transform the world.

As with Jacob, our imagination can provide the necessary first step toward transforming our world and ourselves.

⁙

Parashat Va-Yetze/He Went Out
Take 2

Dust Thou Art

To what can we compare the Jewish People? Our history and our influence are unique among the peoples of the earth. When stripped of their autonomy and their sovereignty, other peoples slipped off the stage of history. Only the Jews were able to survive for two thousand years without a homeland, a sovereign government, or a military. Who today claims to be a Hittite, a Phoenician, or an Edomite? But held together by our religious civilization—a blend of beliefs, rituals, laws, and learning—we Jews maintained our identity throughout the lands of our dispersion.

Despite how small in number we have been, our ideas have helped shape the history of the world: the connection between worship and ethics, the belief in the unity of God, the idea that God is passionate about justice and that all human beings are reflections of the Divine Image.

This Torah portion does not compare us, therefore, to another people in history. Instead it compares us to . . . dirt.

Fearing the anger of his brother, Esau, our ancestor Jacob is heading toward his distant family in Haran. Somewhere north of Beersheva, he falls asleep and dreams. There is a ladder on which angels descend to the earth and climb up to heaven, and God announces that Jacob and his descendants will inherit the Land of Israel. "Your descendants shall be as the dust of the earth," God says in Jacob's dream.

What does it mean to be like the *dust of the earth*? Couldn't God have picked a loftier image? "You shall be like drops of crystal blue water in the sea"? "Gusts of cool air in the sky"? Or, as in an earlier section of Genesis, as "the shimmering stars in the heavens"? Dust is so . . . well . . . *dirty*!

The *Midrash B'raisheet Rabbah* offers several possible explanations for this unflattering choice. Reflecting on our long and sorry history of persecution and oppression, the *midrash* provides a message of hope amidst the grains of dust:

> Just as the dust of the earth wears out all utensils even of metal, yet itself remains forever, so will your children outlive all and exist forever. Just as the dust of the earth is trodden upon, so will your children be downtrodden beneath the powers.

For centuries the people of Israel, descendants of the prophets and sages, were "downtrodden beneath the powers." We were victims of hatred wherever we lived: Europe, Asia, Africa. Even today in much of America, Jews all too often feel constrained to mask their identity lest they be thought "too Jewish." The sad truth is, having been underfoot so often, we do resemble the dust of the earth.

But dust *lasts*. And like the dust, we have outlived the most mighty powers of the world—arrogant Alexander of Macedon, the cruel Roman Empire, the haughty Byzantines. All claimed eternity, and all disappeared. We, like the dust, are still here.

Dust is also ubiquitous. Just as the dust of the earth is to be found in every part of the globe, so, too, are Jews everywhere. On every continent, in every place where people dwell, there are Jews—still affirming our glorious history; still advocating the revolutionary insights that permeate Torah, Talmud, and Jewish religion; still insisting that we can do better, that *humanity* can do better.

After all, dirt has a way of getting under your nails, of clinging to your skin. And, truly, dirt makes the world a more reasonable place: Thanks to dirt, we have sites for gardens and playgrounds for children. It was inspiring to be compared to the "shimmering stars in the heavens." But it paradoxically feels even more ennobling to be compared to the dust.

Parashat Va-Yetze/He Went Out
Take 3

This Time I Shall Praise the Lord

We all dream about our lives, our families, our individual destinies. Born into a world we did not create, motivated by hope, energy, and drive, we spend our childhood and adolescence absorbing wonderful stories of adventure, heroes, and fantasies.

And we dream.

We dream of achieving the highest ideals of our fantasy life . . . of being brilliant successes, traveling the world, becoming famous, or wise. Venerating a galaxy of admired adults, we imagine ourselves as one of them, as one of the best of them.

In the fantasies of children, life has no end; only possibilities, no limits.

We are not alone in spinning those dreams. Children aggrandize themselves with the active consent and encouragement of their parents, grandparents, teachers, and a supporting cast of thousands. We urge our children on, at the same time as we implicitly ask them to "take us with you," and fulfill all of *our* unaccomplished dreams. We drive our children to ballet, music lessons, ballparks; we urge them on with their science projects and religious school.

And we hope in the process that they will become what we dreamed of becoming and abandoned. Often without even being aware of our own fantasies, we impose them on our children. We seem to make peace with our own limitations, but in actuality project our own ambitions on our children: "I won't ever be a concert pianist, but my child might."

This pattern of reality disappointing one generation, causing it to transfer its hopes and dreams onto the next generation, is as old as humanity itself. We catch a glimpse of it as Leah realizes that her husband, Jacob, doesn't love her as much as he loves his other wife, her sister Rachel.

Wrestling with the pain, anger, and disappointment of rejection, lonely in the face of her husband's disinterest, Leah—the one with the soulful eyes—is also the one with tremendous hopes. In the depths of her misty pupils, one can see the pining for a passion she would never know; in the drops of her tears, her pent-up caring and affection leaking away.

Each of her sons, one after another, embodies yet another desperate attempt to win her husband's love. Each one is, therefore, loved not for himself, for being a beautiful infant. Instead, her children represent hope deferred and aspiration transferred.

Reuben is so named because "the Lord has seen my affliction" and "now my husband will love me." Shimon, "because the Lord heard that I was unloved and has given me this one also." Leah calls her third son Levi because "my husband will become attached to me, for I have borne him three sons."

Each one of these boys embodies yet another cry of pain and grief, another unsuccessful attempt to win Jacob's affection. Ironically, all three sons will, as adults, disappoint and anger their father, producing tragedy for the aged patriarch.

With the birth of her fourth son, Judah, Leah finally achieves the inner strength to stop craving her husband's approval. Now she no longer lusts after his concern. She is able to stand on her own. Judah is a source of pure joy, in and for himself: "This time, I shall praise the Lord." The renowned commentator Rabbi Ovadiah Sforno notes that this is the first child in the Torah whose name contains that of God! Like God, Judah is himself a source of joy, not merely a tool toward accomplishing some other goal.

Rabbi Abraham ibn Ezra observes that Leah's choice of a name is a confession that "I will praise God because I do not desire more." "Therefore she stopped bearing."

In her own process of growth and maturation, Leah came to recognize her own worth independent of Jacob's opinion. While grieved by his rejection, she accedes to the reality of the present, without having to impose her dreams on her sons.

In our own lives we, too, face disappointments and the need to relinquish our childhood ambitions and dreams. Like Leah, we can grow to accept ourselves and reality without saddling the next generation, our children, with the unrealized fantasies of their parents.

And only then are we in a position to truly praise, to thank, and to love.

VA-YISHLACH/He Sent

Genesis 32:4–36:43

Jacob prepares to face his brother at Seir. Attempting to assuage his brother, Jacob sends servants in advance, who report that Esau is with four hundred men. Fearing violence, Jacob divides his retinue into two separate camps, hoping that at least one of them might survive. After praying to God for safety, Jacob sends a large selection of animals from his herd to his brother as a gift. These he sends in droves, hoping to propitiate Esau. Then, Jacob spends the night alone by the River Jabbok. A mysterious man wrestles with him all night, wrenching Jacob's hip at the socket. Jacob refuses to release the stranger without a blessing, and the other renames Jacob as Israel, "for you have striven with beings divine and human, and have prevailed." From that day on, Jacob limps, and the children of Israel do not eat the meat around the sciatic nerve. When the brothers reunite, Jacob and Esau embrace and weep. Jacob tells his brother, "Seeing your face is like seeing the face of God." Esau invites Jacob to travel with him, but Jacob and his retinue venture alone to Succoth and then to Shechem, purchasing land from the local ruler.

Dinah visits with the local women, attracting the attention of Shechem, son of Hamor the Hivite, who rapes Dinah, and then asks his father to arrange a marriage. Hamor invites the Israelites to intermarry with the Hivites, and he asks for Dinah for his son. Jacob and his sons are outraged by the assault. Speaking with guile, they insist that the Hivite men must become circumcised, which they do. While the Hivite men still hurt, the Israelites attack, killing the males, taking the women and children captive, and gathering the livestock as booty.

Jacob is outraged by his sons' behavior and he moves on to Bethel, instructing the members of his household to purge themselves of any idols. Jacob builds an altar at the very site where God first was revealed to Jacob. At Bethel, Rebekah's nurse, Deborah, dies, and God confirms Jacob's new name, promising, "The land that I assigned to Abraham and Isaac I assign to you; and to your offspring to come will I assign the land."

Rachel struggles in labor, and dies giving birth to a second son who she names Ben-oni ("son of my suffering"). Jacob renames him Benjamin ("*son of my right hand*"). *Rachel is buried on the road to Ephrat, near Bethlehem.*

Reuben, Jacob's son, sleeps with Bilhah, his father's concubine, and Jacob discovers the betrayal but does nothing about it. Isaac dies at the age of 180, and Jacob and Esau bury him. The parashah *ends by listing Esau's descendants, including Edom.*

Parashat Va-Yishlach/He Sent
Take 1
Wrestling with Ourselves

Can people change? Or is it more likely that human beings' fundamental characteristics remain constant throughout their lifetimes?

Both viewpoints claim vociferous adherents. Yet to assert that people cannot transform themselves is to accept our flaws and shortcomings and to resign ourselves to society's inconsistencies.

Judaism insists that people are dynamic. Throughout our lives we struggle to determine what kind of person we wish to be. "Who is strong?" asks the *Mishnah*. It answers, "One who controls his own impulses."

Through *talmud torah* (study), both Jewish and general learning, we deepen our understanding of the world and of human beings. Through *mitzvot* (commandments) that strengthen our awareness of God and those that engender love between people, we apply what we have learned in study to remake our world and ourselves. And through *tefillot* (prayer and contemplation), we cultivate our ideals of our world and ourselves as they ought to be.

That threefold program for improving our world and ourselves implies a vision of human beings as creatures who grow and develop throughout their lifetimes. As dynamic creatures, we play a significant role in determining what values to embody and how to express those values in deeds.

Committed to a view of people as both dynamic and responsible, Judaism requires a commitment to the long haul. Nowhere is that commitment better expressed than in today's Torah-reading. We see our ancestor Jacob returning to apologize and make amends to his brother, Esau. His thoughts must certainly have focused on a flaw in his own character: that of pursuing his own self-interest to the detriment of his older sibling, and misusing his own intelligence as a tool to hurt other people.

As he approached the fateful meeting with Esau, he must have wondered what it would take to change himself, to prevent a recurrence of his own deceitful arrogance.

At night, left alone, Jacob suddenly finds himself wrestling with someone whom he cannot identify. Is this a person or an angel, or is it the embodiment of his own doubts and failings?

We never learn the answer to that question. But we do learn what it takes to remake one's own character—the ability to hold on. Jacob refuses to let go and he wrestles the stranger throughout the night. Only in the morning does Jacob agree to let go, and then only after receiving a new name, a renewed identity.

Jacob becomes a deeper, more mature person. True, he now limps. Our struggles in life, with others and with ourselves, leave scars. But they also produce growth and change. Jacob is no longer the wily, shrewd, and obnoxious child he once was. Instead, through the process of introspection, remorse, and a commitment to confront his own failings, Jacob is able to make himself into a better, more empathetic individual.

Jacob is able to find the inner strength to apologize to his brother and to change the way he relates to other people.

All it takes is effort, time, insight, and commitment.

Parashat Va-Yishlach/He Sent
Take 2

We Have Nothing to Fear ... Or Do We?

"Being religious would have one advantage. I wouldn't have to be afraid anymore."

Those sentiments may sound familiar. Many thoughtful people, themselves not religious, assume that a principal benefit of Judaism and other religions is that of no longer having to fear life's hazards: loneliness, loss, pain, death. Many religious spokespeople offer the same opinion. If you would only *truly* believe, the claim goes, you would realize that all of life is in God's hands. There is no need to worry.

A nice idea, isn't it? Believe in God with enough intensity and you will never feel anxious again. Inner peace is a general anesthetic, dulling your nerves into a stuporous quiet.

Life, though, doesn't seem willing to cooperate. Rather than providing religious Jews with amiable families, smooth careers, and a healthy old age, life treats everyone equally. The good and the wicked, the believers and the skeptics—all suffer the same losses and enjoy the same pleasures. All grow old and lose loved ones. Everyone eventually dies.

Is fear a denial of God? Does anxiety mean that you really don't believe in God, or that you reject God's loving covenant with the Jewish People?

Let's look to the patriarch Jacob for a resolution to that dilemma. Returning from Haran, Jacob discovers that his brother, Esau, is preparing to meet him, accompanied by four hundred men! Jacob concludes that Esau is still angry, and has organized an army to attack him as soon as possible.

Now Jacob is an extraordinary person. God has explicitly told him that he is under Divine protection and that God will be with him throughout his life. Jacob, in turn, loves God so deeply, and is so eager to enter into the *brit* (the covenant with the Divine) that as a youth he engineered receiving the birthright and was willing to fool his father and deceive his brother in order to inherit his father's blessing. Jacob's love for God is profound, and God's special affection for Jacob is clear. Yet when Jacob first hears of Esau's approach, the Torah relates that "Jacob was greatly frightened."

Midrash B'raisheet Rabbah comments, in Rabbi Reu'ven's name, that "two people received God's assurances, yet they were afraid: the chosen one of the Patriarchs (Jacob) and the chosen one of the Prophets (Moses)." This, despite the admonition to "trust in the Lord with all your heart" (Proverbs 3:5). Thus, according to the *midrash,* the Jewish People in later moments of panic could justify their own fear: "Israel deserved to be destroyed in the days of Haman [for losing hope], but they defended their attitude by that of their ancestor, saying, 'If our ancestor Jacob, who had received God's assurance, was nevertheless afraid, how much the more are we justified in feeling fear?' "

The example of Jacob shows us that fear is fully compatible with the deepest faith. The greatest figures of the Torah, and later Jewish leaders as well, all experienced moments of terror and despair.

Judaism is not an antibody that will ward off the experience of fear. But what Judaism *can* do is offer a faint ray of light that can ultimately illumine even the densest darkness. When all appears hopeless, it is natural to feel overwhelmed. But the comfort of God's love and the covenant between God and our People can allay that sorrow, allowing meaning to be rebuilt and strength restored.

Judaism cannot prevent depression or worry. But it provides the perspective with which we can endure and survive. In the words of the prophet Isaiah, "They who trust in the Lord shall mount up with eagles' wings."

Though we may face troubles, we can still be uplifted, and even fly.

Parashat Va-Yishlach/He Sent
Take 3

Truly Present to God and People

Throughout the ages, religious thinkers have pondered this question: How do people have the audacity to stand in the presence of God? Finite in power, wisdom, and longevity, human beings are paltry and insignificant when compared to a supernova or to a galaxy; how much more so to the eternal Creator who fashioned those marvels? Is it not unconscionable temerity to place ourselves before God, to address God, and to argue with God?

The same question might be asked about the paradox of standing in the presence of another human being.

Each of us is a universe in miniature, replete with our own depths and eddies, our hidden doubts and fears and talents. No one can ever fully know himself or herself, let alone claim to truly know another person. So how do we summon the nerve to address each other with intimacy and familiarity? The inexpressible depth of one human soul exposed to the unfathomable profundity of another, the encounter of unknown meeting unknown, ought to silence the entire universe.

It is a marvel that we can reach each other at all. It is a paradox that finite human creatures can presume to call to God.

Today's Torah portion expresses a similar dilemma, contrasting the encounter of two human beings with an encounter with the infinite Holy One.

On his way back to *Eretz Yisrael,* Jacob finally reestablishes contact with his brother, Esau. Years before, Jacob had deeply offended his brother, and now, as an adult and a sage, he hopes to restore some familial connection between them. But how can he communicate across the silence of acrimony, hidden hurt, and lost years?

Jacob's words are instructive. He presents his brother with a series of gifts, and then says to Esau, "To see your face is like seeing the face of God, and you have received me favorably."

What a remarkable comment! Jacob compares greeting his brother with theophany itself, as if exchanging words with his once-estranged brother is nothing less than revelation! So problematic was Jacob's linking of his brother and "the face of God" that generations of Jewish scholars backed away from his bold claim. In tenth-century Babylon, Saadia Gaon interpreted Jacob's remark as comparing the vision of Esau to "the face of the prominent." In twelfth-century Spain, Abraham ibn Ezra insisted that Jacob didn't really mean God; he meant an angel. And a hundred years later in France, Radak, most boldly of all, argued that Jacob mentioned seeing the angel in order to intimidate Esau, thinking, if Esau thought an angel was present, he would refrain from harming his saintly brother.

What can we do with Jacob's shocking comparison? A starting point is to note that Jacob compares Esau to God in two ways. He says that seeing one is like seeing the other, a reminder that even Esau is made in God's image. And, second, he demonstrates that one serves both in the same way: As the Ramban notes, just as Jacob brought gifts and offerings to placate his aggrieved sibling, so one brings gifts and sacrifices to worship God.

Perhaps what the Torah and the Ramban are pointing out is that we communicate best not by relying on the superficial devices of words and thoughts, but rather by allowing our deepest selves to respond to the presence of the other. Because encountering another person is like seeing the face of God, we approach that person with reverence and warmth. Like an offering to the Divine, we show openness to her concerns and her fears. In so doing, we affirm the unique marvel of each individual.

Just as God asks not to be approached empty-handed, so, too, we can approach one another with offerings of respect, affection, and wonder. And then, like Jacob, we may feel ourselves encountering God in everyone we meet.

VA-YESHEV/He Dwelt

Genesis 37:1–40:23

We meet Joseph as a seventeen-year-old who tattles on his brothers. Jacob favors Joseph, presenting him with an ornate, colored coat. This contributes to the brothers' jealousy, as do Jacob's recurrent dreams in which his entire family bows down to Joseph. Oblivious to the fraternal hostility, Jacob sends Joseph to report on how his brothers are faring while shepherding the flocks. A mysterious man directs Joseph to Dothan, where the brothers are gathered. When they see him approach, they plan to kill him, but Reuben persuades them to throw him into a pit instead. They strip Joseph of his coat and throw him into the pit. Then, sitting to eat, they spy a band of Ishmaelite and Midianite traders passing by. Judah suggests selling Joseph into slavery rather than letting him die, and Joseph is sold for twenty pieces of silver. Jacob refuses to be comforted over the supposed "death" of his son, saying, "No, I will go down mourning to my son in Sheol." In Egypt, the Midianites sell Joseph to Potiphar, the chief steward of the pharaoh.

Meanwhile, back in Canaan, Judah marries a Canaanite woman, Shua, and they have three sons, Er, Onan, and Shelah. Judah marries his eldest son to Tamar, and when Er dies childless, marries Tamar to the next son, Onan. God kills Onan, too, and Judah hesitates before giving son number three. He tells Tamar to return to her parents' home and wait. Some years later, Judah's wife having died, he goes to Timnah. Tamar dresses like a prostitute and sleeps with Judah, demanding his staff and his ring in lieu of payment. Months later, when he hears that she is pregnant, he orders her execution when she presents his own emblems to him. He realizes that she is more in the right than he is, and she gives birth to twins, naming one Perez (the ancestor of King David and the Messiah) and the second Zerah.

Joseph, in Egypt, quickly gains the favor of his new master, becoming his assistant in the house. There, Potiphar's wife lusts after Joseph, trying to force herself on him. When she fails, she accuses him of trying to rape her. Potiphar imprisons Joseph, but even there the chief jailer favors him.

Some time later, Pharaoh's baker and his cupbearer are imprisoned.

Each has perplexing dreams, which trouble them. Joseph says to them, "Surely the Eternal One can interpret dreams," and when they recount their dreams, he informs the cupbearer that Pharaoh will soon pardon him. He then tells the baker that Pharaoh will find him to be guilty and will execute him.

Events occur exactly as Joseph predicts, but the cupbearer forgets about Joseph and his abilities as soon as he is restored to high office.

❧

Parashat Va-Yeshev/He Dwelt
Take 1

The Proud and the Lonely

The Torah portrays a bittersweet lesson about the loneliness of pride as it recounts for us the story of Joseph's character and the events of his life.

At first glance, there seems to be no reason for Joseph to feel lonely. After all, he is his father's favorite child. He is surrounded by eleven brothers in the midst of a bustling and energetic family. Joseph seems to have the potential to fill his life with friendship, family, and love.

Yet Joseph becomes increasingly isolated from his own kin, for he needs to feel preeminent. He needs to belittle his brothers in order to glorify his own talents, to stand out.

The Torah hints at the extent of Joseph's pride from the very start. "Being seventeen years old," says the Torah, "Joseph was still a lad." The rabbis of the ancient *midrash* struggle with that last phrase. After all, if Joseph is seventeen, they ask, how can the Torah consider him just a lad?

Their response is to suggest that the Torah is telling us that Joseph behaved like a young boy; he "penciled his eyes, curling his hair, lifting his heel." In other words, Joseph thinks that if he invents a false and glamorous image of himself, the world will recognize his worth. Even more pitiful, he feels compelled to put others down in order to be noticed and appreciated.

This desire to be better than everyone else is even expressed in his dreams. Twice, he dreams about his family bowing down before him. Both times, he tells his family about those dreams, his visions of his own superiority.

Hurt and enraged by their sibling's arrogance, the brothers sell Joseph into slavery. The result is that Joseph experiences the depths of despair as an Egyptian slave and as a prisoner in an Egyptian jail.

It is only in prison that Joseph is able to overcome his arrogance and learn how to sympathize. He learns that even prisoners are human beings, and that one can excel without having to belittle the talents or interests of other people.

Only in prison does Joseph learn to accept a fundamental principle of Jewish living: *kol Yisrael areivim, zeh ba'zeh*: We are all responsible for one another.

As the Torah shows us, Joseph's interest in the dreams of a lowly fellow prisoner, a deposed butler and baker, is exactly what enables his own eventual restoration; only here does his future glory begin to unfold. He learns through suffering that his own talent can thrive only when it is accompanied by caring for another's well-being.

Far from being a threat to us, the happiness of acquaintances, friends, and relatives forms a supportive environment in which each of us can blossom. By living in community, we can support one another to be the best that we can be. That is one of the ways, this Torah portion teaches us, that we can all hasten holiness on earth.

Parashat Va-Yeshev/He Dwelt
Take 2

God Be with You!

So often, with our focus on building large edifices, increasing synagogue membership, or cultivating contributions for a deserving charity, we forget the original purpose of Jewish identity. We were not called to be Jews in order to spread Borscht Belt humor, or to convince everybody to eat bagels, or to provide a voice for the Jewish Federation's solicitations once a year.

We were called—and are enjoined still—to be a people of priests, and a holy nation. Our mission to the world is to embody a communal life of holiness, sensitivity, learning, and justice, and in this way to testify to the One God who made the heavens and the earth. In the words of the *Shabbat* morning prayer, we are summoned to be "servants of the Holy Blessing One."

How does a Jew *serve* God when our leaders and teachers are so uncomfortable talking *about* God? How many times have you heard "the Torah commands . . ." and "our tradition teaches . . . ," as if a book could give an order, or an inheritance could conduct a class! We are more comfortable talking about the latest political outrage than talking about the spiritual issues at the core of our communal existence.

Who are we as Jews? What is our role in the world? What are our ultimate values? Modern Jews rarely discuss these questions, so essential to a meaningful identity as bearers of God's covenant. Consequently, many of our people look elsewhere; they associate Jewishness with history and heritage, and Eastern religions or cults with ultimate questions and a relationship with divine reality.

Joseph provides a role model of a different, more complete, type of Jew. After being sold into slavery in the household of Pharaoh, we are told that "the Lord was with Joseph." The ancient rabbis were puzzled by this strange phrase. Wouldn't we assume that God was with Joseph all the time? Being the son of one of the patriarchs, a hero of his own biblical tale, Joseph is obviously one of God's intimates. Why else would he play such a prominent role in the Torah? Evidently, the phrase "the Lord was with Joseph" must mean something else.

One possible meaning is provided in *Midrash B'raisheet Rabbah*. According to Rabbi Huna, the phrase means that "Joseph whispered God's name whenever he came in and whenever he went out." It is not that Joseph received the special attention of God, but that Joseph cultivated his own consciousness of God's presence. By continually repeating God's name to himself and regularly invoking God's love and involvement, Joseph trained himself to perceive the miraculous in the ordinary, to experience wonder in the mundane.

Significantly, according to Rabbi Huna, Joseph *whispered* God's name. He kept quiet about his own religious experience, and taught the love and power of God not through words but through deeds. By performing *mitzvot* and acts of love, Joseph testified to God's love with his own example.

Rashi provides an alternate way to read our phrase. According to that medieval commentator, "the name of God was often in his mouth." For Rashi, Joseph spoke often *about* God, not merely *to* God. A willingness to share his ardent love of God, and eagerness to serve God and to let others know that he was serving God, forced those around him to consider their own relationship to God, to morality, and to the *mitzvot*. By speaking about God without discomfort or insensitivity, Joseph challenged the conventions of those around him, provoking others into rethinking their own assumptions.

Both interpretations, one of quiet piety and another of a willingness to speak of God openly, have their place in Jewish religion. Sometimes we best testify to God's loving care simply by embodying that love and involvement. By visiting the sick or caring for the homeless, we demonstrate God's faithfulness far better than any sermon could. A hospital bed is no place for a theology debate, and a homeless shelter is not the location for a lesson in morality. In such instances, our hands can speak more eloquently than our mouths.

There is also a time for speaking about God. Inside our synagogues, Torah study groups, adult education classes, and religious schools, we need to think together about how we conceive of the Divine, and how our Judaism can vivify and concretize our ancestral love affair with our Creator and our Liberator.

Ana avda de-Kud'sha b'rikh hu: We are the servants of the Holy Blessing One.

Parashat Va-Yeshev/He Dwelt
Take 3

The Evolution of a Mitzvah

The majority of American Jews are unaware of the centrality of *halakhah*, Jewish law, and live without recourse to its guidance. At the other extreme, a core of Jews are committed to a static notion of the commandments. Both groups presume that Jewish law is monolithic, unchanging, and driven by concerns of ritual and impurity; they simply differ about whether or not to accept that law as binding.

Both of these positions ignore a central truth about Jewish law: Its history has developed throughout the millennia to incorporate new insights and moral vision, while expressing God's commitment to compassion and justice. The engine that drives the Torah's concern is morality, the passionate commitment to righteous living. Because of that unwavering focus, a *mitzvah* may shift in its expression from biblical times into the Talmudic era and then through the medieval period before it reaches the modern age. What remains constant throughout time is the pursuit of sanctity and justice.

Found in today's Torah portion, *levirate* marriage, *yibbum,* is such a *mitzvah.* Its origins precede the Torah itself. We have evidence of the practice in Hittite, Assyrian, and Nuzi law codes. In each of those cases, however, *yibbum* asserts the ownership of the woman by the husband's family. She is to be inherited like any other property.

Jewish law seems to start with that assumption as well: When Judah's son Er dies, Judah transmits Tamar, his daughter-in-law, to his son, Onan. When Onan dies, Judah hesitates before giving her to his third son, fearful that she was the source of death for his elder boys.

We see legal development within the Torah itself. In Deuteronomy, the law presumes that a brother will provide the semen necessary for his late brother's widow to produce a son who will in turn carry on his father's name. If a brother refuses to marry the widow, he is to be shamed in the humiliating ceremony of *halitzah.*

The rabbis of the Talmud had qualms about this forced marriage, however, particularly since Talmudic law permits marriage only with the woman's consent. A sage of the *Mishnah* asserts that *yibbum* is objectionable, and in some cases, the equivalent of incest. To restrict the possibility of this forced marriage, the Talmud adds new requirements: If the widow has borne a daughter to her late husband, not just a son, the need for this liaison no longer exists. Other limitations, moreover, make it difficult for *yibbum* to take place.

With the passage of time, the priority shifted from *yibbum* to *halitzah,* from intercourse to a public ritual. Whereas the Torah calls for the widow to spit in the face of the brother who won't marry her, the rabbis direct her to spit in his presence but not on him. At the end of the *halitzah* ceremony, the judge is required to voice the wish "that the daughters of Israel shall have no need to resort to either *halitzah* or *yibbum*." In Ashkenazic Jewry, *halitzah* replaced *yibbum,* when, in 1950, the Chief Rabbinate of Israel made *yibbum* illegal. What originated as a way of ensuring family continuity became objectionable because the ancient notion of women as chattel was replaced by a growing recognition in rabbinic Judaism of women as responsible adults. As the implications of the Torah's morality constantly unfold, as Jews are better able to integrate the Torah's values into their social lives, *halakhah* also evolves to codify that evolution.

Dynamic law is the way Judaism has always maintained consensus among our people, established standards to which we can all aspire, and instilled a sacred passion for justice among all-too-fallible folk. Dynamic law—*halakhah*—is what will sustain our people and our covenant, now and in the ages to come.

MIKETZ/At the End

Genesis 41:1–44:17

Pharaoh dreams that seven sturdy cows are grazing by the banks of the Nile when they are swallowed by seven thin cows. He has a second dream in which seven healthy ears of grain are consumed by a stalk of seven parched grains. In a panic, Pharaoh seeks the meaning of his dreams, though none of his magicians or wise men can decipher them. It is then that the cupbearer remembers Joseph, and tells Pharaoh of the Hebrew youth who can explain dreams. Pharaoh summons Joseph from jail, and relates his two disturbing dreams.

Joseph explains that both dreams are one, foretelling seven years of abundance, followed by seven years of famine. Joseph then offers some unsolicited advice to Pharaoh: Find a man of discernment and wisdom to administer Egypt, so that the people can survive the next fourteen years. Pharaoh likes the plan, and realizes that he won't be able to find another like Joseph, in whom Pharaoh senses the spirit of God, so he appoints Joseph as his prime administrator, giving him the name Zafenath-paneah and a wife, Asenath. During the years of plenty, Joseph and Asenath have two sons, Manasseh and Ephraim.

The famine begins, and is no less severe in Canaan, so Jacob sends his sons to procure food from the new vizier in Egypt. Joseph, now aged thirty, recognizes his brothers, although they do not seem to know him. He accuses them of being spies, and he tells them that to prove their innocence they must bring their youngest brother, Benjamin, to Egypt. He imprisons the brothers, and then offers to let them all go free if one remains in the meantime. The brothers realize that they are being punished for their treatment of Joseph, and Joseph, overhearing their recognition, goes off to cry in private. He keeps Shimon in prison, and the rest go home, discovering their returned money in the sacks of grain on the way.

At first Jacob refuses to let them take Benjamin, but the severity of the famine forces him to relent. When they arrive in Egypt, Joseph takes them into his house and gives them a lavish feast, offering double portions to Benjamin. Again Joseph cries in private.

He then has his servants place his silver goblet in Benjamin's sack of grain. Once they set out for home, Joseph instructs his soldiers to pursue them, to accuse them of stealing the cup, and to search the sacks. Benjamin is caught, and Joseph threatens to enslave him, despite Judah, who steps forward to plead on Benjamin's behalf.

✦◆✦

Parashat Miketz/At the End
Take 1

Two Kinds of Intelligence

Pharaoh has endured a night of terrible dreams. To make matters worse, neither he nor any of his ministers understand what the dreams mean. The only person able to interpret those dreams is a Hebrew prisoner in an Egyptian jail, Joseph.

After hearing the dreams described, Joseph announces that Egypt will enjoy seven years of abundance, followed by seven years of universal famine. He argues that Pharaoh should appoint someone *navon vehakham,* "discerning and sage," who will store enough food to ensure the survival of the population.

Why did Joseph use *both* words, "discerning" and "sage"? Wouldn't either one have sufficed to describe the type of person needed?

Our traditions regard each word of the Torah as necessary; any apparent redundancy must be there to teach a specific lesson. Thus each of those words, our rabbis taught, refers to two different kinds of knowledge. The Ramban, Rabbi Moses ben Nahman, comments that the two types of knowledge apply in different spheres of learning. "Discerning," he suggests, refers to knowing "how to support the people of Egypt from his hand with bread . . . how to accumulate wealth" for Pharaoh.

In other words, the first category of knowledge pertains to social policy. A government official must understand how to develop programs that will actually accomplish their stated goals without bankrupting the government in the process. *Discerning,* in this case, reflects the ability to match goals with the appropriate means of achieving those goals. Good intentions are not enough, nor are mere pronouncements. A vision of how to relate policy with purpose and action is the key qualification for any level of leadership.

The second category, *sage,* according to the Rambam, Rabbi Moses ben Maimon, refers to a knowledge of "how to preserve the produce so that it should not rot." According to this standard, the prospective bureaucrat had to know more than just how to govern. He also had to have expertise in his field; in this case, how to store grain for seven years without any loss. To lead a people, one must know about more than power. The realities of human life, the concerns that fill our daily schedules and plague our nights, must be familiar to anyone who would represent a community and seek to direct its affairs.

A broader approach to these categories may be built on the understanding of the Ramban. The first category applies to human learning and human structures; the second, to natural phenomena and properties. To be considered discerning and sage requires education in the humanities, the social sciences, and the natural sciences as well. A fully educated human being must know not only about himself and his community, but also about the larger world.

There is, finally, a third way of understanding the text. Perhaps the two categories refer to the importance of both Jewish and secular learning. Many Jews today know the writings of Shakespeare, Freud, and Hawkings, but are unfamiliar with the works of Yehudah Ha-Levi, Moses Maimonides, and Abraham Joshua Heschel. That form of illiteracy—ignorance of Jewish religious thought and education—limits us to an impoverished relationship to Judaism.

Similarly, to know only Jewish religious sources—Torah, Talmud, and *Midrash*—represents no less a shortcoming than not knowing them at all. In the words of the Talmud itself, if you have only Torah, then you don't have even Torah.

Learning, both Jewish and secular, is essential if we are to become fully human, to become, indeed, discerning *and* sage.

Parashat Miketz/At the End
Take 2

Having a Cow over Hostility

Have you ever noticed that the most contented people seem to deal with deprivation better than others who are less happy? That those people who feel the most lovable are also best able to perceive criticism as an opportunity for their own transformation and growth? The ability to transform negative into positive has to do with one's orientation toward others, the ability to trust other people, and willingness to define one's own advantage in terms of communal prosperity and well-being.

Today's Torah portion teaches that lesson through the saga of the two flocks of cattle.

That great dread sovereign, the most powerful man in the ancient world, the pharaoh of Egypt, dreams of seven cows "beautiful of appearance" who were swallowed by seven ugly cows.

Why are we told that the first group of cows is beautiful while the second is not? And why are the second cows hostile while the first are not?

Rashi explains that the phrase "beautiful of appearance" intimates "the days of plenty, when creatures appear pleasing to each other, for the eye of one creature is not envious of the other." In other words, looking sturdy is a symbol of inner plenty. When we feel a sense of inner richness and love, we tend to see others in a loving and positive light. Self-hatred, on the other hand, translates into misanthropy.

Additionally, Rashi alerts us to the correlation between contentment and envy. If we are satisfied with what we ourselves have, we will not be threatened by the prosperity of someone else. This insight corresponds to a teaching found in the *Mishnah*: "Who is rich? One who is content with his portion." Wealth, then, is not simply a number in a bank account, it is an *attitude* toward one's possessions.

Feeling envious of others is thus often a warning sign of our own inner poverty, of the need to enhance our own sense of worth and belonging.

How much of the hostility among the different movements within Judaism is motivated by worry over the shallowness or insularity of one's own Jewishness? Is it possible that claims of "fanaticism" or "lack of standards" are really projections of our own fears of inadequacy, dogmatism, or loneliness?

Charges that some groups are "tampering with the tradition" or that some are "blindly clinging to the past" may reflect more than merely differing approaches to Jewish living and to Jewish values. Perhaps the anger and passion of those attacks reflect a fear of becoming isolated in the Jewish world, without allies or friends to support one's own spirituality.

The proper response is that of the sturdy and beautiful cows. Content with their own wholesomeness, they were not threatened by each other's successes. Consequently, they could act as a united herd, each cow sharing the others' blessings as their own.

Kol Yisrael areivin zeh ba-zeh: All Jews are responsible for each other. We owe each other responsible criticism and careful dialogue about our differences. But at the same time *haverim kol Yisrael,* all Jews are companions and friends. We also owe each other love, respect, and support.

Just as our covenant with God was given to our entire people, so our love for each other must extend to our entire people.

Perhaps if we show each other enough love, each group within our people will feel secure enough that the disproportionate anger will drain from our disputes. We will not always agree. But if our disagreements can remain within a context of affection, and if our disputes are with an eye toward learning from each other and refining each other, the vitality and unity of our people will be significantly enhanced. Then, and only then, will we have the surplus love to fulfill God's charge to be a "light to the nations."

Our role models are cows. The beacon of light is love.

Parashat Miketz/At the End
Take 3

Dreams into Blessings

Our age is entranced by the hints and possibilities encoded in dreams. Rapt and eager, we attend the modern priests of the subconscious, the analysts and therapists; we sit at their feet, lie on their couches, flash their interpretations as beacons to illuminate our depths. We are convinced that the secrets of our inner lives, the hidden byways of our childhoods and our troubled yearnings, are all addressed in our dreams, if only we had the key to unlock their secrets.

Dreams have fascinated people throughout the ages. In antiquity, philosophers and magicians made a great art of the interpretations of dreams. The Babylonians composed a book of dreams, listing what dreams had which meanings ("If you see a cat crossing your path . . ."). The Egyptians, the Greeks, and others focused on the dream as a guide to what the fates held in store for the hapless sleeper. Dreaming was understood to be the portal of communication to a higher world.

In the modern age, the two great dons of dreaming are William James and Sigmund Freud. James sees the subconscious as the bridge connecting the physical world, accessible through our senses, and the realm of the sacred. For James, dreams represent a secret message from a higher order of being. His theory recapitulates the consensus of mankind throughout antiquity and the Middle Ages.

In a break with that inherited tradition, Sigmund Freud insists that dreams reveal not the future, but the past. Dreams represent the efforts of the human mind to make sense of its own experience, to meet the unmet needs of the heart. We dream, says Freud, because, while awake, we "can't get no satisfaction."

Jewish tradition has also paid homage to the dream.

One of the great dream stories in the Torah is that of Joseph in jail. Imprisoned falsely, he wins his freedom by artfully interpreting the dreams of two Egyptian prisoners, correctly predicting which one would be released and restored to his former employment. According to Rabbi Hisda, "a dream which is not interpreted is like a letter which is not read." Because of his spiritual rigor, Joseph is the only one capable of deciphering the message of the dream.

The sages of the Talmud, Rabbi Hisda among them, recognize that dreams reveal not only something about the future, but something about the character of the person who is dreaming. They understand that there is no exact correspondence between a dream and the future. "While a part of a dream may be fulfilled, the whole of it is never fulfilled." Rabbi Hisda goes even further, suggesting that perhaps the significance of the dream lies in its contents itself, not in any possible predictive powers: "The sadness caused by a bad dream is sufficient for it, and the joy which a good dream gives is sufficient for it."

The rabbis of the Talmud were united in the understanding that dreams possess a power to prompt introspection and to provide new insight into human behavior and its consequences. For that reason, a bad dream was more highly esteemed, because it could inspire repentance and self-improvement.

Our own age differs from the rabbinic estimates of dreams in two regards: Our experts discount the possibility that dreams reveal the future; similarly, they remove any moral element from dreams and their interpretation. But we may well ask, even granted that the subject matter and raw material of dreams are our own experiences, longings, disappointments, and urges, doesn't that lead to night thoughts about what we want from the future? Isn't wish fulfillment possible to attain only in the future? In that sense, then, dreams *do* speak of our tomorrows, alerting us to our own unresolved conflicts and their desired resolution.

How we treat those aspirations, and how we align our behavior to our needs—whether in a way that increases others' dignity and our own, or in a way that reduces us to pleasure machines—is very much a matter of ethics.

Remembering that, we can join our ancient sages in their prayer to God: "Turn our dreams into blessings."

VA-YIGASH/He Came Near

Genesis 44:18–47:27

In an act of great integrity, Judah steps forward and explains that he will allow himself to become a slave so that Benjamin will not have to do so, because their father so loves Benjamin that losing his favorite son, to whom his soul is bound, would kill him. Joseph is so moved by this clear evidence of Judah's repentance that he reveals himself to his brothers, crying so loudly that it can be heard even in Pharaoh's palace. Joseph explains that it was God's plan to send him to Egypt to make sure the family wouldn't starve during the famine, "so it was not you who sent me here, but God." He tells his brothers to hurry back to get their father, and invites them to all live in Egypt, in the region of Goshen.

Pharaoh is pleased to learn of the reunion of Joseph's family, and he, too, invites them to move to Egypt. The brothers prepare to fetch Jacob, and Joseph instructs them to not be quarrelsome on the way.

Jacob and his family sleep in Beersheva overnight, and God visits Jacob one more time, assuring him that he need not fear going down to Egypt, for "I Myself will go down with you to Egypt, and I Myself will also bring you back." Jacob descends on Egypt with a party of seventy people. Joseph rides his chariot to greet his father, and the two men embrace and weep, as Jacob says, "Now I can die, having seen for myself that you are still alive."

Joseph instructs his family to claim that they are shepherds, whom the Egyptians abhor, since this will allow the Israelites to dwell apart in Goshen. Indeed, when Pharaoh has an audience with the brothers and Jacob, he does grant them the region of Goshen. When Jacob appears before Pharaoh, he tells him, "the years of my sojourn [on earth] are 130. Few and hard have been the years of my life, nor do they come up to the life spans of my fathers during their sojourns."

During the remainder of the famine, Joseph sustains his family and manages Egypt for Pharaoh. Under his guidance, Pharaoh acquires all the land in Egypt, as well as its people, who sell first their real estate, and then themselves, in exchange for sustenance.

Parashat Va-Yigash/He Came Near
Take 1

Don't Be Quarrelsome on the Way

In the *Parashat Va-Yigash,* Joseph finally reveals his true identity to his brothers. He loads them with all sorts of riches from Egypt and tells them to return with their families so they can settle in Egypt and survive the famine under his supervision.

In the midst of his brothers' newfound wealth and security, Joseph gives them a strange piece of advice: "Do not be quarrelsome along the way."

Why would Joseph say that? And why, especially, in the middle of a joyous reunion, amidst unexpected wealth and success?

Rashi suggests that, on the way home, each brother might blame the others for having sold Joseph into slavery years before. Joseph, understanding how guilt and denial operate, anticipates his brothers' need to blame each other, and he therefore instructs them not to engage in recriminations about the past. In effect, Joseph tells his brothers that they will never agree about the past, but that they can still live in harmony despite that disagreement.

That advice is no less precious today. Conflicts within families are often magnified by our propensity to remember the past in a way that is most flattering to ourselves. As a result, two loving relatives end up disagreeing not only about the *meaning* of what happened, but even about the facts themselves. By focusing on those areas of disagreement, we lose sight of a shared desire to be part of each other's lives. Joseph's advice still rings true—in such times, it may be best simply to agree to overlook the past, and start afresh in the present.

A second possibility, also raised by Rashi, is that Joseph instructs his brothers "not to engage in arguments of Jewish law (*divrei halakhah*), lest the road become unsteady for you."

We Jews have always argued about our beliefs, and we have always mined our sacred traditions to articulate visions of how the world is structured and how we should live our lives. According to Rashi's second understanding, Joseph's brothers, like Jews throughout time, would spend their time on the road arguing about questions of *halakhah.*

Caught up in the passions of their discussions, they would lose their way religiously as well as geographically.

Our Jewish obsession with ideas contains a potential danger: that we will become so excited by the ideas themselves that we will lose any sense of a connection to reality. The ideas will justify themselves, regardless of how they work in the world, and whether or not they conform to our views of reality.

Judaism has always reflected this tension between the adherence to timeless standards and the renewal of those standards in the light of developing communal understandings and ongoing social needs. We must take care never to curb our passion for ideas, but we must also be on our guard, lest our ideas cease referring back to reality, to questions of how to live a moral, holy, fully *human* life.

A third possible reading of Joseph's warning is that Joseph sees that his brothers are now wealthy because of his gifts. Wealth often brings unexpected tensions. Worried that his brothers might feel the pressures of their wealth, and therefore begin to quarrel about how they live together, Joseph urges his brothers not to allow money to divide them.

We, too, face that challenge. American Jewry is a generally comfortable community. As one consequence of our wealth, we have raised up many different organizations, movements, and institutions, all vying for our attention, our energy, and our resources.

Can we see those different movements and institutions as complementing one another, contributing to a communal life that is multilayered and profound? Or will those movements and institutions perceive each one another as competitors, and waste a great deal of energy trying to impede the growth and health of each other's ways of being Jewish?

As we travel on the road, we do well to remember Joseph's advice: "Do not be quarrelsome on the way!"

Sheep, Shepherds, Egyptians, and Us

Why is it that so many conflicts divide humanity? Shouldn't we all be able to recognize our common identity as people, regardless of our race, nationality, gender, or religion? Why is it that our labels, which ought to represent our most beautiful ideals, so often seem to create conflicts and divisions where previously none existed?

Apparently, part of our self-definition relies on forming borders or limits, where our own identities stop and those of others begin. Knowing who *I* am requires knowing that *I* am not *you*. From that simple distinction, however, it is a small step to feeling threatened by a different way of being. If my form of identity is right for me, then why shouldn't it be right for you, too? And if you have another form of identity, doesn't that challenge the nature of who I am? Too often, groups of people view the differing characteristics of other groups as threatening to their own integrity and survival.

While there is no way to cultivate identity without making distinctions, the danger of distinctions is that they may breed contempt for others. That disdain confronted our ancestors when they moved into ancient Egypt, where Joseph reported to his brothers that "all shepherds are abhorrent to Egyptians."

Many groups remained on the periphery in the hierarchical society of ancient Egypt. It is not surprising that Egyptians hated shepherds. While we can accept the fact of their scorn, Joseph never explains *why* the shepherds were the objects of Egyptian hatred.

Several medieval commentators attempted to provide plausible reasons for this animosity. In developing these explanations, the *parshanim* (commentators) explore how social groups respond to those beyond their own self-understanding.

Rashi asserts that the sheep in the flock represented Egyptian divinities. So he sees the Egyptian abomination of shepherds as reflecting a resentment of power. Hizkuni builds on Rashi's construction, claiming that "they [the Egyptians] feared that their destiny depended on them [the shepherds] and that they were slaves of the flock."

Hizkuni's answer posits a sophisticated theory of powerlessness. The Egyptians felt helpless in the face of the divine sheep. They resented the control that the sheep could exercise over their lives even as they feared their potency. One way to live with their fear was to find someone who was even less in control than the Egyptians were. Since the shepherds cared for the flocks, the Egyptians could view them as the slaves of their gods. This bolstered their own sense of security at the expense of the shepherds.

Rabbis David Kimhi, the Radak, and Rabbi ibn Ezra suggested a completely different motivation for hatred. They assumed that the Egyptians were vegans, that they refrained from eating meat as well as any products derived from animals (though Radak held that the Egyptians did drink milk). In this reading, the source of Egyptian hostility toward shepherds was that they saw no personal benefit from keeping sheep.

Indifferent to whether other societies benefited from herding flocks, the Egyptians looked only to their own profit. Seeing no gain for themselves, they despised the shepherds for their seemingly fruitless endeavor.

What is striking here is that the Egyptians claim the right to judge what is and is not useful for all humanity, not merely for their own society.

Finally, one *parshan,* Rabbi Shmuel ben Meir, known as the Rashbam, avoided trying to find a specific reason at all. Rather than trying to justify hatred, the Rashbam said simply that the Egyptians found the shepherds abominable because they hated them. Simple in its scope, the Rashbam's insight is that hatred is the product of *a priori* prejudice, not of ideology. Only after fostering a need to hate do we develop reasons to justify our hatred. Stripped of the hatred, the reasons are revealed as irrelevant.

Emerging from insecurity and a sense of weakness, hatred is an illegitimate tool for empowering ourselves. Rather than turning our distinctions into occasions for bigotry, let us see them as opportunities to learn from each other's different cultures, styles, and histories. The light of God's abiding love shines most vividly in the full and variegated rainbow of humanity.

Parashat Va-Yigash/He Came Near
Take 3

What's Love Got to Do with It?

We are in love with love in this country. We speak so often of love these days that it has become a postage stamp. Valentine's Day, which used to be a religious festival for a Christian saint, is now a pageant of tinsel love. July 4th is for love of country; Thanksgiving, love of freedom. Mother's Day, Father's Day, and even Grandparent's Day are commercial opportunities as much as they claim to be chances to express love.

With all these celebrations, one would assume that Americans are the most affectionate people on earth, secure in our network of love, generously encouraging one another to be the very best. Alas, the evidence for this is questionable. Do we set aside specific days for love so it won't get in our way the rest of the time? Our cities are too dangerous for random strolls at night; our children absorb record levels of violence on television and movies and then beat each other to shreds during recess; married couples split up faster than paramecia.

How *do* you measure true love?

Today's Torah portion contains one of the most sublime comments about love. In discussing Jacob's passionate love for his youngest son, Benjamin, in three short words we are told that *naf'sho keshurah benaf'sho*, "his own life is bound up with his soul."

The biblical word for self, *nefesh,* came to mean "a soul" in later rabbinic and philosophical Hebrew. Is the Torah telling us that true love occurs when one's own essence becomes inextricably linked with another's? *Keshurah* is what a knot is: tied, bound. The two souls, of father and son, are as firmly interwoven as the threads of a tightly tied knot.

According to Harvard philosopher David Nozick, love is the attempt of two people to expand their own definition of themselves to include the other person. Rather than thinking of ourselves as a discrete "I," we now consider ourselves to be part of a "we."

Perhaps that same insight motivated the Radak when he explained this verse to mean that, because of the great love that Jacob bears for Benjamin, Jacob's "soul will leave him" if the brothers return from Egypt without Benjamin. It is as though Benjamin is now a part of his father's very life, so that any injury to the one is a blow to the other as well. Similarly, any goodness done to the son is also a kindness to the father.

Love, then, means rethinking our own sense of who we are. No longer simply individuals, we grow to incorporate the needs, desires, and hopes of those we love. A spouse, as lover, is more than the person we live with, more than our sexual partner. Our spouses are really another manifestation of this new creature, a "we." Harm the one and the other cries. In the explanation of the Rashbam, because their souls are bound together, when he sees that the youth is missing, Jacob will die.

Love is not merely who you want to live with or how you like to spend your time. Love is what we are willing to die for. Nor is love a matter of choice. We don't choose to feel pain when a loved one suffers, but we suffer that pain whether we want to or not.

Jacob understood the high cost of love. Married and bereaved at an early age, he spent the rest of his life mourning his lost Rachel. Her two sons, Joseph and Benjamin, were particularly precious to him because they were gifts from her, remnants of her life. When Joseph was lost to him, too, Jacob suffered a double loss, surrendering his son—and his wife yet again. His loneliness was the sorrow of a "we" severed into two, longing for its other half.

In growing to see ourselves as incomplete without another—without spouse, without children—we open ourselves to great pain, to the possibility of loss and disappointment. At the same time, we make possible the kind of growth of soul, the integration of another *nefesh* with our own, that is as close as we can come to glimpsing the divine.

VA-YEHI/He Lived
Genesis 47:28–50:26

Jacob is ill, and Joseph takes his two sons and visits his ailing father. Jacob tells Joseph that he wants to claim Joseph's two sons, Ephraim and Manasseh, as his own, because of Rachel's early demise. Joseph brings them to his father's bedside, and Jacob embraces the boys, telling Joseph, "I never expected to see you again, and here God has let me see your children as well."

He then crosses his arms, blessing the eldest with his left hand and the younger with the right. When Joseph tries to correct him, Jacob insists, saying that the younger brother shall be greater than he. Jacob blesses the boys, saying, "By you shall Israel invoke blessings, saying: God make you like Ephraim and Manasseh." Jewish parents use this same blessing for their sons to this day.

Jacob then summons his sons, and offers them each a blessing in one of the Bible's finest poems. In his blessing, he does not omit areas of disappointment, such as Reuben sleeping with his concubine, or Simeon and Levi's violence against the residents of Shechem. Jacob assigns sovereignty to Judah—"the scepter shall not depart from Judah,"—and interrupts his message to his sons to exclaim, "I wait for your deliverance, the Eternal One."

Jacob concludes by asking to be buried with Abraham and Isaac in the Cave of Machpelah. When he dies, Joseph gets permission from Pharaoh to bury his father in Canaan, which he does with the entire court, and there he observes Shiva, the traditional seven days of mourning. Afterward, the brothers fear that Joseph will seek retribution, but he tells them, "Am I a substitute for God?" and assures them that they need not fear him.

Joseph lives to be 110 years old. Prior to his death, he extracted a promise from the Israelites that they are to carry his bones from Egypt and bury him in Eretz Yisrael, when God brings them up from Egypt to the land promised to them.

Unlike the patriarchs (Abraham, Isaac, and Jacob), Joseph is buried in a coffin, following Egyptian custom.

Parashat Va-Yehi/He Lived
Take 1

Looking at the Larger Picture

Remember the *midrash* of the blind people and the elephant? Each one touched a different part of the animal and then described the elephant based on his own particular perceptions. One compared the elephant to a long, powerful tube. A second portrayed the elephant as an enormous barrel. A third, feeling the elephant's ears, depicted it as resembling large drapes. Everyone described what they knew and thus accurately characterized part of the elephant, but were incapable of representing the animal as a whole.

That same discrepancy between individual perception and objective reality occurs every day. We each view the world through our own eyes, listen to its sounds through our own ears, and analyze what we see and hear through our own blend of personality, culture, and training. The world we live in—a filtering of external fact through subjective perception and collective history—is literally one of our own making.

We often do not recognize the larger import of events, because we are chained to our own particularity. We plan our behavior from our own perspectives, and we analyze its consequences from our own viewpoints. The result is that we often fail to perceive the harmony and unity that link everything that exists to everything else and provide coherence by pointing to the Source of all existence.

That same inability to see the larger picture is exemplified by the fears of Joseph's brothers. Recall that the entire family—the patriarch Jacob and the eleven remaining sons—moved to Egypt on Joseph's recommendation. They settled in Goshen and busied themselves with herding sheep. Throughout this time, the courtier Joseph treated his family with great honor and love. But with the death of Jacob, Joseph's brothers become terrified that there are no longer any restraints on their powerful sibling. Perhaps, they reasoned, Joseph was kind to us and protected us for our father's sake, out of respect for his feelings. Now that our father no longer lives, our brother will seek revenge on us for all the evil we did to him.

From the perspective of the brothers, what they did to Joseph was unforgivable. After all, they discussed killing him, and only later decided to sell him into slavery. All of Joseph's suffering as a slave in Potiphar's house and in the Egyptian prison was the fault of his brothers in Canaan. From their perspective, and from his, Joseph had every right to be furious with them.

Yet Joseph's position as a religious role model emerges from his response to their fear. Rather than restricting his perspective to his own subjective position, Joseph struggles to understand what happened from God's vantage point. So he says,

> Have no fear! Am I a substitute for God? Besides, although you intended me harm, God intended it for good, so as to bring about the present result—the survival of many people. And so, fear not. I will sustain you and your children.

According to Rashi, Joseph is struck by the fact that although his father may no longer be living, the God of Israel still lives, and still commands moral behavior. The standards of Israel's God, embodied in the Torah and in later rabbinic sources, retain a commanding voice because Israel's commander still speaks. From the human perspective, Joseph's brothers sold their sibling into slavery. From the divine perspective, they initiated a process that would assure the survival of countless human beings many years later.

We cannot know the consequences of our deeds. Like Joseph's brothers, we must be responsible for our own actions from our own perspective. But like Joseph himself, we also need to look to a higher, more encompassing vision of what life can be. Joseph's response is a vivid reminder that we do not assign ultimate meaning. God does.

May your perspective, too, reflect God's vision of a world redeemed.

Parashat Va-Yehi/He Lived
Take 2

Immune to Despair

The last century was one of the greatest disappointments in human history. More people died in warfare in the twentieth century than in all others combined. Racial hatred rose to unprecedented heights. Despots plunged to new depths of ruthlessness and efficiency. Epidemics, illiteracy, and bigotry, our inheritance from times past, continued. Our environment began to crumble. Democracy forgot that it was to be humanity's last, greatest hope: whether a nation conceived in liberty could long endure. The nation does endure, but liberty has taken a backseat to pleasure, ambition, and materialism.

We Jews are no strangers to disappointment and to tragedy. While the last century witnessed the miraculous migration of Jews from Eastern Europe and many other countries to North American freedom and the rebirth of the State of Israel, it also saw the murder of the largest Jewish population of its time, the savage attack against Jewish populations throughout the Middle East, and the sweet poison of indifference and assimilation in our newfound freedom in America.

It is almost enough to drive a person to despair.

Yet we Jews know that the prime commandment is never to despair.

So often in our past, when our trials seemed endless and our pain unbearable, we have witnessed the miracle of hope, the resilience of our sacred purpose. After every devastation, we have renewed ourselves and rededicated our energies to the establishment of God's justice and love on earth. Other nations rise and fall, and the Jews remain vital, rolling up their sleeves to work to redeem the world, to vindicate our God. Our stubborn resistance to despair is itself an unexplainable miracle.

But a Jew who doesn't believe in miracles, it has been said, is not a realist.

As Jacob lay on his deathbed, surrounded by his sons and daughters, he, too, must have been seduced by despair. In an alien land, far from his beloved Israel, surrounded by sons whose moral fiber and past behavior were hardly the pinnacle of pious living, he must have been tempted to sigh, shrug his shoulders at the hopelessness of it all, turn his face to the wall, and die, drenched in his own tears.

Yet in the midst of blessing his troublesome boys, Jacob exclaims, "I hope for Your deliverance, O Lord."

What inspiration! Expecting despair, Jacob insists on hope. *Midrash B'raisheet Rabbah* recognizes the power of that exclamation:

> Everything is bound up with hoping. Suffering is bound up with hoping, the sanctification of God's name with hoping, the merit of our ancestors with hope, and the desire for the Coming World with hope. Grace comes through hope, and forgiveness comes through hope.

Rabbi Isaac tells us that hope is the spice that keeps life delicious. Hope is the essence that makes for courage and resilience. Hope borrows from our dreams to transform our reality. It imposes our highest aspirations on our most mundane or painful necessity.

To be Jewish is to hope. When we recite the *Sh'ma,* we proclaim that there is a God in the world, one who summons us in partnership to mend the world and to testify by our lives to God's love and God's holiness.

By committing ourselves to Jewish living, now with the pathetic and bloody twentieth century behind us, we affirm the need for hope, and we channel its power, confident that the new century we live in can be different, better.

For Your deliverance, O Lord, we hope. And we roll up our sleeves, and work.

Parashat Va-Yehi/He Lived
Take 3

Hearkening, O Israel

Put yourself in Jacob's place. Laying on his deathbed, he is filled with apprehensions about the special way of understanding God and the world that his grandfather, Abraham, established. It wasn't so long ago, he must have mused, that everyone worshiped a multiplicity of deities, that people sacrificed children to their gods, that some gashed themselves with knives in religious fervor, that cultic prostitution was an integral part of worship.

By recognizing that the diversity of nature is only apparent, and that beneath that variety is an underlying unity, Abraham was able to recognize that all things are linked to that one Source of life, and that that Source, God, demands justice, morality, and compassion. He and Sarah were able to transmit that heritage to only one of their sons, Isaac. Then, Isaac and Rebekah were able to pass this vital truth on to only one of their sons, Jacob, known also as Israel. And now, nearing the end of his life, the weary patriarch must have feared for the future of this precious insight.

His twelve sons were unlikely religious heroes. Marred by their propensity toward violence, their explosive tempers, and their jealousy, they had given Israel abundant cause for alarm. Could he trust them to hold fast to the central legacy of Judaism, to the God who is passionate about ethics, who infuses moral fervor with ritual profundity?

Just before he is about to die, Jacob summons his children to gather around his bed. He tells his sons, "Come together that I may tell you what is to befall you in days to come." Then, rather than begin his list of predictions, he interposes the comment, "Assemble and hearken, O sons of Jacob; *ve-shim'u el Yisrael avikhem* (hearken to Israel, your father)."

The rabbis were struck by the unexpected disruption. Why didn't Israel simply continue with his predictions for each son? They also noticed that the language of his digression strongly echoed one of the most famous declarations of Judaism: "*Sh'ma Yisrael Adonai Eloheinu Adonai Echad.*" And they believed it was scarcely coincidence.

Midrash Devarim Rabbah makes explicit why Israel digresses, and why this verse echoes the lines of the *Sh'ma*:

> From where did the Jewish People merit to recite the *Sh'ma*? From the death of Jacob, who called all the tribes and said to them: "Perhaps after I perish from the world you will worship other deities?" The sons responded to their father, "Hear, O Israel, *Adonai* is our God, *Adonai* alone."

The *midrash* then goes on to develop a dialogue between the patriarch and his descendants. Fearful that his sons feel loyalty to Judaism only out of deference to him, Jacob asks whether they will turn away from Judaism once he has died. In unison, the sons respond, "Listen, Dad,

Adonai—the God our great-grandfather recognized as the exclusive sovereign of the world—is our only God. We'll stick with it, not for your sake, but for our own and for God's."

Responding to his sons' fidelity and conviction, Jacob exclaims, "*Barukh Shem Kevodo l'olam va-ed*: Praised be God's glorious sovereignty throughout all time."

The *midrash* thus transforms the *Sh'ma* prayer into a living drama: The latest generations of Jews promise those who have come before us that our loyalty is undimmed by the years, and that our faithfulness to the covenant of Abraham and Sarah, Isaac and Rebekah, Jacob, Rachel, and Leah, still informs our identity and motivates our deeds.

How many Jews remember keeping a kosher home out of respect for an observant grandparent or parent? How many have allowed those precious practices to evaporate, the inheritance of millennia past vanishing in the short space of a single lifetime?

Now is the time to stand with the children of Jacob, swearing our renewed loyalty to the Jewish calendar and the sacred deeds and practices of our ancient heritage, to renew our loyalty to the God of Israel. Can we conjure with integrity the memories of Bubbes and Zeydes, of childhood rabbis and the great scholars, martyrs, and leaders of our people throughout history, and tell them that their God is still our God, that their legacy is apparent in the food we eat, the rituals we observe, and the deeds of loving-kindness that we practice?

Let us give Israel the same assurance and comfort that his twelve sons were able to provide.

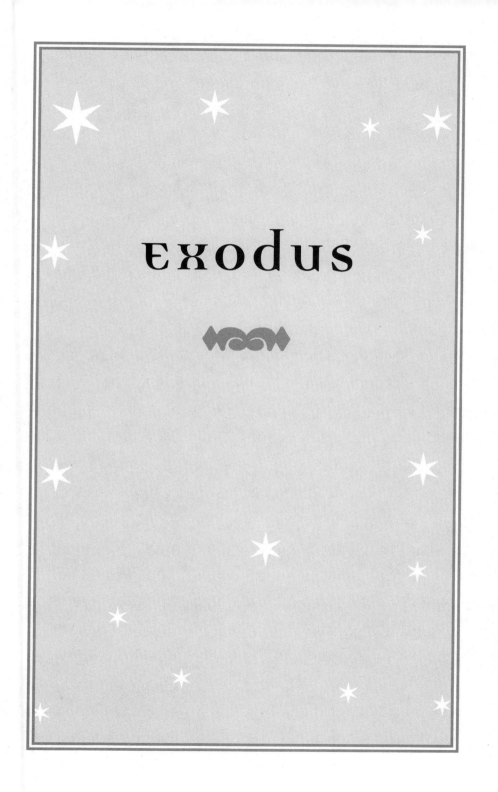

Exodus

SH'MOT/Names
Exodus 1:1–6:1

A new king arises over Egypt who does not know Joseph, and fears that the Israelites pose a threat to his power. The new pharaoh forces them to brutal labor, building the garrison cities Pithom and Raamses. Despite the bitterness of slavery, the Israelites continue to thrive, so Pharaoh orders the Hebrew midwives, Shiphrah and Puah, to kill any Jewish boy at birth. The midwives are pious, however, and they don't follow Pharaoh's order. Pharaoh then orders every Egyptian to throw the Israelite boys into the Nile to drown them.

A Levite woman, Yocheved, bears a son and hides him for three months. She then fashions a wicker basket to float her son down the Nile, hoping that he might survive. The baby's sister, Miriam, follows on the shore, and sees Pharaoh's daughter take the child as her own. Miriam offers the services of her mother as wet nurse. Pharaoh's daughter names the child Moses.

When Moses is an adult, he walks among the slaves, seeing their oppression. He is so outraged by the sight of a taskmaster beating a slave that he kills the Egyptian. The next day, he tries to stop two Hebrews from fighting, and one accuses him, "Who made you chief and ruler over us?" Pharaoh tries to kill Moses, who flees to Midian. By a well, he defends the seven daughters of Jethro, the priest of Midian, against other shepherds, and the women invite him home. He stays, and marries one of the daughters, Zipporah. They have a son whom Moses names Gershom, meaning, "I was a stranger in a strange land."

Pharaoh dies. God determines to free the Israelites. Moses sees a bush that burns, but is not consumed. God calls from the bush, commanding Moses to remove his shoes, since he is standing on holy ground. Then God tells Moses that he is to go to Pharaoh and insist that he let the Israelites go. To bolster Moses's credibility, God reveals the special divine name, Ehyeh-Asher-Ehyeh, I will be what/that I will be. God instructs Moses to turn his rod into a snake, to convince the people of his authenticity.

As Moses sets out for Egypt, God tells Aaron, his brother, to meet him in the wilderness. They assemble the elders of Israel, and the people, who are now convinced. Moses and Aaron then appear before Pharaoh, demanding, in the voice of the Holy One, that Pharaoh "Let My People Go that they may celebrate a festival for Me in the wilderness." Pharaoh refuses, and orders the taskmasters to make the labor even more onerous. The stage is set for the stark confrontation between God and Pharaoh.

✦❦✦

Parashat Sh'mot/Names
Take 1

These Are the Names: Where Is Yours?

In many ways, *Sefer Sh'mot,* the Book of Exodus, is the most Jewish book of the Torah. It begins with the origins of the Jewish People as a nation, newly liberated from Egyptian slavery by the God who created the Universe, and led to Mount Sinai, where that same God establishes an eternal covenant with the Jewish People. The remainder of *Sefer Sh'mot* details the content of that covenant in the many *mitzvot* that comprise Jewish practice, and then authorizes the building of a place of worship, the *Mishkan* (Tabernacle), so that God can dwell amidst the Jews.

Sh'mot has it all—a wonderful story of God's saving love, extensive *mitzvot* so that Jews can reciprocate and concretize that love, and a form of worship through which God and Jews can celebrate their relationship together.

With all those great details, why would *Sefer Sh'mot* start with a long list of names?

The book begins, "These are the names of the sons of Israel who came to Egypt with Jacob, each coming with his household . . ." The narrative then lists each of those children, even though the list already appeared throughout the Book of Genesis.

In fact, this is not the only place in the *Tanakh,* Hebrew scripture, where a long list of names appears, and these boring lists are the first to go whenever *Reader's Digest* or some other user-friendly group tries to streamline the Holy Book!

Why are there so many of them? Why start an otherwise promising book with one?

Jewish commentators offered several answers to that problem. *Midrash Sh'mot Rabbah* asserts that listing the names "adds new praise for the seventy souls who are mentioned, indicating that all of them were righteous." In this interpretation, listing names is a way of affirming the worth of each individual listed.

In a similar vein, the same *midrash* equates the importance of the people of Israel with the stars in the heavens, noting that the same Hebrew word, *sh'mot* (names), is used to apply to both. Rashi summarizes these *midrashim* when he informs us that "even though they were recorded during their lifetimes by their names, the Torah returned and recorded them after their deaths to proclaim how beloved they were."

Lists matter only if those listed matter. All of us can remember reading an author's lengthy list of acknowledgments at the beginning of a book, or can recall enduring a retirement or Bar Mitzvah speech during which a long list of names consumed endless time, as in "I'd like to thank my Uncle Milt and Aunt Esther for flying all the way from Atlanta to be here today." For the family involved, and for those whose names were read, the time passed pleasantly and quickly. Only those who didn't know the people being thanked experienced the list as excessively long.

Certainly when one is singled out for special praise, one enjoys having one's name publicly announced. Look at all the plaques and dedications festooning our synagogues, community centers, and federation buildings. Those names are there because the honorees and those who love them care about seeing people who perform good deeds recognized by the community.

In precisely the same way, the long lists of the Torah represent an assertion of human worth. We may not care about every name listed there, but the author of the Torah does, and wants us to learn to care as well. Those names teach us that more people are involved in our lives than we choose to acknowledge, that we are more deeply embedded in our society than we will ever know.

Just think, for a moment, about all the people who have had an effect on who you are today. Your parents, siblings, grandparents, and close family members may be only the beginning. Consider your preschool teachers and classmates. Add the parents of your preschool friends, all your teachers and friends in grade school, your favorite TV characters and books, and then the names of many people you don't even know—the authors of those books and the producers of the television shows. Include those special teachers of your religious school days, culminating in your Bar/Bat Mitzvah teacher and your childhood rabbi and cantor. In high school, the list broadens to include even more authors and thinkers who may have influenced your life: athletic coaches, drama instructors, art teachers, people who gave you summer and afternoon jobs, those who ran your summer camp or organized your vacations. And of course, don't forget your first romantic partners. A lengthy roster already, and this one goes only up to high school!

Clearly, a list of people who contributed to who you are today would be tremendously long. To other people, your list would probably be boring. But each of us cherishes such a private list of gratitude, since that list represents the many facets of our own personality.

By insisting that we endure several such lists, the Torah opens us to recalling our own dependency on others, and also spurs us to be such influences for those people whose lives we can touch.

Whose lists are you on? How many lists *could* you be on that you have simply not bothered with—getting involved with your synagogue, donating blood to the Red Cross, becoming active in teaching religious school, or working with a homeless shelter, an important charity, a political campaign, or an art festival?

There are so many lists waiting to be assembled. All of them have a space available for your name, and only you can place your name where it should be.

We depend on each other to be able to blossom into the best that we can be. Not only as human beings, but as Jews—a small minority wherever we live—the deeds that we do for each other, the energy and insight we give to building a sensitive, caring, and stimulating Jewish community, the ways we demonstrate our love for our fellow Jews and for all humanity—such deeds can bless innumerable lives in unpredictable ways.

"These are the names." Where is yours?

*Parashat Sh'mot/*Names
Take 2

The Bush Is Still Burning

The Torah recounts that Moses "came to Horeb, the mountain of God. An angel of the Lord appeared to him in a blazing fire out of a bush. He gazed, and there was a bush all aflame, yet the bush was not consumed."

How odd—a bush ablaze, yet the flame doesn't destroy the bush!

Sh'mot Rabbah, an ancient *midrash,* remarks that "just as the bush burns with fire but is never consumed, so Egypt will never destroy Israel."

A simple bush that is constantly under attack, yet which thrives nonetheless—an unimpressive plant that became the preeminent symbol for our people throughout our long and remarkable history.

What an apt symbol it is.

Like the bush, we, too, are very small. One out of every four people on the globe is Chinese. The Christian and Muslim populations constitute half of humanity. Jews are a mere twelve million, less than $1/300$th of the world's population.

A tiny people, we have suffered the attacks of every major Western and Middle Eastern power: Egyptians, Assyrians, Babylonians, Greeks, Romans, Byzantines, Arabs, and the nations of Europe all have taken their turn oppressing, expelling, or murdering Jews.

Yet, like the burning bush, we were not consumed. Instead, we continue doing what we Jews have always done to implement our sacred covenant with God, working to make the world more ethical, more compassionate, and more godly.

Despite our lack of numbers, our relative poverty, and our powerlessness, we have cast a healing beam of light on humanity. Our articulation of ethics—embodied in the Ten Commandments and in the Holiness Code of Leviticus—are common knowledge throughout the world. The Jewish idea of *tikkun olam*—repairing the world—inspires countless numbers of people, Gentile as well as Jew, to spend their lives giving to others of their time, their energy, and their resources.

We have, through our daughter religions of Christianity and Islam, spread the message that God is passionate about justice on a social level, and forgiving and loving to individuals.

The notions that all are "created equal" and "endowed by their Creator with certain inalienable rights" which undergird democratic theory spring out of the Torah, with its insistence that all are made in the Divine image.

The bush is still burning, still giving off light. In our generation, we have been blessed to witness the revival of our ancient language (Hebrew) in our ancient land (Israel). The lesson of the burning bush is a lesson about the shining light of being Jewish. Rooted in its own soil, illumined by the burning presence of God, the humble little thornbush became the catalyst for the liberation of Egypt's slaves.

As the people of the burning bush, we—if we cherish our ancient heritage and live its values—can do so, too.

Parashat Sh'mot/Names
Take 3

Standing on Holy Ground

Every place is not the same. Intuitively, we have a sense that there are distinctions of space that are just as fundamental to human identity as are distinctions in time. When we enter the elevated vaults of a Gothic cathedral, marvel at the staggering beauty of the Grand Canyon, or shrink under the lofty heights of a New York skyscraper, we respond distinctly to different spaces.

Is the distinction between one place and another something intrinsic to the place itself, or the result of perceiving different meanings in different places? Would there be different places if there were no different viewers?

Today's Torah-reading contains the first biblical example of a sacred space, and thereby provides a view of how Judaism approaches the notion of distinction in space. Having fled from Egypt and his execution of a cruel taskmaster, Moses arrives in Midian and attaches himself to the family of Jethro, a local patriarch. One day, while caring for Jethro's flock, Moses approaches a mountain where he sees a strange phenomenon: It looks like a burning bush, although the bush appears to be impervious to the fire.

His curiosity aroused, Moses approaches the flame. Suddenly, the holy voice of God commands, "Do not come closer. Remove the sandals from your feet, for the place on which you stand is holy ground."

Is the ground holy because there is something special and unique about that particular place, or is its holiness contextual, deriving from its special use at that moment?

What makes a place holy?

The great Ga'on, Saadia, was one of the earliest to recognize that holiness is not intrinsic to any one particular site; rather, holiness is the result of what we do, and the meaning we can focus into a particular moment or a special ritual on that site. In commenting on the words "holy ground," Saadia explains that the phrase means "made holy." The sanctity of that site derives from what God and Moses do there, not from the nature of the place itself.

Similarly, Ramban recognizes that "even though [the site] is distant from the bush, take care with it, because the descent of God's presence sanctified all of the mountain." Hizkuni notes a similar description elsewhere in the Bible: When Joshua is commanded to circumcise the Israelites, he is told that he should remove his shoes because the place is sacred. When the priests ministered in the Tabernacle's Holy of Holies, they did so barefoot. Why? The Ramban explains, "because in every instance in which a sign of God's presence precedes prophecy, there you find the place 'sanctified.'"

Judaism wrestles with the tension created by the unequal natures of God and humanity. We are finite and tangible. We perceive reality through our senses, and we experience meaning through our emotions. God, according to Jewish teaching, is beyond body, beyond limit or understanding. How can two such different orders of being meet in a relationship? How can the infinite and the universal accommodate the needs of the moral and the individual? How can God and humanity ever encounter one another?

From the perspective of human need, sacred space is real and essential. In the words of religion professor Jonathan Smith, we require "a focusing lens for meaning"; that lens is the function of sacred space. In that space, *made* sacred because of what we do and experience there, we can explore our spiritual depths, encounter the holiness of life, and reaffirm our sacred identity as Jews. In our synagogues and houses of study, we can encounter God.

But God does not need sacred space. If God is everywhere, then all space is equally sacred, presenting equal insight into God's presence and promise.

Sacred space is religion's accommodation to human beings. Our finiteness, our need to witness the special signs of sanctity—the Torah scroll, the *Tallit,* or the *Shabbat* candles—to hear the sounds that recall religious fervor—the shofar call or the chant of *Kol Nidrei*—all contribute to our sense of meaning and connection.

God may not need our rituals, but being fully human requires establishing reliable tools to focus our attention, to help us concentrate on who we are and what we value, to link us to the universe and its Creator.

Moses stood on sacred soil because, in that context, he was in the presence of God and he knew it. We, too, stand in a sacred place any time we are aware of the lofty potential of that moment and of all moments.

Perhaps that is the ultimate mission of the Jew: to transform every moment into a sacred moment and every place into a sacred place. Then, in a world of ritual profundity, ethical rigor, and social justice, we, too, will remove our shoes in reverence—the better to savor God's awesome embrace.

VA-ERA/He Appeared

Exodus 6:2-9:35

God summons Moses to demand that Pharaoh free the Israelites, and to establish a unique relationship: "I will take you to be My people, and I will be your God." Moses objects that he has a speech impediment, so God appoints Aaron to be the spokesman. God explains that Pharaoh's heart will be hardened to demonstrate the extent of God's might to the Egyptians. Moses and Aaron appear before Pharaoh, and cast down Moses's rod, turning it into a snake. Pharaoh's magicians are able to replicate this wonder, although Moses's snake swallows those of Pharaoh. Pharaoh still refuses to listen. The next morning, Aaron and Moses go to the banks of the Nile. They strike the water with the rod, and the Nile turns into blood, and all the fish in it die. Again Pharaoh's magicians seem able to replicate this wonder, and Pharaoh refuses to concede.

After seven days, God tells Moses to threaten Pharaoh with a plague of frogs. There come to be so many of them that they cover the entire land, and Pharaoh asks Moses to plead with God to remove the frogs. Moses agrees to do so in order to show Pharaoh that there is none like the Lord our God. The frogs die, yet Pharaoh still refuses to heed God's will. Aaron holds out his arm, striking the dust with his rod, and a plague of lice swarms throughout Egypt. This time, the magicians' attempt to replicate this action fails completely and the magicians recognize that this is indeed the finger of God.

Pharaoh still refuses to relent.

Moses threatens a plague of locusts, which devour the crops. Pharaoh summons Moses and Aaron, permitting the people to leave and sacrifice to God if they will but plead with God to remove the insects. Once this is done, however, Pharaoh reneges on his agreement to let the Israelites go.

The next day, the plague of pestilence wipes out the Egyptian livestock, while the livestock of the Israelites remain healthy. Pharaoh still refuses to free the slaves.

Moses and Aaron throw up handfuls of soot, which becomes a fine dust throughout Egypt, causing boils on the people and the remaining animals. This inflammation is so severe that it strikes the magicians themselves, but Pharaoh's heart remains hard.

Moses announces that the next plague will be hail, and those Egyptians who revere God take their slaves and livestock inside. The hail is so heavy, fire flashing in its midst, that it wreaks widespread devastation.

There is no hail in Goshen. Pharaoh asks Moses to intervene, but once the hail stops, he again refuses to liberate the slaves.

✤☙◑✤

Parashat Va-Era/He Appeared
Take 1

The Importance of Playing God

Once again, Moses prepares himself to enter Pharaoh's court. Raised there from childhood, and having fled the court to avoid Pharaoh's anger, Moses now returns to demand the liberation of his people. Formerly a slave to the Egyptians, and adopted grandson to the Pharaoh, Moses must transform his inner nature to stand in a new role in court. Moses is summoned to grow in stature before he meets with the earthly king.

In preparing Moses for his mission, God tells him, "I place you in the role of God to Pharaoh, with your brother, Aaron, as your prophet."

Ordinarily, such a claim would be the height of arrogance. The act of "playing God" implies assuming powers or feigning a certainty which is beyond the proper purview of any human being. Certainly, pious Jews throughout the millennia have worked hard to cultivate their own humility, their own sense of being "mere dust and ashes." Yet God instructs Moses to "play God" as a necessary step in our historic liberation from slavery.

The rabbis of antiquity, in *Midrash Sh'mot Rabbah,* understand this verse as evidence of God's uniqueness. Most rulers, they point out, prohibit any other person from using their staff of office, wearing their crown or robes, and, most especially, assuming their names: "One must not call himself by the name of a mortal king, Caesar or Augustus, for if one assumed his name, he would be executed; yet God called Moses by His own name." Other sovereigns are finite in their power and their wisdom. Perhaps because they are all too aware of their own limitations, they become jealous of the emblems and titles of their rule. God, on the contrary, is without limits. Not needing to fear running out of goodness or majesty, God willingly imparts holiness and dignity to all of creation.

Perhaps the verse hints at an insight that extends beyond the unique example of Moses and Pharaoh. Perhaps Moses and Pharaoh provide a lesson in seeing God in every encounter with another human being.

After all, *Braisheet,* the first book of the Torah, reminds us that all people are made in the Divine image. And the Book of Psalms tells us that we are "made little lower than the angels."

If God's image is found reflected in the humanity of other human beings, then each encounter with another person is potentially an encounter with God. Each conversation, each opportunity to interact with someone else, with anyone else, is no less than an act of revelation.

Rabbi Abraham Joshua Heschel, for many years a professor at the Jewish Theological Seminary, used to criticize the popular idea that Judaism prohibited images of God inside synagogues. In fact, he would say, if you look around during a *Shabbat* service, you will see that God's image fills each occupied seat. The assembled worshipers are themselves images of God!

To experience revelation, however, takes a certain inner openness. All of us have the ability to come face to face with God in our contacts with each other. The *midrash* tells us that Moses had to confront Pharaoh so that the self-obsessed monarch would be able to look upon a former slave and say, "This is God."

Can we, in the weeks ahead, teach ourselves to regard our fellows and to say the same?

Parashat Va-Era/He Appeared
Take 2

Liberation Proceeds in Stages

One of the characteristics of youth is impatience: While older adults are tempered by the realities of human passivity and inertia, young people agitate for immediate change and progress. Unwilling to concede that society moves very slowly, unable to accept human suffering and callousness, young people, in their eagerness to translate their dreams of a redeemed humanity into living reality, often grow angry with the plodding cautiousness of adults.

That same impatience must have struck young Moses as well. Watching his people suffer under the strains of Egyptian slavery must have been a tortuous agony. We know that Moses, in his youth, was passionate about his people and about justice, and that he did not hesitate to intervene to redress grievances and to assist the weak and the needy.

Like so many moderns, Moses must have often despaired of divine assistance. After all, the Jews had been slaves in Egypt for four hundred years, and there was no sign of the Egyptian dynasty relenting at all.

In the midst of this youthful zeal, Moses encounters God, the ancient Holy One. In the process of liberating the Jewish people, God also teaches a lesson in persistence. Permanent change in human nature requires time, patience, and determination. Liberation comes in stages, not all at once. Cosmetic alterations may come easily, but permanent and significant growth emerges over a long period and only with great effort.

In today's Torah portion, God tells the Jewish people, "I am the Lord, I will free you from the labors of the Egyptians and I will deliver you from their bondage. I will redeem you with an outstretched arm and through extraordinary chastisements. And I will take you to be My people and I will be your God."

These four verses of liberation, "I will free you . . . I will deliver you . . . I will redeem you . . . I will take you," became the single paradigmatic emblem of Jewish redemption. According to *Midrash Sh'mot Rabbah*, "the Sages ordained four cups to be drunk on the eve of *Pesah* to correspond with these four expressions, in order to fulfill the verse, 'I raise the cup of deliverance and invoke the name of the Lord' " (Psalm 116:13). Thus, each cup of wine at the Seder represents a different aspect of the process of liberation.

According to the Ramban, each aspect of deliverance marks an advance toward the goal of complete freedom. Thus the first step, "I will free you," refers to the cessation of external bondage. The *sine qua non* for any human freedom is an end to external oppression. The absence of outside pressure is not itself freedom, however. The next step, "I will deliver you," refers to leaving the sovereignty and control of the former oppressors. Remaining under their influence, even if no longer under their servitude, precludes true liberation.

The third stage of freedom, "I will redeem you," involves a reorientation of values. It is through the mighty acts which accomplished the exodus from Egypt, the signs and wonders, that the Israelites came to understand that human pomp and pretension were unable to provide ultimate meaning and value. The temptations of Egyptian society were, in the final analysis, mere glitter and distraction from what made life ultimately significant. The moment of redemption was that time when Israel realized that ultimate worth—the goal of the religious endeavor—came in serving something ultimate, rather than furthering any human conceit.

The fourth stage of freedom, "I will take you to be My people," refers, according to the *Bekhor Shor,* to the meeting of God and Israel at Mount Sinai.

Ultimately, freedom is much much more than the absence of external restraint. Freedom is the ability to assume responsibility for one's own life and for one's community as well. We are most free, most fully human, when we help ourselves and others to live up to our best potential as caring human beings and as serious Jews.

Thus, the freedom of Torah—the only true freedom that Jews can enjoy—is a call to responsibility, toward spiritual adulthood. By assuming responsibility for the *mitzvot,* by taking our place in the unbroken chain of Jewish observance, tradition, and transmission, we renew the ancient process of liberation that our ancestors experienced in Egypt.

When each of us proceeds through the stages of liberation, we exchange the modern-day Pharaoh of materialism and the contemporary idolatry of the self, for the purifying service of the Holy Blessing One, and acts of love toward our fellow human beings.

The process begins anew today. It calls to you.

Parashat Va-Era/He Appeared
Take 3

Bearing Fruit Even in Old Age

Most of our lives are darkened by the shadow of aging. We are made uncomfortable by the aged, made nervous by their physical conditions; we may find ourselves joking about being in wheelchairs, in convalescent homes, in hospital beds. Old age may be associated with the incompetent, with a state of permanent boredom and irrelevance. By bleaching our hair, lifting our faces and breasts and calves, liposuctioning off our fat, and dressing in the gaudiest way possible, we hope to "stay young" forever.

Our fear of age trails us everywhere, urging middle-aged women to undergo cosmetic surgery and middle-aged men to find a mistress. It whispers to us of "our last chance"—whatever the vice in question. There is a frenzied quality to our recreation, our relationships, and our acquisition of property, since we expect all of them to ward off the inevitable: death.

There is one way to ward off death, but it doesn't lie in the distractions and the stuporifics offered by today's fashion magazines. We can ward off death, prevent its encroachment into the realm of life, only by truly living each and every day, only by refusing to see the elderly as the walking dead, or to view aging as equivalent to dying.

We can put off death by honoring the old among us.

Look, for a moment, at how our Jewish tradition speaks of age. In today's Torah portion, Moses and his brother, Aaron, receive God's command to appear before Pharaoh to demand the freedom of the Jews. In what looks like an unnecessary digression, after discussing the conversation between the brothers and God, the Torah records that, "Moses was eighty years old and Aaron was eighty-three, when they made their demand on Pharaoh."

Why does the Torah stoop from the drama of statecraft and diplomacy at the highest levels to reveal something so mundane, so irrelevant as the age of these two leaders?

According to Rabbi Abraham ibn Ezra, this reference to advanced age is unique: "We don't find prophets anywhere else in Scripture for whom the text points out that they prophesied while elderly, except here." Only for Moses and Aaron does the Torah go out of its way to tell us that they were old. Why?

Rabbi ibn Ezra explains:

Because it attributes greatness [to Moses and Aaron] beyond all other prophets, for only to them did God appear . . . for only to them was the Torah given, and thus through their hands do the righteous inherit the Coming World, while all other prophets either chastise or predict the future.

Rabbi ibn Ezra notices a distinction in the functions of these brothers and all subsequent Jewish prophets: Only Moses and Aaron transmit new teaching to the Jewish People, and their teachings become our portal to eternal life and higher purpose. All the other prophets, as great as they indubitably were, worked to remind us of the ethical and spiritual core of the Mosaic revelation. While Rabbi ibn Ezra's insight is itself remarkable, for our purposes what stands out is his evaluation of age. He sees the statement of Moses and Aaron's old age as highly complimentary. Not only do they not hide their age, but it is a source of pride. In the words of the Talmud, "at eighty—the age of strength."

What is the strength of eighty years? Surely a teenager is stronger physically, and a child can run farther and exudes more energy! The acumen of a forty-year-old is more quick and deft, and a sixty-year-old is more cognizant of the ways of the world.

The strength of eighty is the wisdom that comes from experience and completion. Having run much of the course of life, having seen the follies and passions of the human heart rise and subside, having seen his own dreams and limitations and achievements and those of his friends, an adult of eighty is finally able to look at the human condition with compassion and some skepticism. At eighty, we need no longer serve either passion or ambition. Rather we can review our lives, taking stock of how those who cared for us as children paved our paths through life, for good or for ill.

The Talmud relates that Rabbi Hanina used to say that one was regarded as healthy, "as long as one is able to stand on one foot and put on and take off one's shoes." Rabbi Hanina reportedly was able to do so at the age of eighty. He remarked that "the warm bath and oil with which my parents anointed me in my youth have stood me in good stead in my old age."

In our youth, each one of us was cared for by someone older. As links in the chain of generations, we also care for others who depend on us to transmit what they need to establish lives of purpose, accomplishment, and belonging.

Judaism is the warm water and Torah is the oil with which to anoint our children and ourselves, the bath to keep away the chill. Then, even in old age, we will flourish like cedars. Planted in the courtyards of our God, we shall bear fruit even in old age.

BO/Go
Exodus 10:1–13:16

Sending Moses to Pharaoh again, God clarifies the pedagogy behind the plagues: "that you may know that I am the Lord." Moses and Aaron tell Pharaoh to free the Israelites or face a plague of locusts. By this time, Pharaoh's courtiers are disheartened, and they, too, entreat Pharaoh to relent. Pharaoh is willing to let the men go to worship God, but insists on keeping the women and children, to which Moses responds, "We will go, young and old. We will go with our sons and daughters." Pharaoh refuses to permit the entire people to go.

Moses holds out his rod, and God brings an east wind, which covers the entire land with locusts; they devour every remaining plant, fruit, grass, and tree in Egypt. Pharaoh summons Moses and Aaron, admits his guilt before God, and asks Moses to intercede. When Moses does, God removes the locusts, but Pharaoh's heart is hardened and he refuses to let the Israelites go.

Moses then stretches out his arm and God brings a plague of darkness, so thick it can be touched. It covers the land for three days, while all the Israelites enjoy light in their dwellings. In a panic, Pharaoh is willing to permit the people to go, but insists that the flocks and herds remain behind. Moses refuses, and Pharaoh kicks him out, saying that if he sees Moses again, Moses shall die. Moses responds that his words are confirmed above; the two will never again meet. God turns the hearts of the Egyptians to the Israelites, and Moses is himself highly esteemed by the Egyptian people. The Israelites "borrow" objects of silver and gold from the Egyptians, who willingly give them over.

The final plague is the death of the firstborn.

The establishment of the festival of Pesah (Passover) interrupts the progression of plagues. On the tenth day, each household selects a lamb (or joins with other families and shares a lamb). When the lamb is slaughtered, its blood is spread on the door posts, and it is roasted and eaten in its entirety that same night, with matzah (unleavened bread) and marror (bitter herbs). Throughout the week of Pesah (Passover), the Israelites are to eat only unleavened bread and remove all traces of

hametz *(leaven) from their possession. This celebration is for all generations: "When your children ask you, 'What do you mean by this rite?'
you shall say, 'It is the Passover sacrifice to the Eternal One, because
God passed over the houses of the Israelites in Egypt when God smote
the Egyptians, but saved our houses.' "*

*In the middle of the night, God strikes down the firstborn Egyptians
(and the firstborn cattle, as well). The outcry of the Egyptians is so great
that even Pharaoh awakes, and he summons Moses and Aaron and tells
them to leave with the entire Israelite people and their flocks and herds.
The Egyptian people also urge the Israelites to hurry. Along with the
Israelites, other peoples, too, flee into freedom. The night of their journey
into freedom has been commemorated throughout the ages.*

✦◗◖✦

Parashat Bo/Go
Take 1

A Once and Future Freedom

The central story of the Jewish People is our story of liberation. The
exodus of Israel from *Mitzraym*—leaving the bondage of slavery under
Pharaoh to become a free people in our own land—has stirred the souls
of countless peoples around the globe, as they, too, have struggled for
independence and freedom. One of the most profound gifts of the
Jews to the world has been just this recognition that God sides with
slaves and intervenes on behalf of the downtrodden.

How ironic, then, that the tale of freedom which inspired, and still
inspires, millions should be incomplete. Our liberation from Egypt, the
great paradigm of freedom, is flawed by the very haste with which freedom was achieved. Instructed about the first paschal offering, the Torah
relates:

> This is how you shall eat it: your loins girded, your sandals on your
> feet, and your staff in your hand; and you shall eat it hurriedly.

Why must the slaves eat the *Pesah* lamb hurriedly? Because "you
departed the land of Egypt hurriedly" (Deuteronomy 16:3).

That first liberation was rushed. Huddled in their homes while the Destroyer struck down the Egyptian firstborn children outside, the Jews ate their meal in haste, fearful for their own safety and excited by the prospect of freedom, and pressed to leave Egypt before the oppressive Pharaoh changed his mind yet one more time. So, the twelfth-century Bekhor Shor comments that they ate in haste like people who rush to be on their way.

However, a rushed liberation is bound to be incomplete. To be free physically does not necessarily mean one's spirit is free, nor is society as a whole free. While the slaves' bodies were taken away from their servitude, such a hasty freedom left both their souls and the larger society unaltered. The liberation from *Mitzraym* was unfinished.

On one hand, the liberation on *Pesah* was a reminder that human freedom is a real possibility, that slavery is not forever. In our own lives, chained by social pressure, imposed expectations, or our own inner drives, we hasten toward rare moments of freedom and escape. Yet our hurry itself testifies to the abiding power of those oppressive forces. Fearful that the moment might pass us by, we rush before the chance to escape eludes us forever.

On the other hand, true liberation never follows an external schedule. Faithful to its own nature, inner liberation unfolds at its own pace, until total liberation is achieved. In that unfolding, ideal liberation doesn't leave pockets of suffering, or aspects of reality still unredeemed.

The rabbis of antiquity saw the liberation from slavery in *Mitzraym* as a model for an ultimate, more complete liberation to come in the future, beyond the reaches of human history. Thus, *Midrash Sh'mot Rabbah* says that our ancestors rushed through the exodus from Egypt, but "in the messianic era, we are told, 'You will not depart in haste, nor will you leave in flight' " (Isaiah 52:12).

The future liberation will unfold at an unhurried pace in order to be thorough, equally concerned with inner peace and outer justice. Ultimate liberation—the messianic age desired by so many generations of Jews—only begins when human suffering abates, when human caring and sharing initiate a new age.

The *Pesah* liberation was our first demonstration that human beings could and should be free. But that liberation of the past, as with all liberations within human history, remains partial, a response to either specific political situations or to the issues faced by the individual psyche.

That limited reality—of gradual political progress and partial psychological adjustment—represents faint footsteps toward the messianic future.

Our ideals outstrip our ability to realize them; our dreams soar beyond our plans. The end of days, the messianic vision of Judaism and the Jewish prophets, is a call for us to transcend those limitations, to stretch the muscles of spirit and body toward a better day.

Yesterday's march to freedom is still incomplete. Can you hear the advancing steps? Are you ready to join the ascent?

✦✦✦

Parashat Bo/Go
Take 2

With Our Young and Our Old . . .

Pharaoh and Moses are locked in a conflict between two opposing worldviews. Pharaoh stands at the pinnacle of a society that is organized in a strict hierarchy—a world in which everybody is assigned a place below someone else, in the service of the vast aristocracy of the state. In contrast, Moses and the Torah mark the beginning of a society dedicated to limited government and the rule of law under God.

The difference could not be clearer, the choices more stark.

In this Torah-reading, one more difference emerges, a difference that also sets the two worlds of values in radically opposing contexts.

Pharaoh makes an attempt to buy Moses's acquiescence to slavery. Moses has insisted that Pharaoh let the entire people go. Pharaoh realizes that such an action would end the slavery of Israel in Egypt. So he makes a counteroffer: The men may go out to the wilderness to worship God, but the women and the children must remain behind in Egypt.

Pharaoh was speaking the normal language of politics, in which opposing camps compromise in order to reach agreement. Neither side walks away completely satisfied, but each is able to claim some concession from the other. Ever the consummate politician, Pharaoh offers a sweeping compromise which allows him to retain what he wants—Hebrew slaves—while simultaneously permitting Moses to claim a significant victory. After all, Moses would be able to assert that Pharaoh had acceded to his demand to worship God in the wilderness.

The distinction between a good politician and a great one is the ability to know when a compromise is inappropriate. Moses was a great politician.

Moses knew that the one area in which he could never compromise was his insistence on including all the people. Pharaoh wanted to restrict worship to the men, and Moses's rejection is immediate and total: "With our young and with our old, we will go; we will go with our sons and daughters . . . for we must observe the Lord's festival."

Judaism would not be simply the preserve of one caste, one sect, or one gender. Old and young, male and female—all of us together form the community of Israel, and all of us together are God's people.

That spirit of inclusion began at the very beginning, in the heated arguments between Moses and Pharaoh. And from the start, Moses taught us that a Judaism that cannot make room for all Jews is no Judaism at all.

As we continue the journey initiated by our ancestors so long ago, it is well worth focusing on the adamant insistence of our first teacher, Moses: "With our young and with our old . . . our sons and daughters . . . we will go."

Parashat Bo/Go
Take 3

Ready for Renewal

We live with a great uncertainty. While we ransack the past and its accumulated wisdom for guidance, we also know that the degree of change today in every aspect of our lives is without precedent. Groping in the dark, treading uncertainly down a road never before taken, humanity is unaware of its destination today and isn't even sure it is enjoying the trip.

We have good cause for our doubts.

Consider the amount of change witnessed by the last century alone. At the turn of the twentieth century, wars were fought using foot soldiers, ships, and bullets. Tanks, planes, missiles, nuclear bombs, space satellites, submarines: All of these modes of mass slaughter characterize the modern era. We think nothing of e-mailing anywhere in the world;

we schedule a flight halfway around the globe and arrive, all things being equal, within hours. If we like something we read, we download and print it—no big deal.

When I was a freshman in college, only wealthy students had electric typewriters. Today, most students have access to the latest PCs on the market.

Advances in science have extended human life but have also burned a hole through the ozone layer. We have used both penicillin and Agent Orange. We expend enormous skill and energy to teach developmentally disabled children, but we abandon pregnant teenage girls to their own resources.

At the turn of the century, men were secretaries and women stayed at home. Now both may be secretaries and no one is at home. Women vote, but many women politicians act just like their male colleagues.

Men and women no longer have an unwritten code telling them how to behave with one another. The divorce rate is at a record high, which just might also mean that unhappy marriages are at a record low.

In every area of human life, we find murky transitions—we don't have the comfortable consensus and social standards that guided our grandparents a hundred years ago.

That same situation faced Moses and the children of Israel when God commanded them to leave Egypt.

Slavery was unquestionably a source of suffering. The Hebrews were not allowed to have male children; the work was oppressive. Yet slavery was also a pattern of life that had endured for four hundred years. As slaves, the ancient Hebrews experienced no surprises, no unpredictable moments.

The offer of freedom interrupted their lives. To be free means being able to choose, and also means having to choose from a confusing and paralyzing number of options. Life would become more interesting, but it would never be as simple.

"We do not know with what we are to worship the Lord until we arrive there," Moses announces to Pharaoh. He intends that remark as a way of keeping Pharaoh in the dark. Ironically, however, Moses himself isn't sure where his people are to worship God.

Uncertain of where they are going or what they are to do when they get there, the Hebrew slaves have to be willing to live with the burden of freedom—the power to make choices and to take responsibility.

Ultimately, freedom is the ability to take responsibility for life and its direction.

In our own generation, we face that same crossroads. The traumas and opportunities of our lives can both excite and terrify us, beckon us with the enticements of new possibilities, and chasten us with complexity and confusion.

No matter. The future is ours if we are willing to throw ourselves into the task with our hearts, minds, and hands. We *can* build a vibrant Jewish future, but it will take effort. One kind of effort involves supporting institutions of our communal life: our places of worship, synagogues, afternoon religious schools, day schools, and Jewish universities and seminaries, for they are essential to help us fashion Jewish lives in the future.

For our communal life to have vitality, we also need the perspective of the "seeking Jew": A willingness to wrestle with difficult questions, with imponderable mysteries, and with the marvel of life itself nourishes spiritual Jewish growth. It takes perseverance to enter a synagogue and to return there, week after week, to learn the service. It takes courage to sign up for an adult education class or to meet with a rabbi. But in the words of the great philosopher Franz Rosenzweig, "The Jewish individual needs nothing but readiness."

Are *you* ready?

BE-SHALAH/He Sent
Exodus 13:17–17:16

Liberated from bondage, the Israelites begin their march toward their own land. God leads the people to the Sea of Reeds (the Red Sea). Marching with the bones of Joseph, the Israelites follow a pillar of cloud by day and a pillar of fire by night.

God tells Moses that Pharaoh will pursue the former slaves, and indeed, the king regrets having freed the Hebrews. He orders his chariot and soldiers to go after the Israelites and they overtake the terrified people by the sea. Crying out to God, the people panic, but Moses calms them with the promise that they will see God's work that same day. God scolds Moses, telling him not to cry to God, but to tell the Israelites to go forward. Moses then lifts up his rod, and the sea splits, so that the Israelites may march through on dry land. Behind the fleeing people, the cloud of darkness settles on the Egyptians, preventing them from moving ahead.

The next morning, the Egyptians are able finally to give chase, but a pillar of fire creates panic among the soldiers. The chariot wheels become bogged in the mud, and the Egyptians finally realize that God is fighting for the Israelites. God instructs Moses to extend his rod once more, and the sea crashes over the Egyptian army, drowning every one of the once-proud soldiers. So great is their joy at seeing this miracle of liberation that Moses and the Israelites sing a song to God: "Who is like You, O Lord, among the mighty?" Miriam takes up a timbrel, and she and the women dance and sing in celebration.

From the sea, the Israelites move on into the wilderness. For three days, they find no water, and begin to criticize Moses. With another miracle, Moses is able to make bitter water sweet, until they finally arrive at an oasis at Elim. A few days later, the Israelites again grumble, this time complaining of hunger. God responds by making manna and quail fall from the sky. The Israelites are commanded to gather the manna each day, and on the sixth day to collect double so they won't need to violate the Sabbath by working on that day. The people are instructed to remain in their places inactive for the Sabbath day, and to remain inactive on that holy day.

From the wilderness of Sin, the Israelites move on to Massah and Meribah, again quarreling with Moses over water. God tells Moses to strike the rock with his rod, and when he does, water shoots forth.

Finally, the evil Amalekites launch an attack on the Israelites at Rephidim. Moses sits between Aaron and Hur. They hold up his arms and Israel prevails under the military leadership of Joshua.

◄◄●●►►

Parashat Be-Shalah/He Sent
Take 1

Judaism: The Cliff Notes

One of the ironies of modern Judaism is that so many of us consider the sermon to be the high point of the *Shabbat* service. In fact, a sermon in the spoken language of the congregation is a relatively recent addition to the service, and our tradition, as a whole, minimizes the significance of preaching. The Torah prefers to teach through the concrete examples of people's lives, or through the presentation of rules that make for a sacred and compassionate society.

Today's Torah portion is no exception to that general premise. Here, in very clear terms, the Torah presents a concise description of biblical and rabbinic Judaism: "Heed the Lord your God diligently, doing what is right in God's sight, giving ear to God's commandments and keeping all God's laws." From the liberation of our ancestors from Egyptian slavery to the present moment, the central focus of Judaism has been the translation of Jewish values into *acts* of sacred obedience. As the *Mishnah* insists, "It is not the explanation that is essential, but the deed itself." Hardened on the forge of actual living, refined in the bellows of daily practice, Judaism is thus able to provide guidance and comfort in moments of crisis or despair.

In the very fact of our having been commanded, the rabbis of antiquity recognized a special kind of love between God and the Jewish People. According to the *Mekhilta,* it is through providing the *mitzvot* to the Jews that God "bestowed greatness upon them." High standards are only demanded from people or issues that matter in one's life.

The *Mekhilta* continues by explaining just what those standards are, interpreting the above passage in the following way: "The voice of the

Lord" refers to the Ten Commandments; "what is right in God's sight" refers to praiseworthy conduct which is apparent to all humanity; "give ear to God's commandments" refers to decrees that stand to reason; and "all God's laws" refers to those practices which have no other rationale than that the tradition requires them.

How striking, then, is the range of Jewish responsibility! We are accustomed to think of Judaism in terms of specific rituals—lighting *Shabbat* candles, or keeping the dietary laws of *kashrut*—but the rabbis here explain that those decent practices which all humanity insists on—not murdering, fair business practices, not stealing—these too are a part of the fabric of Jewish living.

Just because a deed or an insight is not unique to Jews does not mean it is not essential to Judaism. At the same time, those deeds which cannot be explained simply according to logic may be among the most essential. Civilizations cultivate and signify belonging through practices that are largely arbitrary. Why wear a tie around the neck? Why smear bright-colored paint only on the lips? These practices demonstrate belonging and associated values—their justification has little to do with reason and everything to do with community. So, too, says Rashi, with those commandments in the Torah that appear to have no basis in reason. The commandments not to mix linen and wool in the same garment and to refrain from pork, for example, provide Jews with a common identity and a set of symbols which can remind us of the values and moral impulse underlying all of Jewish practice. Those inexplicable practices are the very foundation of Jewish civilization, the ongoing training grounds for Jewish belonging.

Judaism—a network of sacred deeds—provides a path to holiness and goodness through the tangible acts of moral and ritual living. By cultivating the practice of *mitzvot,* the Jew learns to identify with a glorious and ancient history, to exemplify caring and a rigorous morality, and to demonstrate reverence and obedience to the God who liberates slaves and who has chosen us in love.

That same God calls to us now. Will you *do* something about it?

Parashat Be-Shalah/He Sent
Take 2

When Miracles Are Not Enough

Surely this Torah-reading contains some of the most dramatic and well-known scenes in all of written literature. The liberation of the Israelite slaves by God, the pursuit of the fleeing Hebrews by Pharaoh and his army, the splitting of the Red Sea, with Israel crossing safely beyond and Pharaoh's forces drowning in the waters—these scenes indelibly shaped the consciousness of the Jewish people throughout our tumultuous history.

We are who we are precisely because we recall our origins as a slave people, for so much of Jewish practice is designed to remind us that we owe our freedom to a God of love and justice.

The story of the liberation from Egypt is thus the cornerstone of Jewish existence. Or is it?

Read the *parashah* again, and you will find that what is most striking is not the miracles, wondrous as they may be. What is particularly noteworthy is how quickly the Israelite slaves forget about their extraordinary redemption.

Barely have they crossed to freedom when the people begin to complain to Moses and to God. They complain about a lack of water, they complain about a lack of goods, and they complain simply about no longer being surrounded by good, old, familiar Egypt.

No wonder the *Midrash Sh'mot Rabbah* challenges them: "Have you forgotten all the miracles which God performed for you?"

Miracles, clearly, seem to be an ineffective way of inculcating a consciousness of God. In fact, the entire Bible can be read as a book about the consistent inability of God to teach the Jews to be grateful.

Consider the following. First, God tries an idyllic garden. Adam and Eve disobey anyway. Then God sends a flood. That fails also; people continue to act violently. God then enslaves the Jews, sends a liberator, and redeems them from Egypt. After ten miraculous plagues and a split sea, the Jews still act truculently. God gives a Torah of instructions; the Jews ignore it. God sends prophets of insight; the Jews rebel against them.

The Bible seems to indicate that miracles don't work. People marvel at them while they are taking place, and then forget about them the moment they are finished.

To reform human character takes much more than "special effects," no matter how divine their origin. To transform human behavior requires instead constant and gradual education, reinforcement, discipline, and community. The shift from biblical to rabbinic Judaism also reflects the emerging divine insight that the way to mold a sacred people lies not in external miracles but in inner transformation.

That transformation is accomplished through small, prosaic progress. By gradually incorporating *mitzvot* into our lives—by moving a step at a time toward making *Shabbat* and *tzedakah, kashrut* and social justice, prayer and study, a regular part of our existence—we can, with time, remake ourselves in the image of the Divine. Such a transformation is much more difficult than merely splitting a sea. It involves a tenacity and openness that must be continually cultivated.

But the reward of such a transformation is precisely what God sought more than three thousand years ago at the shores of the Red Sea—a Jewish community which puts God at its center through the study, practice, and development of our sacred heritage.

Parashat Be-Shalah/He Sent
Take 3

What Becomes a Legend Most?

All of Pharaoh's Hebrew slaves were scurrying through their homes and gathering their possessions in preparation for their march out of Egypt, toward freedom. Collecting their pots and pans, clothing, children, animals, and meager property, the Jews rushed to be ready to leave when the moment of liberation finally arrived.

And Moses? What personal objects did he collect?

> Moses took with him the bones of Joseph, who had exacted an oath from the children of Israel, saying "God will be sure to take notice of you: then you shall carry up my bones from here with you."

While the other Jews strain to gather their things, Moses meticulously gathers the remains of the ancestor of the Jews, and makes sure that he brings Joseph's bones with him as he begins the march to *Eretz Yisrael*.

The *Midrash Mekhilta* understands this care as a natural reflection of the greatness of both men involved. Just as Joseph oversees the burial of his father, Jacob, in Israel, so he deserves to have the same care taken with his remains. Later, the remains of Moses, in turn, will be cared for by none other than God! Both Moses and Joseph achieve greatness because they regard their own personal desires as secondary to the needs of their community and the commandments of God.

How do we learn the proper way to relate to others? Are human beings intrinsically kind, thoughtful, patient, and generous? Or are those values in need of social reinforcement and constant training?

The philosophers of the Enlightenment and Romantic periods of the eighteenth and nineteenth centuries asserted the inherent goodness of humanity and the consequent inevitability of progress. According to these European thinkers, in "the state of nature," each individual is noble and self-sacrificing. The constraints and burdens of civilization and religion corrupt that inherent goodness, producing competition, greed, and cruelty. The obvious cure, then, is to leave people alone to pursue their own self-interest as they define it.

Traditional Judaism never accepted that lovely delusion. Believing that human beings are neither intrinsically good nor intrinsically evil, Judaism insists that people must be taught both what is good, and how to embody that righteousness in their lives. The Torah and the Talmud contain a myriad of *mitzvot,* commanded deeds, which channel human energy toward compassion, justice, and holiness. It is precisely through these teaching tools, inculcating the habit of discipline and morality, that we grow to be fully human, reflecting the Divine image of God.

We teach others how we want to be treated by offering them practical lessons through how we care for them; not by imposing our own desires on others, but by *refraining* from what we ourselves don't like. In the words of the first-century sage, Hillel: "Don't do to others what you don't want them to do to you." By treating others with respect, dignity, and kindness, whether deserved or not, we demonstrate how human beings should be treated.

Moses taught that lesson by taking the time to worry not about possessions but about human fidelity. He knew that the Jews had made an oath to Joseph. While some might argue that since Joseph was dead, promises to him were no longer important, Moses demonstrated that commitments to others don't stop at the grave.

What had Joseph done to deserve this loyalty? The *Mekhilta* records that the ark carrying Joseph's bones was transported next to the ark containing the Ten Commandments. "The nations would say to the Israelites: 'What is the importance of this coffin that it should go alongside of the ark of the Eternal One?' And the Israelites would say to them: 'The one lying in this coffin has fulfilled that which is written on what lies in that ark.'"

Joseph, too, had filled his life with *mitzvot*. He demonstrated a fidelity to others by using his ability, energy, mind, and heart to provide for the hungry during a terrible famine and by securing his family's safety at the same time. Through loyalty to the Ten Commandments, Joseph had made himself into a human replica of the two tablets.

Deeds of goodness, acts of fidelity, and embodiments of sanctity are the building blocks of the Jewish tradition—and the stuff of which real people are made.

YITRO/Jethro
Exodus 18:1–20:26

Jethro, the father-in-law of Moses, hears of the miracle of Israel's liberation, and he brings Moses's wife, Zipporah, and their two sons, Gershom
and Eliezer, to the Israelites' encampment. Moses goes out to greet his
family, escorts them into his tent, and recounts the many wonders that
God performed against Pharaoh for the sake of the Israelites. In joy, Jethro
blesses God and offers a burnt offering, joined by Aaron and the elders.

The next morning, Moses works as judge for the people from early
morning until late at night. Jethro is horrified, telling Moses that this
seeming act of kindness is actually an imposition on the people, and
that he will wear himself out. Jethro organizes a hierarchy of judges, culminating in Moses as Chief Judge, thus allowing the people to have
access to justice and Moses to rest. Once Moses establishes this judicial
order, Jethro bids him farewell and returns home.

Three months after the Exodus, the Israelites arrive at the wilderness
of Sinai. God offers a special covenant confirming the unique relationship between God and the Jewish people: "If you will obey Me faithfully
and keep My covenant, you shall be My treasured possession among all
the peoples."

When Moses reports this offer to the people, they respond in unison,
"All that Adonai has spoken, we will do!" For three days the Israelites
purify themselves. On the morning of the third day, they hear thunder
and lightning, see a dense cloud on the mountain, and hear a loud blast
of the shofar. Moses ascends to the mountaintop as God descends. God
tells Moses to return to the people, and when he and they are together,
God speaks the words of the Ten Commandments.

1. I am Adonai your God.

2. Worship no idolatrous images.

3. Do not swear falsely by the name of God.

4. Remember the Sabbath and keep it holy.

5. Honor your father and mother.

6. You shall not murder.

7. You shall not commit adultery.

8. You shall not steal.

9. You shall not bear false witness.

10. You shall not covet.

The people are so awed by this revelation that they ask Moses to inter-cede and record the rest of God's word while they remain at a distance. God concludes by prohibiting idolatry, establishing animal sacrifice in "the place where I cause My name to be mentioned," and prohibiting the use of hewn stones in the altar.

❖❖❖

Parashat Yitro/Jethro
Take 1

The People Chosen for What?

At the textual summit of the Book of Exodus is the encounter between God and the Jewish People at Mount Sinai. Here, God and the Jews meet and exchange promises of loyalty and love. Here, God and the people embrace the Ten Commandments—the first articulation of our sacred, mutual *brit,* our covenant.

Immediately preceding this momentous event, God speaks to Moses, contextualizing the ensuing revelation. For the first time, God clearly articulates a notion of the Jews as the Chosen People: "Indeed, all the earth is Mine, but you shall be to Me a nation of priests and a holy nation."

This one sentence indicates the tension inherent in the concept of "chosen people": How can the God of the Universe choose just one people? If God is truly omniscient, isn't the restriction of God's choice to one particular people an act of xenophobic idolatry? Doesn't God love everybody equally? The impetus behind these questions has caused some observant Jews to renounce any claim to chosenness.

They argue that chosenness is an arrogant claim that denigrates the rest of humanity.

Is that appraisal the only way to understand this central biblical claim? After all, the Bible itself presents this assertion as the contextual underpinning for the Ten Commandments, and for all the profound teachings that follow. Doesn't denying the context result in uprooting the values and heroic figures of the biblical tradition?

Rather than rejecting such a pivotal idea, we would do well to try to understand it in a way that is consistent with both the divinity of all humanity, and of the uniqueness of the Jews. Viewed in that light, we must quickly echo the words of the Bible that the "chosenness" of the Jews is consistent with the assertion that God loves and cares for each human being. We are all precious.

But chosenness implies a uniqueness, a particular purpose. The statement, "I was chosen today," is incomplete unless I specify what it is I was chosen for. Similarly, *Jewish* chosenness is a sentence fragment. It is grammatically and theologically incomplete.

What completes the chosenness of the Jews is the assertion that Jews were (and are) chosen to embody the life and values of the Torah and rabbinic tradition. By living a life centered on *mitzvot* and by constantly growing as Jews, we *choose* to be chosen. We allow the *brit* to live by the way we conduct our lives. As with any love relationship, both partners have the power to affirm or to rupture that relationship of their own free will. The idea of *brit* places that enormous responsibility in our hands, no less than in those of God.

In the words of the *Mekhilta,* the ancient rabbinic commentary to Exodus, the phrase "and you shall be Mine" means "you shall be turned to Me and be occupied with the words of the Torah." God doesn't love Jews better; God loves us differently.

By immersing ourselves in the study and practice of Torah, we Jews renew our unique relationship with God. By living lives centered on God and *mitzvot,* we justify the claim, not of being God's *only* love, but of being God's first.

And in building communities of holiness and love, we assist our non-Jewish neighbors in cultivating their love relationship with God as well—joining hands together to build a world that is just, compassionate, and worthy of God.

Parashat Yitro/Jethro
Take 2

All Aboard for the Shabbat Cruise!

Much of our culture is materially opulent and spiritually starved. Throughout American communities, lavish homes and well-furnished schools provide our children and ourselves with abundant physical comforts. Some of us have all the possessions we can imagine.

Our richness in *things* is counterbalanced by our poverty in time. According to a study in *Time* magazine, the average American workweek has increased from forty-one to forty-seven hours, with many adults working far longer hours. With both members of most couples employed, many of us are able to pay for lovely homes, beautiful cars, active children, and elegant evenings out. But we rarely have the time to enjoy these luxuries.

We undervalue time and overvalue possessions. But happiness is to be found not through ownership, but through relationship. Contentment emerges from meaningful living. As Rabbi Abraham Joshua Heschel said, "Things are the shore, the voyage is in time."

Learning to bask in time, rather than to squander it trying to keep up with our possessions, is the fundamental task facing millions of Americans today. In teaching ourselves how to effectively utilize time, to remember the art of resting and renewal, we can strengthen ourselves to confront our finitude in time and our loneliness as solitary souls.

The solution to our thirst for time is *Shabbat,* the Day of Rest. While the remainder of the Ten Commandments focuses on matters of theology or of interpersonal ethics, *Shabbat* is the *only* ritual that merits a place in these highly charged words:

> Remember the Sabbath day and keep it holy. Six days you shall labor and do all your work, but the seventh day is a Sabbath of the Lord your God: you shall not do any work—you, your son or daughter, your male or female slave, or your cattle, or the stranger who is within your settlements. For in six days the Lord made heaven and earth and sea, and all that is in them, and God rested on the seventh day; therefore the Lord blessed the Sabbath day and hallowed it.

Shabbat is the fundamental building block for all of Judaism and all of Jewish values. It is our portable home in time, a movable tabernacle that travels with the Jewish People through our journeys in history. Once each week, Jews can put aside chores, obligations, and distractions—the activities that rightly claim our attention during the week—and reassert our sovereignty over work. For twenty-four hours each week, Jewish families are guaranteed quality time together, time to focus on their relationships, on learning about their Jewish heritage, on building a Jewish community enriched by their participation and their worship.

A Judaism that does not make time for *Shabbat* is a mere religion. A Judaism centered around *Shabbat,* consecrated for quiet, meditation, celebration, study, and play, is one that can outlast the ages. Such a Judaism can infuse our lives and our communities with a sense of balance and perspective, sanctity and wisdom, which our age—so rushed and frantic—sorely lacks.

Every Jew is invited to a weekly cruise. All embark on Friday night. Once on ship, there is no need to work, since all the preparations are already complete. Instead, the voyagers can finally focus on refreshing their tired spirits, their strained hearts, and their distracted minds. An opening service involves poetry, song, and discussion aimed at thanking the Captain and crew for preparing such a restful and pleasant voyage. A lavish dinner follows, complete with candlelight, sparkling wine, and a bread so rich it tastes like cake. People retire early for private time and for restful slumber. The next morning, the voyagers gather for a light breakfast, and then spend the morning together, reading and thinking about their goals in life, where they've come so far, what their history has taught them, and what kind of people they want to be. At noon, another festival meal, no less wonderful than last night's dinner, is served. In the afternoon, some walk the deck, some play ball, some read, while others sleep. At the end of the day, as the cruise returns to shore, all gather for a candle lighting ceremony and farewell. Renewed and energized, the participants are able to face the new week with anticipation and zeal.

Such a cruise is available to you each week, and has been departing every Friday night for over three thousand years. The good ship *Shabbat* is as seaworthy as ever; all it needs is passengers—no advance reservations required.

All aboard!

Parents Make It to the Top Ten

Each of us is descended from parents.

A man and a woman were involved in your inception and birth, and generally, in your childhood, teen years, and early adulthood as well. How are we to respond to these people, how should we adjust to our own increasing powers of understanding, physical strength, and financial ability in the light of the gratitude and respect we owe our parents for the care we received at an earlier age?

That we owe our parents honor and reverence is a given in Jewish tradition. The *mitzvah* of *kibbud av va-em,* honoring the father and mother, is the fifth of the *Aseret Ha-Dib'rot,* the Ten Commandments, standing halfway between the first four, which deal with the Jewish relationship with God, and the last five, which establish standards of social morality. That placement expresses the insight that parents represent a bridge between God and the world, between our own personal drama of Creation and our entry into the world of human interaction and expectation.

The Talmud teaches that three partners are involved in the birth of every person: God, mother, and father. One of the roots, then, of our obligation to honor our parents is their role as a preeminent source of life.

Parents represent God not only for their role in our inception and birth, but also on a psychological level. Ideally, parents teach, through their raising of children, that the world is reliable and basically good. Each time a mother comforts a screaming baby, each time a father offers a bottle to a hungry infant, the child receives a concrete lesson that she is not abandoned in a meaningless void, that needs are met, that compassion and love are real and potent. In nurturing their children, parents establish the emotional base for a subsequent relationship between child and the sacred.

As we would expect in any instance in which we are given a gift without having earned it, showing gratitude is an integral part of a child's relationship to parents. No one does anything to deserve being born. Each of us is gratuitously created and nurtured for countless hours, through illness, temper, and the normal self-absorption of childhood. As adults ourselves, we honor parents to demonstrate gratitude for those years of service.

There is also a specifically Jewish component to honoring parents. Parents provide the tangible link to our sacred past and our covenant with God. The childhood memories of lighting Hanukkah candles, the smell of warm loaves of *hallah* on a newly set *Shabbat* table, the joy and love of a Passover Seder, all of these connections to our Jewishness are through our parents and grandparents. Even in those families in which the child's Jewish commitment is more consuming or elaborate than that of the parents, the core of the child's identification as a Jew is still a product of who the parents are, and of the nature of their family and friends.

If parents are so central, why doesn't the Torah or the Talmud mandate the love of parents?

The lack of such an imperative is the result of a recognition that there is no relationship as complex, multilayered, and deep as that between parent and child. Experiences of dependency, of rebellion, of increasing similarity, are all commonplace between the generations. Spouses can divorce, and friends can separate, but a parent is forever.

Given the profound complexity of our emotions toward our parents, it would be impossible to mandate our feelings toward them. But our *behavior* is another matter.

Thus, Jewish tradition does not tell us what to *feel,* but what to *do.* It places a great emphasis on *kibbud,* honor, and *yirah,* reverence, toward parents. As the people to whom we owe life itself, as the people who provided years of care, and as transmitters and links to Judaism and the Jewish past, our parents merit our honor and respect.

MISHPATIM/Ordinances
Exodus 21:1–24:18

This parashah is known in Hebrew as Sefer Ha-brit, the Book of the Covenant. It contains the first body of laws in the Torah. These rules, a combination of moral imperatives, social standards, civil and criminal injunctions, and rules for proper worship, are all recognized as the will of God, the embodied consequence of the distinct relationship between God and the people Israel.

Beginning with laws concerning slaves, the Torah establishes a kind of indentured servitude for a fellow Hebrew, who must go free after seven years of enslavement. If the eved Ivri, Hebrew slave, wishes to remain with master, wife, and children, he is taken to a door and his ear is pierced with an awl, after which he is a slave for life. The Torah also establishes procedures for the female slave, the amah.

In a section on criminal legislation, the Torah lays out three capital offenses: murder, injuring parents physically, and kidnapping. The punishment for crimes of bodily injury caused by human attack is limited to no more than an equivalent loss: "an eye for an eye." A homicidal beast is to be killed. A thief is to repay the lost object and four (for an ox) or three (for a sheep) more animals as restitution. Responsibility to care for loaned items is enforced, whether these items are fixed property or an animal. Seducing an unmarried woman forces the seducer to pay her bride price or to marry her.

A second section of Mishpatim lays out a variety of categorical laws, known as apodictic laws: prohibition of sorcery and idolatry; justice for foreigners, widows, and orphans; extending loans for the poor; respect for God; honesty in courts; humane treatment of one's enemy; and a series of agricultural laws. Mishpatim then lays out the calendar of the three festivals of Passover, Shavuot, and Sukkot. God reiterates a promise to protect the Israelites during their wanderings, and commands the Israelites to remain distinct and true to their covenant.

Finally, Moses and the elders repeat all the commands and rules of the Lord aloud, and the people affirm their loyalty to the covenant and its commandments with one voice. As the elders and people celebrate the *new partnership with God, Moses goes up to the mountaintop to receive the stone tablets containing God's inscription of the laws and rules. Moses remains hidden in the clouds for forty days and nights.*

Parashat Mishpatim/Ordinances
Take 1

Pull Them from My Altars!

Our society offers an array of temptations to titillate every taste. Sex, money, power, fame—all beckon and entice. We are so accustomed to the corruption of our leadership that we are no longer surprised when a new escapade hits the headlines. Our newspapers routinely inform us of legislators who accepted bribes or who intervened on behalf of disreputable but wealthy supporters. Even the lives of movie stars and rock musicians provide grist for a cynical view of human beings as motivated by lust, addiction, and celebrity.

We no longer expect the prominent or the powerful to embody nurturing and moral ideals. With few role models left, is it any wonder that our children don't aspire to great heights, or that our culture has so few real heroes?

The Torah portion this week includes a message that addresses the fallen standards of our age. In *Parashat Mishpatim,* the Torah notes, "When a man schemes against another and kills him treacherously, you shall take him from My very altar to be put to death." In other words, taking refuge even at the altar in the Holy Temple in Jerusalem did not immunize a criminal from receiving justice! Claiming sanctity is no cover for corruption, and the love of God is no excuse for human disregard. Thus, no matter how acceptable a certain corrupt behavior may have become within one's profession, the timeless claims of justice and equity cannot be swept aside without great cost to our entire community and nation.

Rashi makes this point explicitly when he quotes the Talmud: "Even if he were a *Kohen* (priest) and he intended to perform the sacrificial service in the Temple, take him away to be executed." According to the *Mekhilta de-Rabbi Ishmael,* "the punishment of murder should set aside the Temple service."

A career in religion or the calling of public service, medicine, law, business, or indeed of any other human endeavor, is a credit to those who pursue it with integrity and human kindness. Such conduct provides support to needy human beings and cultivates our ability to help each other and to elicit the highest potential of each member of our community.

To pervert these professions into excuses for human abuse, for transforming people into manipulated objects, is to deny all that is good and decent in human potential. In the face of this kind of callous cynicism or shameless greed, the nobility of these callings is neither shield nor cover. A murderous priest is removed from God's altar, even if preparing to perform the sacred service there. And corrupt politicians, adulterous clergy, and abusive entrepreneurs should expect no less.

Judaism insists that the God of Israel is passionate about justice and honesty: "The seal of the Holy Blessing One is truth." To hide behind the Source of truth in the pursuit of evil is to deny the authority of God and to scorn membership in human society.

Only under the healing light of integrity and morality can we all thrive.

Parashat Mishpatim/Ordinances
Take 2

On Peaks and Plains

In seeking spiritual highs, people often travel to exotic locations or seek moments of emotional intensity. Spirituality is imagined as involving a jolting transformation, an overwhelming sense of God's presence that is different than ordinary experience.

Such moments occur in biblical and rabbinic Judaism as well—Moses at the burning bush, the people at the foot of Mount Sinai—such moments are rare. The pursuit of spiritual "peaks" can reflect a hedonism no less compulsive and damaging than those sought through physical indulgence.

Periodic peaks are essential if we are to be reinvigorated, reoriented, rededicated. But we do not live on the peaks—the air is too thin, the winds too brisk to sustain human life, family, community. So we need a religious orientation that sustains us on the plains, amid our concerns for security, education, and relationship. Life begins *after* the revelatory moment passes, when the high is over.

And there, too, Judaism must dwell.

Parashat Mishpatim expresses precisely that kind of spirituality, and teaches us to look for God not with closed eyes but with hands engaged; not with a mantra, but with involvement.

We find God in the world by making the world more godly—through labor, compassion, and justice. *Parashat Mishpatim* is a collection of laws pertaining to living our daily lives: laws of marriage, employment, lost property, integrity, and financial practices. Why the focus on such mundane detail? Judaism has always insisted on translating philosophy into action.

Ideology without action becomes anemic and self-serving. Action without conviction becomes mechanistic and insincere. The balance between deed and creed is the realm of *mitzvah*—where God's will and human integrity meet in practice.

Today's Torah portion insists that our deepest convictions find articulation in deeds and cooperative behavior. By training ourselves to perform *mitzvot,* we school ourselves anew in the values and perspectives of Judaism. We transfer an aspect of the original peak experience, a spark from the original flame, into the remotest aspects of our daily lives.

With the light of those sparks, we warm our fellow human beings and ourselves. We illumine our lifelong journey, invigorating ourselves, our traditions, and our God.

Parashat Mishpatim/Ordinances
Take 3

Here Comes the Judge!

At its deepest core, America prides itself on the rule of law, the insistence that no individual, however wealthy, influential, popular, or powerful, is above the rules that govern human conduct. Our body of laws translate general principles into legal guidelines for harmonious living.

The superiority of the rule of law was not always the case in America. The West, with its frontier ethic, the South with its racial hatred, and the

Northeast with its violence against labor unions, often acted against this national commitment to the rule of law. When told of a decision of the Supreme Court that he opposed, as great a president as Andrew Jackson responded, "They've made their decision, now let them get their own troops to enforce it!" Certainly, in our own time we have also witnessed presidents claiming immunity from various laws because of their high office.

In spite of all the times that Americans fail to live up to the principle of law, that ideal still remains a potent force for justice and equality in our society. It allowed the Reverend Martin Luther King Jr. to fight entrenched racism, and women, as well as the disabled, to fight for justice in our courts.

We inherit the commitment to the supremacy of law from our Bible. In part, the Torah itself is a book of law, presenting the Jewish conviction that the will of God is translated into action through law. By using the metaphor of law to frame Jewish religious obligations, our tradition raises goodness beyond the tenuous level of preference or mood, establishing the rejection of evil and the pursuit of righteousness as a mandate at all times and places.

The Torah argues for the rule of law both through its overall structure and also explicitly in today's portion: "In all charges . . . the case of both parties shall come before judges." Establishing courts of law in which disputes can be resolved is an indispensable requirement for religious society, in the Torah's view.

According to rabbinic understanding, this obligation to establish courts of law applies for all time, not only for the period in which the Temple stood in Jerusalem. And it is binding in all places, not only in the Land of Israel. As the thirteenth-century Spanish author of the *Sefer Ha-Hinnukh* recognized, the absence of a legal system and of open trials "causes ruin for the land, since a country cannot be civilized except by law." That perception echoes the claim of the *Mishnah* that "the world stands on three things," one of which is law.

This *mitzvah* is binding on Jews, as well as on all peoples, according to rabbinic tradition. Out of the 613 biblical commandments, only 7 pertained to the *b'nei Noah,* all of humanity. These laws were of such import that no person could claim to be civilized or fully human without embracing them. For the rabbis, establishing courts of justice was a fundamental human act, one which allowed for the values of ethical monotheism to extend to everyone, regardless of their religious affiliation or social status.

Ours is a religion of law. Take away the force of law and Judaism becomes merely a series of helpful suggestions. Just as one cannot claim to embrace American values without adhering to American law, so, too, one cannot distinguish Jewish values from Jewish law.

But the point here goes beyond the structure of our faith, beyond a definition of what it means to be an American. By insisting that the establishments of law courts are part of the laws of *b'nei Noah,* our tradition reminds us that the key to human potential and harmony is adherence to a legal system that is accessible, fair, speedy, and just.

As Jews, as Americans, and as human beings, we all have an interest in that.

TERUMAH/Offering
Exodus 25:1–27:19

The Torah now records the instructions for the building of the Mishkan, the Tabernacle, which will house the Ark of the Covenant, with the tablets of the Ten Commandments. The Tabernacle becomes a symbol for God's Presence among the Israelites, and its mobility allows that Presence to follow the Israelites throughout their wanderings. It was stationed at the center of the encampment, a token of national unity for the entire people.

It is striking that, just as the story of the Creation unfolded on six days, each of which began, "And the Lord said . . . ," so the instructions for building the Tabernacle are found in six sections, each of which begins, "The Lord spoke to Moses." The seventh section deals with the laws of Shabbat. What this suggests to us is that building the Tabernacle marks a second Creation—this time, the Creation of the Jewish People.

The people are to bring gifts for the construction of the Mishkan voluntarily. God shows Moses the pattern of the building, and commands that the Israelites build it so "that I may dwell among them."

They are to fashion an ark to house the two tablets of the Decalogue, and to make poles so the ark can be transported as the people themselves move. Above the ark is the kapporet, a slab of gold with a cherub on each end of the top. God promises to speak to Moses from between the two cherubim. These are the contents of the most sacred space, the Holy of Holies.

In the second region, the Holy Place, is a table of acacia wood overlaid with gold. This table will be used to hold the lechem panim, showbread. Near the table is the menorah, the seven-branched lamp stand. Permeated with plantlike traits (cups, calyxes, and petals), the menorah is a symbolic Tree of Life, providing light in the Tabernacle at night. Layers of woven cloth are used to cover the Tabernacle, and wooden planks form its outer walls. Separating the inner and outer courts is a hanging tapestry, the parokhet.

The outer courtyard has the sacrificial altar at its very center. The altar is to be square, with hornlike protrusions at each corner. The parashah ends with instructions for making the enclosure for the outer courtyard.

Parashat Terumah/Offering
Take 1

The Menorah: Let Your Light Shine

Everyone knows that the principal symbol of Judaism is the six-pointed Star of David.

But did you know that the *Magen David* became a Jewish symbol only in the Middle Ages? Despite its prominence on *kiddush* cups and on the flag of Israel, the *Magen David* is a rather late representative of Judaism and the Jewish People.

For most of our history and throughout antiquity, the preeminent symbol of the Jewish religion was the menorah: the seven-branched candlestick found first in the Tabernacle of Moses and later in the Temple of King Solomon in Jerusalem. That menorah is mentioned for the first time in today's Torah-reading, when God tells Moses to "make a lamp stand of pure gold . . . its base and its shaft, its cups, calyxes, and petals shall be of one piece. Six branches shall issue from its sides."

Reading the description of the menorah can be confusing; the details are so complex that one can easily despair of visualizing it correctly.

That same confusion must have overwhelmed Moses as well. An ancient *midrash* recorded in the Talmud states that "three things presented difficulties to Moses, until the Holy Blessing One showed Moses . . . the menorah, as it is written, 'and this was the work of the menorah.' " According to another ancient tradition, the angel Gabriel drew a picture of the menorah so that Moses could see the image God was portraying in words. Yet another tradition, found in *Midrash Bamidbar Rabbah,* holds that Moses kept confusing the details each time he returned to the camp. After Moses forgot for the third time, God told him not to worry, because the details would be remembered correctly by the artist Bezalel (as indeed they were).

Why did Moses find the details of the menorah so difficult to retain? After all, according to one tradition of how the Torah was recorded, Moses memorized the whole Torah—and according to *Mishnah Avot,* he also remembered the Oral Teaching! How could such a skilled and gifted mind have trouble remembering the details of the menorah?

Perhaps the Torah is telling us that even the most gifted among us has both strengths and weaknesses. Moses was a brilliant role model for our entire people, yet he, too, was imperfect. The gifted artist Bezalel, whose name is never mentioned in relation to Jewish law or literature, nevertheless was essential to the establishment of a Jewish symbol, and thus of Jewish religious expression.

Each of us has a special ability or gift that is our unique strength. No matter how impressive other people may seem, you bring your unique perspective and insight and talents to life in a combination that no one else can produce. In the words of the *Mishnah,* "there is no one who doesn't have their hour, and nothing which does not have its place."

Each one of us can add something irreplaceable and unique to the luxurious weave of humanity. Each individual person, like each glistening thread, makes the cloth shimmering and durable. No one can replace you.

Perhaps that is also why the menorah has so many lights. Each one of the seven lights shines in its own uniqueness. In fact, the only thing that can make a menorah *treif,* ritually impermissible, is if the lights are not all on the same level—precisely even—so that no two lights can be confused as one.

The Talmud teaches that replicas of the Temple menorah may no longer be made or displayed. Perhaps this, too, is an assertion of the unique importance of each individual. For just as the Temple menorah cannot be replaced, so, too, every human being is ultimately irreplaceable.

Instead, those seven burning flames testify to the unique shining light within each human being—"the human soul is the lamp of God."

The light of God's love, justice, and concern can illumine the world only through the individual light that we shine through our deeds, our communities, and our performance of *mitzvot.*

Like the menorah of old, we can illumine the world.

May your light shine brightly.

Parashat Terumah/Offering
Take 2
"I Will Dwell Among Them . . ."

Parashat Terumah focuses on the construction of the *Mishkan,* the Tabernacle, a portable tent filled with sacred objects used in early Jewish rituals.

What is the purpose of this building? Why would Israel want a portable building, or any building at all? Isn't a *brit,* a covenant, with the God of the universe sufficient? Apparently not.

We all yearn for transcendence of some sort. For some, transcendence involves pursuing an ideal of the good or the beautiful; for others, it is a sense of awe at the workings of nature and the subtleties of the human mind; for still others, transcendence subsumes both of these categories in a striving for the holy.

Our human nature seeks relationship, so we search for ways to enter into relationship with the unreachable. We launch rockets into space, plumb the depths of the oceans, and look deep into human history and human emotion to grasp a sense of identity with transcendence in all its starkness.

From the very beginning, the Jewish sense of transcendence has displayed a personality. We call the transcendent "God." And we seek, through community, value, and action, to build a relationship with God—a relationship that simultaneously respects God's transcendence while accommodating our need to love and to be loved.

The *Mishkan* was a representation of that love. Moses and the Jewish People built a building in which they could concretize their lofty conceptions of the living God. The voice of God could be sought in the *Mishkan,* just as it had reverberated during the encounter at Sinai.

Rabbi Moses Nachmanides articulates that insight when he writes, "the secret of the *Mishkan* is that the glory which abode upon Mount Sinai openly should abide upon it in a concealed manner."

The *Mishkan* is a portable, internalized Sinai. With the portable Tabernacle, Jews could carry a representation of their bond with God throughout their wanderings. In each place, they could see a physical emblem of their special *brit* with God.

What about us? At what do we gaze to remember that same special *brit*? Our generation has to look no further than our own bookshelves, our own communities, and our own homeland.

Do you want a reminder of your love for God and of God's love for you? Pick up a Jewish book. The Torah, with commentary, is a good place to start. Involve yourself in a synagogue, where the people of the covenant can help to activate the spark inside of you. Visit Israel, where our ancient, holy language lives in the mouths of our own people.

We are loved; and we can share that love.

❧

Parashat Terumah/Offering
Take 3

One Relation: Visible and Under God

Every February, Americans send each other cards with fat, little, winged babies and big, red hearts. The babies flutter around, shooting silly-looking arrows, while the cards often float on boxes of chocolates or bouquets of flowers. Valentine's Day is more than an annual celebration of romance; it's also a big industry, when you care enough to spend the very best.

Where did the idea of chubby boys with wings come from, and why is that a symbol of love? One source is the idea of Cupid, the mythical son of the Roman goddess Venus, whose arrows caused instant passionate love to burn in the heart of the target. The hunger that Cupid's arrows implanted produced a heartburn that never went away.

Not so the Jewish notion of a cherub. The Torah, and the rest of the Hebrew Scriptures, mentions the cherubim several times. Their most prominent role occurs in this week's *parashah,* in which the Torah relates God's instruction:

> Make two cherubim of gold—make them of hammered work—at the two ends of the cover. The cherubim shall have their wings spread out above, shielding the cover with their wings. There I will meet with you . . . from between the two cherubim that are on top of the Ark of the Pact.

What were these statues doing in the middle of biblical religion? And why were they in the most awesome of all possible places, right in the Holy of Holies, just above the Ark of the Covenant? Didn't the Ten Commandments prohibit fashioning any image of anything in the heavens or on earth?

In fact, cherubim were common throughout the Ancient Near East. The Akkadian word *kuribu,* originally meaning "to pray," was used to describe creatures which were part human, part beast, and part bird. Statues and portraits of these cherubim guard the entrance of pagan temples to petition the deities on behalf of the worshipers.

The image of the cherubim troubled our medieval sages. Interested in the mechanics of their involvement, Rashi (Rabbi Shlomo ben Isaac) explained, "a voice descended from the heavens between the cherubim . . . and was heard by Moses in the Tent of Meeting." For Rashi, these images were tools for focusing to help Moses recognize the Divine source of his instructions from God.

The Rashbam was more interested in a psychological facet, recalling the words of the Talmud, which explained that these cherubim had faces like children (*ke-rabbiya*). In that sense, the cherubim are close to God (the word *cherub* is related to the Hebrew word for *close*) because they symbolize that purity, goodness, and trust of the world found primarily in young children.

Most insightful, however, is the remark of Hizkuni that the cherubim are permissible, even though they appear to violate the prohibition against statues, because they are made not to be worshipped, but rather to symbolize God's invisible, glorious throne.

The cherubim point to a higher truth: the invisibility of the God of Israel. Showing the *base* of the throne highlights the impossibility of portraying the throne itself, much less the God whose Presence fills it. The physical image of the cherub, then, draws our attention to the absence of an image for God.

Why does the God of Israel have no image?

To portray is to limit, to encompass, to comprehend. That path leads to the trap of excessive intellect, of human arrogance, to the mistaken idea that expertise or knowledge can replace faithfulness or goodness. God is always *ain sof,* "without limit." Less interested in being understood, God passionately seeks commitment, being, and involvement.

Prayer, in the Tabernacle of old or in the synagogue of the present, is less a recital of words, or an exercise in self-expression, than it is a response of wonder, gratitude, and love.

God and love dwell not in Cupid's arrows, but in humanity's heart, invisible, and for all.

TETZAVEH/You Will Command
Exodus 27:20–30:10

This parashah *picks up where* Terumah *leaves off. Having concluded the instructions for building the* Tabernacle, Tetzaveh *begins with commands about providing fuel for illumination; in this case, olive oil. Aaron and his sons are to set up these lamps in the* Ohel Mo'ed, *the Tent of Meeting, where they will burn from evening to morning.*

The Torah *now moves to establish the* Kahunah, *the priesthood, through Aaron and his sons: Nadav, Avihu, Eleazar, and Ithamar. They are provided with special dress to distinguish them from the other Israelites and to mark them for sacred service.*

The Kohen Gadol, High Priest, *is unique in his golden attire. He wears eight special objects, among them:*

1. *The* Ephod, *or apron*

2. *The* Hoshen, *or breastpiece, which uses twelve colored stones to signify the Twelve Tribes of Israel*

3. *The* Urim ve-Tummim, *devices used to discern the will of God*

4. *The robe made entirely of* tekhelet, *the blue dye also found in one thread of* tzitzit, *and with pomegranates on its hem*

5. *The* Tzitz, *or frontlet, bearing the words "Holy to* Adonai"

6. *The* Kuttonet, *or tunic*

7. *The* Mitznefet, *or headdress*

8. *The* Avnet, *or sash*

The ordinary priests wore four garments.

Tetzaveh *goes on to describe the installation ritual of the priests, a ceremony presided over by Moses, which lasted for seven days (another reference to Creation). The installation ceremony consists of sacrifices of both animals and grain, bathing and cleansing the priests' bodies, robing the priests, and anointing them.*

The portion ends with a summary of the purpose of this elaborate rite: "I will abide among the Israelites and I will be their God. And they shall know that I, Adonai, am their God, who brought them out from the land of Egypt that I might abide among them, I, Adonai, their God."

Parashat Tetzaveh/You Will Command
Take 1

Hear, O Israel,
the Lord Is Lonely

Parashat Tetzaveh uncovers a lengthy description of the *Mishkan,* the Tabernacle, and the sacred garments of the *kohanim,* the priests, who will minister there. At the end of that description, the Torah explains that from God's perspective the purpose of the *Mishkan* is to meet with the Israelites: "And it shall be sanctified by My Presence."

So far, there is nothing remarkable about this passage. Many generations of commentators have noted, in the words of the Talmud, that the purpose of the *mitzvot* found in the Torah is to refine humanity. Consequently, Rashi understands that the *Mishkan* was built to provide for the religious development of Israel. This view assumes that the commandments of Judaism serve a human purpose, reflecting God's concern for the Jewish People and our needs.

But today's Torah portion seems to stand that viewpoint on its head. The passage concludes:

They shall know that I the Lord am their God, who brought them out of Egypt that I might abide among them, I the Lord their God.

This remarkable verse presupposes that the purpose of God's actions to liberate the Jews and to instruct them to build the *Mishkan* was to meet a *divine* need—a need for companionship and for relationship.

This revolutionary shift in perspective drew the notice of several commentators throughout Jewish history. Thus, Rabbi Abraham ibn

Ezra notes that this verse means "the purpose of My bringing them forth from the land of Egypt was only that I might dwell in their midst." Rabbi Moses ben Nahman, the Ramban, observes that this focus on God's need is "a great secret":

> For in the plain sense of things it would appear that the dwelling of the Divine glory in Israel was to fulfill a want below, but it is not so. It fulfilled a want above.

Thus the Torah is telling us that the God of Israel is a passionate God, a God who loves, cares, and gets involved. This is no Prime Mover, which is itself unmoved, no first cause that is beyond causation. While ultimately beyond containment in human language or human concepts, the Jewish notion of God is of one who responds to human needs and desires, who needs a relationship with each one of us.

That notion of God requiring human love and human relationship lies at the very core of Judaism through the ages. God's passion and loneliness find expression and resolution only in the reciprocal love of human beings. It was out of that need for love and commitment that God first created the world and later made a covenant with a particular people, the Jews, before extending that love to all people. The "chosenness" of the Jewish People is a primary expression of God's need for emotional connection and for mutual concern.

It was God's love that created the world. It is our love for God that sustains it and fills our lives and communities with meaning.

How is that love evidenced?

It is shown by the fact that the world is a place where life can flourish, where people are generally able to live and thrive, where children can grow and develop and adults can cultivate their families, their interests, and their virtues.

It is shown by the fact that each of us has a deep-seated need to love and to be loved. It feels *good* to care about another person, to belong to a group of people who share a history, an ethos, and a vision for the future. It feels *good* to help those who need our assistance.

Our tradition teaches us that we are made in God's image: Just as we have been created with a drive to love and be loved, so our Creator, whose image we reflect, needs to give love and to receive it.

Over the millennia, Jewish people the world over have cultivated that special affection through deeds of holiness, through acts of loving-kindness, and through the ongoing study of the accumulated record of our relationship with God, our sacred writings.

The Lover is waiting; the next step is yours.

❈

Parashat Tetzaveh/You Will Command
Take 2
An Eternal Light in Our Hearts

Parashat Tetzaveh opens with detailed instructions about the contents of the *Mishkan,* the Tabernacle, Israel's portable site of worship. The first consideration is for the *Ner Tamid,* the eternal light.

Why should God need a light inside the *Mishkan?* After all, God is not afraid of the dark: The Creator of the Universe can't possibly need external illumination to be able to see.

So what is the reason for the *Ner Tamid,* a light designed to shine from dusk until dawn?

One possibility is that the *Ner Tamid* was ordained not to meet a need of God, but rather to assist the people of Israel. According to *Midrash Sh'mot Rabbah,* God explained that God didn't need the *Ner Tamid,* but wanted it "in order that you may give light to Me as I give light to you."

The *Ner Tamid* becomes a symbol of Israel's eternal relationship of love and loyalty to God, a token of the reciprocity between Israel and God. Its perpetual blaze reminds each Jew of the flame of Sinai.

A related understanding stipulates that the *Ner Tamid* was God's public relations gift to Israel, so that other ancient peoples would say, "Israel gives light to the One who illuminates the whole world." This second perspective reinforces the viewpoint of the first, and directs it outward toward the rest of humanity. The *Ner Tamid* instructs non-Jews about our sacred covenant.

Both explanations are rooted in the idea that the emotional connection between Israel and the Holy One needs a physical representation. But other explanations add entirely new dimensions.

One *Midrash* asserts that the *Ner Tamid* symbolizes the teachings of the Torah: "The words of the Torah emit light to those who study them." Placing a *Ner Tamid* in the center of the *Mishkan* demonstrates our continuing commitment to *talmud Torah,* the study of our sacred writings, cultivating those teachings, and molding our own perspectives around the insights of countless generations of Jewish sages, writers, and communities.

Each time Jews gather to study our sacred writings, the light of Sinai shines anew in our midst.

Yet another understanding asserts that it is *observance* that is symbolized by light: "If one performs a *mitzvah,* it is as if one had kindled a light before God." Each pious deed—whether preparing a kosher meal or assisting the homeless, whether cleaning a city park or praying in a *minyan*—brings holy light into the world and contributes to the collective blaze of Jewish sacred action. Each time Jews perform a *mitzvah,* God's love and sovereignty shine that much more brightly.

A third understanding teaches that each human being is a light, because "the *nefesh* of a person is the lamp of God." God's love and compassion emit light which becomes visible in the feelings, hopes, and needs of another human being. Each time Jews treat another person with care and respect, God's image inside that person shimmers with light.

Through *Talmud torah,* the study of Jewish traditions; *kiyum mitzvot,* the performance of sacred deeds; and *kibbud ha-briyot,* responding to God's image in every person, we too, like our ancestors in the wilderness, can construct and illumine a *Ner Tamid* within the *Mishkan* of our hearts.

Parashat Tetzaveh / You Will Command
Take 3

Holy to God; Holy to People

One of the most colorful figures in biblical religion is the *Kohen Gadol,* the High Priest who ministered in the Temple in Jerusalem. This man, a direct descendant of Aaron, was the highest religious authority during the time of the First Temple (1000–586 B.C.E.) and became the dominant political force in the period of the Second Temple (500 B.C.E.–70 C.E.). His task was to assure the possibility of Israel's atonement and God's forgiveness. Through the elaborate practices of sacrifice, offering, and ritual purity, the *Kohen Gadol* and his associates provided Israel with the comfort of God's renewed love and support.

Perhaps the most dazzling aspect of the *Kohen Gadol* was his physical appearance. The Torah speak of his fantastic apparel—tunic, *ephod,* precious stones, crown, breastplates—each one composed of a multitude of colors and symbolic meaning.

Two, in particular, call for close examination. On his chest, the *Kohen Gadol* wore the *Hoshen* (breastplate), consisting of three rows of four different stones each. On each of the stones was inscribed one of the names of Israel's tribes.

Why would the High Priest wear those stones and carry those names? According to the *Midrash Shemot Rabbah,* they were worn "so that God would look at them and at the garments of the priest as he entered the Holy of Holies on Yom Kippur and be mindful of the merits of the tribes."

In other words, a part of the function of the priest was to remind God of the Jewish People—their striving for holiness, their passion for justice, and their life of sacred deeds. Not only a messenger of God to the people, the *Kohen Gadol* carried a message to God as well, as though God could forget! Or, as though God had a religious need for ritual! In fact, the priest *did* remind God of the humanity, and consequently the nobility, of the Jewish People. Especially on Yom Kippur, the most holy day of the year, the *midrash* recognizes that the responsibility of the *Kohen* included pleading on the people's behalf, acting as their advocate before the Holy Blessing One.

Equally striking is Aaron's second garment, a gold band stretching from ear to ear and two fingers in width, on which was written the words "Holy to *Adonai.*" No hollow ritual, these words required the *Kohen*'s concentration, so much so that Rashi explains that the priest was obligated to kiss them as a way of bolstering his *kavvanah,* his focus.

Thus, it wasn't sufficient for the *Kohen Gadol* to concentrate on representing the people; he also had to represent God before Israel, summoning the Jewish People to renew the covenantal commitment to the values and practices of Torah, *mitzvot,* and loving deeds.

In our own day, we often find the whole of our task difficult to fulfill. Many of us emphasize ethical behavior, filling our time by asserting the values of human belonging and of compassion in the face of perceived need. Others put the emphasis on ritual, pursuing those commandments that relate to themselves and God, whether in the traditional forms of rabbinic observance or the more American form of meditation and retreats.

But both ethics *and* spirituality are necessary. The dual Torah of our God, the multiple mission of our ancestors, was a blend of ethics and spirit that enriched and glorified both. Weaving those two strands together into a single and indivisible cloth was, and is, the special task of the Jew.

We are the people who saw religious service as extending to our care for the weakest among us, to compassion for animals, do the pursuit of peace.

We are also the people who transformed occasions of eating into an encounter with the sacred, who infused the cycle of the calendar with a focus on God, who elevated learning into the ultimate act of piety and self-transformation.

Let the clothing of the *Kohen Gadol* remind all of us of that dual mission. One cannot be religious and yet callous to other living creatures and our fellow human beings. One cannot be ethical or just without applying standards to ourselves that raise us above our own whims and conventions.

Sacred to the Lord and carrying the names of our people, we fuse holiness and ethics for the betterment of both and the repair of the world.

KI-TISSA/When You Take
Exodus 30:11–34:35

Ki-Tissa *begins with a census of Israelite men over the age of twenty, and the assessment of a half-shekel poll tax on each of them. This tax is seen as a ransom to God so the participants will escape plague. The rich do not pay more, nor do the poor pay less.*

God then instructs Moses to construct a copper and bronze laver to be used for washing the feet and hands of the kohanim *prior to their performing sacrifices. (This is still done as a memorial prior to the* kohanim *blessing the congregation during the Days of Awe and the Festivals. Observant Jews still ritually wash their hands prior to eating bread as a gesture of priestly preparation.) Next, God tells Moses to prepare a special aromatic oil and prohibits using it for any purpose other than anointing priests. The contents of the Tabernacle's incense are then detailed, and its use outside is similarly prohibited.*

God appoints Bezalel and Oholiab, two artisans of great wisdom and skill, to do the actual work of building the Tent of Meeting, the Ark for the Covenant, and all the contents of the Tabernacle.

Just as the Tabernacle represents holiness in space, the Sabbath represents holiness in time. God reiterates its observance: "You must keep My Sabbaths, for this is a sign between Me and you throughout the ages, that you may know that I Adonai have consecrated you." Work is prohibited on the seventh day.

God then presents Moses with the two stone tablets, inscribed by God.

Meanwhile, down below in the desert, the people are frantic, because they don't know what has become of Moses. They demand that Aaron make them a god. Aaron takes their gold rings and casts a molten calf, the Egel ha-Zahav. *The people begin to worship it and Aaron makes an altar, which the people use to make a burnt offering. God tells Moses to hurry down and threatens to destroy the people for being "stiff necked." Moses talks God out of this destructive reaction, reminding God of the promise to Abraham, Isaac, and Jacob that their children would become a great nation. Moses then descends from Mount Sinai. As soon as he sees the calf, he smashes the tablets, grinds the calf into powder, throws it in water, and makes the Israelites drink it. Moses calls out, "Whoever is for the Lord, come here!" The Levites rally to him, and they slaughter some three thousand people that day. Moses then returns to God to plead for forgiveness of the people. God relents, but refuses to accompany the people further, at which the people go into mourning.*

Moses continues to meet with God face to face, and pleads with God to resume leading the Israelites directly. God relents, because he has singled out Moses by name. Taking advantage of this favor, Moses pleads to see God's presence. God explains that people cannot see God and live, but agrees to make God's goodness pass before Moses. Moses carves two new tablets, and when God passes by, Moses proclaims, "Adonai! Adonai! A God compassionate and gracious, slow to anger, abounding in kindness and faithfulness, extending kindness to the thousandth generation, forgiving iniquity, transgression, and sin."

God then lays out the prohibition against idolatry, and discusses proper worship, which includes the calendar of the Jewish holidays and festivals, observed to this day.

The parashah concludes with Moses rewriting the Ten Commandments on the new tablets. When he descends the mount, his face is radiant with light, so he covers his face with a veil from then on, taking it off only for private conversation with God.

Parashat Ki-Tissa/When You Take
Take 1

Justice, Community, Tzedakah

Jewish education forms the backbone of our communities. We assure the Jewish People vitality and endurance through the Hebrew studies of our children, outreach programs for those considering conversion, and continuing education programs for other seeking adults. And those programs need our support.

Consider today's Torah portion. God instructs Moses to take a census of the Jewish People in order for each Jew to pay a half-shekel tax to maintain the central communal institution of Jewish learning, the *Mishkan* (Tabernacle).

The *Mishkan,* a Jewish school? Absolutely, since it was there that the entire Jewish community gathered to learn the word of God. And that first school was supported by all. The Torah records,

> Everyone who is entered in the records, from the age of twenty years up, shall give the Lord's offering: the rich shall not pay more and the poor shall not pay less that half a shekel when giving the Lord's offering.

So vital was the necessity of *everybody* contributing to *tzedakah,* a word that literally means "justice" and, by extension, funds for public assistance that, in the words of Rabbi Abraham ibn Ezra, the contribution "atones for a soul." According to the Talmud, "*Tzedakah* is as important as all the other commandments put together." Precisely because of the centrality of giving, the Torah imposes an unexpected obligation on the poor. For this verse insists that the poor cannot give less than a half-shekel. According to Maimonides, "even a poor person who lives entirely on *tzedakah* must also give *tzedakah.*"

Giving *tzedakah* involves the very heart of Jewish responsibility and humanity. To be a responsible Jew implies, among other attributes, supporting the Jewish community. All of us, no matter how rich or poor, are members of a community that provides services to its members. At the center of those services is the need to train Jews to maintain a community. Without knowledgeable and passionate Jews—young and old—there will be no Jewish services to provide since there will be no Jews to provide them. Supporting Jewish education is an act of Jewish responsibility, and an investment in the future.

All of us, even the poor, have a right to be responsible, to feel that we contribute to the maintenance of the Jewish community.

Our claim to humanity and belonging is predicated on our giving *tzedakah.* Our ability to provide Jewish institutions to care for immigrants, the elderly, Israel, oppressed Jewry, civil rights, and a range of other needs depends on the cultivation and continued training of Jews who recognize their obligations and responsibilities as Jews. And that means supporting Jewish education.

Consider a tale from the Talmud. The wealthy Rabbi Tarfon once asked Rabbi Akiva to help him invest his money. Rabbi Akiva took the funds and used them instead to allow poor students to continue their Jewish education. Several days later, when Rabbi Tarfon asked to see his investments, Rabbi Akiva took him to the school and showed him the students as they recited their lessons from the Bible. When they arrived at the verse, "He gives freely to the poor; his righteousness endures forever," Rabbi Akiva pointed to the students and said, "This is the investment I made for you!"

There is no greater investment than supporting places of Jewish learning—our day schools, synagogues, and seminaries. If there is to be a Jewish community tomorrow, it will be a result of the hardworking Jewish educators—rabbis, cantors, teachers, principals, and others—who provide a sense of Jewish identity, piety, and involvement both for children and adults. Without Jewish education, we cannot survive.

And, as today's Torah verse indicates, the responsibility to support Jewish education rests on each one of us.

Rich and poor, together we must assure Jewish survival with our contributions, our involvement, and our hearts.

<hr />

Parashat Ki-Tissa/When You Take
Take 2

Shabbat: A Symbol of Love

Israel shall keep Shabbat, observing Shabbat throughout the ages as a covenant for all time. It shall be a sign for all time between Me and the people of Israel.

Shabbat is the heart of Judaism—quite a claim for a day that is frequently ignored by so many Jews! Yet an examination of our past reveals how vital *Shabbat* has always been in Jewish family life and how central to our spiritual experience. Moreover, an examination of our own age, with its careerism and its bustle, reveals that *Shabbat* is needed more now than ever before.

Ask yourself these questions: Can you guarantee yourself a twenty-four-hour period each week in which you will do no chores? Can you pledge that for an entire day you will simply take pleasure in the company of those you love, unmarred by any need to attend to professional or domestic obligations?

If you are like most modern Americans, you cannot count on it. Like most of our contemporaries, we are deluged by the requirements of maintaining our households or advancing our careers. The luxury of simply enjoying the company of family and friends is postponed until advanced old age. Work comes first; relationships, last (assuming we are still healthy enough to attend to them).

Even our language betrays our trap. Time spent outside of work is time "off," implying that to be fully "on," fully active and creative and involved, we must be working. We have forgotten how to be "on" to each other and to ourselves in any context other than the professional.

Shabbat offers a period of sanity, a time for centering, that is otherwise absent in our culture. *Shabbat* assures each observant Jew that there will be twenty-four hours in which nothing will interfere with spiritual growth, strengthened community, and family. Chores and obligations can wait; cultivating family ties and spiritual values cannot.

Shabbat is a force for sanity in an insane world. In a culture which awards people status based on their income, *Shabbat* places money off limits. In a world in which physical strength and productivity are the pinnacle of human achievement, *Shabbat* asserts that simply *being* is our ultimate source of worth and contentment. In an age of loneliness and alienation, *Shabbat* offers us a dependable haven and a home.

Shabbat is our eternal sign with God, a timely reminder of a timeless bond.

Each week, Judaism presents a recapitulation of the cycles of Creation. Each week culminates in a reassertion of the Divine image inside each person, with the corollary insistence that human relationships and community require (and deserve) our sustained effort.

Shabbat is our time to reorient ourselves to family and friends.

Shabbat is our chance to redirect our technologically oriented culture back to human values and human loves.

Shabbat is our first and earliest source of strength. It is our last and greatest hope.

Seize it.

Parashat Ki-Tissa/When You Take
Take 3
Who Wrote the Book of Love?

One of the arguments separating different contemporary communities of Jews is the contention about who (or Who) wrote the Torah. Is the Torah the direct transcript of the words of God to Moses at Sinai, so that each and every word recorded in that book is the literal speech of God? Or is the Torah a human book, remarkable perhaps, but human nonetheless?

In the first instance, if the Torah is the literal words of God, then everything in it must be obeyed precisely as it was in the past—after all, only a fool would mess with the Creator of the heavens and the earth! But if the Torah is the creation of other human beings, then it is subject to human judgment, ours no less than anyone else's. Consequently, when there is a clash between the Torah and personal will, everyone may legitimately do what they want, even if the Torah prohibits it.

While both of these viewpoints are advanced with great passion and energy, both represent deviations from traditional Jewish understandings of what the Torah really was and is. The answer to the question "Is the source of the Torah human or divine?" is a resounding "Yes!" The Torah is the meeting place of God and the Jews—our loving response to, as well as God's invitation of, love.

In today's Torah portion, Moses receives the two tablets of the Ten Commandments, which were "inscribed with the finger of God." Farther on, the Torah tells us that those tablets were "God's work, and the writing was God's writing." Understood literally, it would seem that the Torah asserts that these specific words are God's, and that God has at least one finger!

Rashi explains that one could indeed understand it literally, but he then quotes the *Midrash Tanhuma,* which says that its meaning is "like the case of one person saying to a colleague, 'all of the efforts of this person are in that work,' so all the delight of the Holy Blessing One is in the Torah." In other words, the Torah is using poetic language to tell us that the Ten Commandments *do* embody divine will.

The Rambam is even more emphatic: The purpose of these words is to tell us that the tablets were "real and not artificial." He points out that the use of a "finger" is just as problematic as saying that God "says" or "speaks," as if God has a mouth and tongue, too! Rather, all this language about God speaking or writing is to affirm that the Torah reflects God's "will and volition."

Countless other traditional commentators reflect this same understanding. The Rashbam says that these words simply teach that "Moses didn't inscribe them" and Rabbi ibn Ezra affirms that even according to the *Mishnah,* the tablets were created before the first *Shabbat* preceding Creation. No one interpreted that phrase literally.

So what is all the fuss about?

If every word of the Torah is literally God's speech, Judaism doesn't change and all should be as it always was. If none of the words in the Torah reflect divine will, Judaism can be anything any Jew wants it to be.

Traditional Judaism refutes both extremes, insisting instead that our Torah is an accurate reflection of Divine "will and volition" (to quote the Rambam) without making claims about literal transmission of speech.

Just as much as there was, and is, a giving of Torah that is active and involves God, so, too, there was (and is) a receiving of Torah that is active and involves the children of Israel. The Torah is at once fully human and fully divine, charged with an electricity that can launch a people into eternity and restore a world to fullness and peace.

VA-YAKHEL/He Assembled
Exodus 35:1–38:20

Moses convenes the entire people. Just as the laws of the Tabernacle end with the laws of the Sabbath, so, too, the process of building it begins with a reiteration of the holiness of the Sabbath, mandating that the people refrain from work and from kindling fire on Shabbat.

Moses then calls for contributions from the people and asks those with talent and ability to participate in the project. The response is so generous and enthusiastic that all the men and women whose hearts moved them to bring anything for the work that the Lord, through Moses, had commanded to be done, did so as a freewill offering. Bezalel and Oholiab take the donations and begin to work, and the donations are so bounteous that Moses has to order the people to stop giving.

The people join in the work of construction, sewing, and building, and Bezalel turns to fashioning the furniture and accessories of the Tabernacle: the ark, the table, the menorah, the altar of incense, the anointing oil and incense, the altar of burnt offering, the laver, and the enclosure.

PEKUDEI/The Accounts
Exodus 38:21–40:38

A tally is made of all the metals used in the construction of the Tabernacle: gold, silver, and copper. The instructions for making the priestly garments are strictly implemented, and the people make the vestments just as God had commanded.

When the work is complete, the people bring each item to Moses for inspection: "And when Moses saw that they had performed all the tasks— as the Lord had commanded, so they had done—Moses blessed them."

God instructs Moses how to now erect the Tabernacle, which is done on the First of Nissan, near the second anniversary of the Exodus from Egypt. Moses does as God commands, and when he finishes the work "the cloud covered the Tent of Meeting, and the Presence of the Lord filled the Tabernacle."

The people rest when the cloud is settled, and move only when the cloud lifts, thus following God's initiative and leadership as they wander toward Eretz Yisrael.

✧✦✧

Parashat Va-Yakhel/Pekudei/The Assembled/The Accounts
Take 1

Seeking Each Other in a Cloud

One of the great mysteries of life is how two people are able to fall in love and build a home together. Think, for a moment, of how difficult it is to know oneself—how many moods, feelings, thoughts, and experiences go into making every single person. The force of our own reactions often surprises us, though we have lived with *ourselves* for our entire lives!

Now, compound that depth of unknown history and unpredictable emotions by putting two people together. Two human beings—worlds unto themselves—are able to nurture each other in a relationship. What becomes astounding is not that there are so many divorces and separations, but that there are so few.

If each person is a little universe, how can two such universes coexist? We are so full of ourselves that there is precious little room left for anyone else, let alone for someone so complex and demanding as another human being!

Today's Torah portion speaks of the miracle of relationship. At the very conclusion of the Book of *Sh'mot* (Exodus), the Torah records that

When Moses had finished the work, the cloud covered the *Ohel Mo'ed,* the Tent of Meeting, and the Presence of the Lord filled the

Mishkan, the Tabernacle. Moses could not enter the Tent of Meeting, because the cloud had settled upon it and the Presence of the Lord filled the *Mishkan.*

Rabbinic commentators were quick to notice a contradiction within the Torah. Whereas this verse says that Moses was unable to enter the *Mishkan* because it was already full of God's Presence, elsewhere the Torah states, "Moses went inside the cloud."

How is it possible that sometimes Moses could enter in the midst of God's Presence, made visible as a cloud, and at other times he could not?

One way to view the image of a cloud filling the *Mishkan* is as a metaphor for the way personality fills a human being, a way of symbolizing the dense and impenetrable quality of our own personalities.

When those personalities are most self-absorbed, it is indeed impossible to enter into a relationship with them. To be able to sustain a friendship, a love, or a marriage requires a willingness on the part of both people to engage in an act of revelation—to open themselves so that their very cores become accessible to those they love. By making ourselves transparent, by opening a path for the explorations of our own prejudices, passions, and opinions, we make love possible.

So, too, with God in the *Mishkan.* The Talmud resolves the contradiction between the two verses by saying that "the Holy Blessing One took hold of Moses and brought him into the cloud." The medieval scholar Joseph Bekhor Shor echoes the Talmud when he comments that calling to the person first must precede any real visit to another. By calling them before visiting, you get their attention, receive their consent to visit, and benefit from their cooperation in making themselves known. The great commentator, the Ramban, adds that "God would call Moses and [only] then would he enter into the midst of the cloud."

It is only by consenting to reveal our own hidden natures, by inviting someone else to share in our inner lives, that relationship becomes a possibility. Opening ourselves to each other's openness is the great miracle of love, where seemingly incompatible universes can meet, explore, and grow. Just as God called to Moses and then permitted him to enter, so God calls today to each of us. The path of relationship is unanticipated, unlikely, and difficult. But without it we are nothing.

Only by making ourselves available to each other and to God, by sharing our joys and our sorrows, by learning and by praying together, can we realize our fullest potential as humans.

Do Clothes Make the Man?

Today's Torah-reading offers an intricately detailed description of the elaborate outfit of the *kohanim,* the priests, in the *Mishkan*. These striking vestments were used both during the forty years of wandering in the wilderness, and later as the paradigm for the priestly robes in Solomon's Temple in Jerusalem. They must have added a powerful sense of majesty and pageantry to the earliest worship of the one true God.

It is only natural that, as the culmination of the rites of the *Mishkan,* the Torah would focus on the human beings who are to serve in that place. But why the emphasis on clothing? After all, isn't it true that what matters most about people is what's in their hearts? Shouldn't we find elaborate descriptions of Aaron's *personality,* rather than lengthy and tedious elaborations of his robes?

Why all this focus on externals?

Clothing is more than simply a way of covering our bodies. In determining how we clothe ourselves, we convey a message to the world about our values, priorities, and relationships.

A few examples will suffice: A woman who paints her lips tells us that she is financially secure and a part of Western culture. That same lipstick, if smeared on her forehead, would communicate to all who saw her that something was amiss.

Similarly, a piece of cloth around a man's neck indicates that he is a businessman, that he identifies with mainstream Western values, that he occupies a certain financial and social position. If he wore that same tie around his head or around his waist, he would be communicating an identification with a counterculture—a rejection of what the exact same tie normally stands for.

So it is that *all* clothing indicates values, revealing with what segment of society we identify and where our aspirations lie.

The elaborate and startling clothing of the *kohanim* indicates how their worldview and their values functioned as well. The fact that they wore intricate and expensive clothing amidst general simplicity, that they wore elaborate jewelry when no one else did so, indicates that biblical

Judaism stressed the royalty of God. Just as God's servants dressed like royalty, so were we to relate to the entire ritual surrounding God as though God were a grand sovereign.

Throughout Jewish history, clothing of the religious leadership indicated how Jews perceived their relationship to God and to each other. The rabbis of the *Mishnah* and the Talmud dressed no differently than any other Jews, stressing the equality of all before God.

In the early parts of this century, many rabbis donned clerical robes and stood on platforms high above their congregants, to emphasize the dignity, majesty, and otherness of God and of the sacred service.

In our own day, Jewish worship has been moving away from a primary concern with decorum and dignity. Instead, we seek community, warmth, and support. The clothing of our religious leaders and the choreography of our services reflect that contemporary emphasis on the *haimish*.

Many rabbis have abandoned formal robes as being too cold, too churchlike. Often, those same rabbis, seeking to foster warmth and community, will leave the isolation of the *bimah* when they deliver their *drashot* (sermons).

Doubtless, the way rabbis and cantors dress will continue to reflect the developing perspectives of future Jewish communities, suggesting how we perceive our relationships to each other, to our traditions, and to our God.

The medium is the message.

Parashat Va-Yakhel/Pekudei/The Assembled/The Accounts
Take 3

If It's Broken, Why Keep It?

Ours is a highly practical society. We pride ourselves on our ability to tinker with gadgets, produce labor-saving devices, and invent fascinating toys that whirl, and spin, and entertain. A range of significant inventions, from the lightbulb to the electronic organizer, typifies this American delight with technology and efficiency.

Doubtless, those inventions have enriched our lives. We are efficient in our work, organized in our homes, and offer a high standard of living to a large number of people. We think nothing of showing a Hollywood movie in the privacy of our own homes, microwaving the pizza of a world-famous chef, and listening to a performance of a renowned conductor on the CD player in our living rooms. All of these conveniences add real pleasure and comfort to the lives of hundreds of thousands of people.

Though we value these trinkets, we throw them out as soon as they break. After all, there is rarely a permanent affection between an owner and a car: One car will do as well as the next. The love is most often with cars in general, not with any specific automobile. Our love for our things is a functional, conditional love: So long as they work, we love them. The minute they stop, we replace them.

Our functional love extends beyond replacing broken items. We even plan their obsolescence, or junk them for the latest model before they have given all the service they could. Clothing, cars, and homes are all "traded in" well in advance of practical need, simply because we have spotted and desired a larger, more sophisticated, or more recent model.

How surprising, then, that we often feel disconnected, lacking in roots or purpose. How can we, when the obsolescence of things often is applied to relationships as well?

Not so the world of the Torah. In today's Torah portion, after the construction of the *Mishkan* has been completed, we are told that Moses "took the Tablets and placed it in the Ark." The rabbis of the Talmud note that the word for tablets—*Edut*—is in the plural. So imagine their interest (and our surprise) to read elsewhere in the Bible, after the dedication of Solomon's Temple in Jerusalem, that "there was nothing inside the Ark but the two tablets." If the word *tablet* is already plural, then two of them must mean that Moses placed in two additional tablets beyond the two tablets containing the Ten Commandments!

What else could Moses have dared to place beside the two tablets of the Commandments?

According to the Talmud, the answer is that "both the *whole* tablets and the *fragments* of the tablets were placed together in the Ark."

Remember when Moses returned to the children of Israel, carrying the first tablets with the Ten Commandments? He was so outraged by the idolatry of the Golden Calf that he shattered the tablets on the ground. After the people had repented of their sin, Moses returned to the peak of the mountain, where God presented a second pair of tablets. So far, the story is typically American—the outmoded commandments were trashed and a new, sleeker model was substituted in their place.

But the Talmud tells us that something very un-American had actually transpired, that the love the Jews felt for that first pair of tablets was not simply because of their function, but something unconditional—bestowed not for their possible use but for what they would always represent.

Think of your feelings about your wedding ring. Chances are strong that in the course of your lifetime you will be able to purchase more elaborate, more expensive rings. Yet your love for that original plain gold band is not simply because it adorns your finger. We love our wedding bands because they remind us of a momentous and happy day in our lives, they signify the most important relationship we will ever have with another human being. Those rings are irreplaceable.

That is precisely our relationship to those first tablets. Moses saved them both, the shattered and the whole, to remind us that not exists for a practical purpose. On the contrary, some of the most important things in life are not especially "useful" in the practical sense. Rather, we treasure those objects that signify happy times, important relationships, or essential values.

Next time you are in a synagogue, or involved in Jewish ritual, don't ask, "What can this do for me?" That's an appropriate question for a lightbulb or a digital camera. Instead, ask, "What values, memories, or deed of loving-kindness can this kindle in my heart?" That is the question to ask of that which endures.

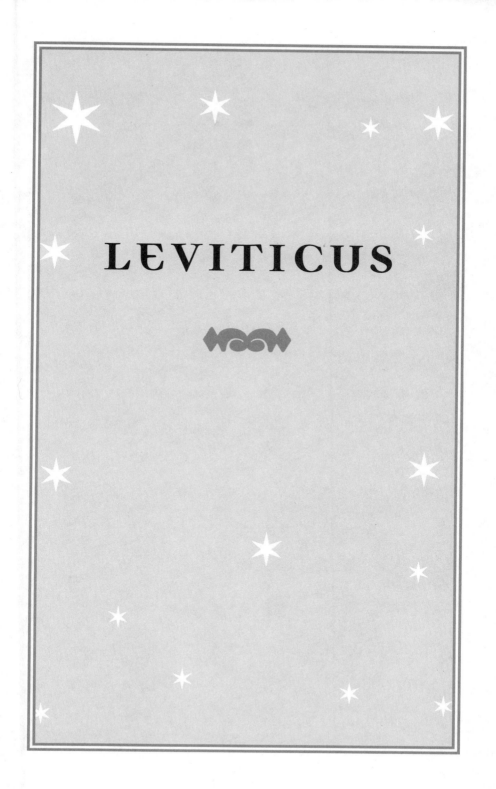

LEVITICUS

VA-YIKRA/He Called
Leviticus 1:1–5:26

The Book of Leviticus is the pinnacle book of the Torah. Located in the very center of the other five, it exemplifies the distinctive fusion of ritual and ethics that has always been the way of Torah. At the center of this central book comes chapter 19 with the Holiness Code, a summary of the entire ethos and norms of a Jewish way of life. Before and after this pivotal section, Leviticus concerns itself with the regulations of the priesthood, the proper performance of the sacrifices, atonement, and righteous living. Each of these facets gives expression to the covenant linking God and the people Israel.

The book begins with three chapters, each of which details the main types of sacrifices that individuals offer. The Olah, the burnt offering, provides a "pleasing odor for God." The Minha, the grain offering, must be without leaven. The fat and blood of the Shelamim, peace or whole offerings, cannot be consumed. These sacrifices serve many different purposes, communal and individual, required and optional.

Chapters 4 and 5 highlight a different kind of offering: the Hattat, sin offering. The Hattat is for the unintentional commission of a prohibited act by a Kohen, the community, the head of the community, or an individual. It is also the necessary ritual response for withholding testimony, touching something tamei (ritually impure), touching human tumah (ritual impariety), or failure to fulfill an oath.

Finally, the Asham, guilt offering, is for robbery or fraud, for me'ilah (the misappropriation of Temple property), and for the unintentional violations of prohibitions.

Parashat Va-Yikra/He Called
Take 1
Your Home Is God's Altar

Most Jews would associate *hametz,* leaven, with the festival of Passover.

After all, it is before that holiday that we remove all *hametz* from our homes, burn some *hametz* and nullify it with a vow on the morning before the first Seder, and appoint a rabbi to be our agent to sell any remaining *hametz* to a non-Jew. During the entire Passover festival no *hametz* is to be found in our homes or in our possession, nor do we eat any *hametz* throughout these eight special days.

The most popular reason given for avoiding *hametz* is found in the Torah itself—that our ancestors left Egypt in such a hurry that they had no time for their dough to rise. As a memorial to their hasty flight, we abstain from *hametz* just as they had to do out of necessity.

Today's Torah-reading provides another possible justification for this traditional practice, linking our avoidance of *hametz* to a broader view of Judaism and Jewish institutions throughout history.

In describing the offerings of the *Mishkan* and later of Solomon's Temple in Jerusalem, the Torah records that "no meal offering that you offer to the Lord shall be made with leaven, for no leaven or honey may be turned into smoke as an offering by fire to the Lord."

Why this peculiar restriction?

According to the Rambam, Rabbi Moses ben Maimon, pagan religion in the biblical period offered meal offerings with leaven and with honey. Since one of Judaism's central struggles was to uproot pagan practices from among the Jews, the Torah here prohibits a practice that Jews would have recognized as idolatrous.

In a sense, therefore, the Rambam avoids the question of why *hametz,* specifically, is forbidden. Instead, he points to a larger opposition to idolatry leading to the general rule that anything they do, we prohibit.

Another attempted explanation was to read symbolic value into the forbidden items. Thus, in the thirteenth century *Sefer Ha-Hinnukh* the author explains that by keeping *hametz,* which is prepared over a long period, away from one's offering, "a person will attain the idea of acquiring the quality of alertness, lightness, and swiftness in deeds on behalf of the Holy Blessing One."

Just as it takes a significant amount of time for leavening to take place, so, too, we might become slothful in fulfilling our religious obligations. By keeping *hametz* away from our offerings, we remind ourselves to act swiftly and with resolution in the service of the sacred and its teaching.

Sefer Ha-Hinnukh offers a second symbolic reading, claiming that we avoid *hametz* "because leaven puffs itself up . . . Hence [leaven was] rejected to imply that 'every haughty person is an abomination to the Lord.' "

Ultimately, however, none of these explanations may be entirely satisfactory. Thus, the Ramban admits that "it may be that there is in all these matters some secret hidden from us," and *Sefer Ha-Hinnukh* concedes that "the reasons from this precept are too hidden to find even a small hint of them."

So what are we left with?

The bottom line is that *hametz* is prohibited in any offerings on the altar of the *Mishkan* or of the Temple. And that same prohibition applies during Passover, the festival that celebrates the liberation of the Jews from slavery and the beginnings of our service to God and humanity as a nation of priests.

Once a year, for slightly more than a week, we elevate our homes to reflect the same level of purity and holiness that characterized the Temple in Jerusalem. Without claiming to know the definitive justification, we fall back on the bedrock values of obedience, loyalty, and identity. Because we are Jews, because our people have always done this, and because the Torah and the Talmud—our links to God's presence in our lives—command us, we remove *hametz* from our homes.

Each year, our table becomes an altar, and our homes become centers of sanctity where God's presence can dwell. By removing *hametz* from our homes, we restore the center—our homes—to that which is central—our heritage, our people, and our God.

Parashat Va-Yikra/He Called
Take 2

The Value of Animal Sacrifices

Sefer Va-Yikra, the Book of Leviticus, is at the center of the Torah, not only spatially, but also spiritually. More than any other single book, *Va-Yikra* sets the tone and establishes the central themes of biblical and rabbinic Judaism throughout the ages.

The central focus of *Va-Yikra* is on establishing a sacred community, "a nation of priests," whose daily deeds perfect the world under God's rule. By establishing an ideal community, *Va-Yikra* recognizes that deeds speak far more eloquently than words, that living in a holy community can provide a sense of God's presence far more pervasive than more ethereal approaches.

So far, so good. Few modern Jews would have any problem, at least in theory, with those general statements.

Our problem starts when we examine how *Va-Yikra* defines the detailed practices of a sacred community. What kind of deeds and activities create the core of *Va-Yikra's* vision?

At the center of this central book lies a preoccupation with animal and vegetative sacrifice, which is far from the worldview of most contemporary Jews, and, for that matter, most contemporary Americans. When we think of religious devotion, we tend to picture silent meditation, appreciation of nature, perhaps even a commitment to ethical living. But the connection between killing animals and serving the Lord escapes us completely.

To understand our own sacred heritage as Jews, to appreciate the religious perspective that emerges from the Torah, the Talmud, and most later Jewish writings, we must come to an understanding of the centrality of Temple ritual and sacrifice.

Objections to animal sacrifices readily abound: It's bloody, it's barbaric, it is too physical, too particular, too ugly. Sacrifice is violent, uncontrolled, and primitive.

All true. But so is life.

And it is precisely in that paradox that we can first recognize the power, if not the aesthetics, of sacrifice.

Life is not neatly packaged, fully controlled, or completely comprehensible. Life includes tragedies of staggering proportions, disappoint-ments of trivial pettiness, jealousies, violence, and rage.

Each one of us is made up of many layers of feelings, drives, and convictions. Only the most superficial layer of our personalities is ver-bal, cheerful, and polite. The deeper layers of the human psyche are nonverbal, contradictory, and impulsive. They include drives toward lust, anger, gratification, jealousy, and safety. Each of us embodies the person we were at every previous stage of development, all previous ages we have ever lived.

All of these competing levels and drives require some mode of expression. If we attempt to deny them, and consequently to stifle them, they will erupt in destructive or inappropriate ways.

For Judaism to be able to assist us in living, it must reflect all of life. Judaism must be the haven in which we can safely channel and express the entire range of human impulses and drives, confront our own sub-conscious, relive our own past, face and share our deepest anxieties. If it cannot be at least this, then it is nothing.

Sacrifice horrifies and stuns precisely because it embodies so many subconscious drives and terrors. We need not reinstitute sacrifice to be able to benefit from recalling this ancient practice in the safe context of a worship service. Are you afraid of death? Confront it by reading about sacrifice. Are you ridden with guilt? Represent and conquer your guilt in the Yom Kippur ritual of the scapegoat and sacrifice.

Our ancestors turned to animal sacrifice because they saw in it a way to express deep rage, feelings of inadequacy, and guilt. They could use the rite of sacrifice as a means of facing their terror of death and the unknown. They could, through sacrifice of animals, see their own frailty, their own mortality, and their own bloodiness.

In our age, a period of sanitized religion and everyday violence, esca-lating drug abuse and rising poverty, the practice of our ancestors has something yet to teach.

And so we read *Sefer Va-Yikra,* and learn to see our fears in the eyes of an animal going to the slaughter, in the cries of the victims of sacrifice.

Parashat Va-Yikra/He Called
Take 3

On Doing Much and Doing Little

"Rabbi, I never joined a synagogue, and we don't practice our religion at home, but I've always had a warm feeling for Judaism in my heart. I know that I've always been a good Jew."

Over and over again, in countless variations, Jews rehearse these lines before rabbis, organization volunteers, and anyone else who holds a position of Jewish responsibility: "I don't show support in any visible way, you can't tell I'm Jewish by any practice in my life, but all of that means nothing compared to the powerful emotional connection I nurture inside. Deep down, I'm Jewish."

This cardiac Judaism of warm feelings in the heart may claim the majority of America's Jews. And, certainly, warm feelings are an important component of Jewish identification and faith. But are warm feelings enough?

Our Torah portion offers a useful distinction between the role of warm feelings and the need for tangible signs and actions that nurture and transmit those feelings across the generations and throughout a community.

The Book of *Va-Yikra* opens with a description of the animal sacrifices that the *kohanim* were to perform in the Tabernacle and in the Jerusalem Temple. One of those sacrifices was the *Olah,* the burnt offering.

The *Olah* was a voluntary offering, brought by a Jew who had a specific need to bring to God's attention. The perceived danger of standing in the presence of God was mitigated through offering a pleasing sacrifice that would focus God's attention on the needy Jew; thus, the Bible elsewhere refers to God as one "who *responds* with fire." The range of possible offerings for this attention getter went from the full-grown cow, which only the very wealthy could afford, to the pigeon, which was easily accessible to anyone. Any one of these animals was acceptable as a burnt offering. Why?

Noting this remarkable commitment that all Jews should be able to use the sacrificial system to gain access to God, the Talmud remarks, "It doesn't matter to God whether one brings much or little, so long as one's heart is directed toward heaven."

Taken by itself, that line in the Talmud appears to justify doing the minimum. After all, if doing a lot and doing a little both count the same, why bother doing a lot? Additionally, this passage seems to place intention above deed, raising the possibility that if a person has the right intention there may be no need for any action at all.

There are many who champion this position today: Religion, we are told, is an affair of the heart; what counts are private feelings. Within Jewish circles, this Talmudic passage is often quoted as the justification for religion stripped of ritual or obligation.

Yet such a view misreads both the Talmud and the role of religion. The Talmud is here speaking about a ritual *bein adam la-Makom,* between humans and God. Few would argue that in the realm of *bein adam le-havero,* ethics or social justice, a little and a lot are the same. There is a big difference between giving 10 percent of one's income to charity and giving 20 or 30 percent. Regardless of one's intentions, it is better to give a lot.

But what about the realm of ritual: of prayer, *Shabbat, kashrut,* and the other *mitzvot* that comprise traditional Jewish expression? Is a little as good as a lot?

If the goal of Judaism were simply the feelings of the individual, the answer would have to be yes. One can feel favorably inclined as a Jew without a lot of Jewish practice. But is that really the only, or even the highest, Jewish goal?

What of the need to instill Jewish values? What of the need to teach self-restraint? What of our ability to improve our society and ourselves by reaching beyond our own perceived needs to a higher level? What of *God*'s warm feelings?

The key phrase of the Talmud is that the *heart must be directed toward heaven.* That doesn't just mean thinking of God as our big buddy in the sky, eager to approve our friendship on any terms. Rather, to quote from the *Mishnah,* it means a willingness to "make God's will your will." In allowing an agenda of holiness and righteousness to replace the drives of the human heart—our own whims, fads, and lusts—we offer our very core to God as a gift. We make of ourselves altars in the service of redemption. What matters is substituting God's agenda for our own, and then participating in the ritual, whether lavishly or not.

You don't have to serve two main courses, but have a *Shabbat* dinner each week. You don't have to eliminate poverty by yourself, but give to charity as much as you can. You don't need two sets of china, but keep a kosher kitchen.

The value of the sacrifice is not its size. But without some sacrifice, there can be no values.

TZAV/Command
Leviticus 6:1–8:36

On the surface, Tzav *appears to repeat much of the previous* parashah. *In fact, the first two chapters instruct the priests how to perform the rituals accompanying the sacrifices described in* Parashat Va-Yikra. *These chapters focus on the priests as officiants and emphasize the care required to maintain a state of* tohorah *(purity). A special focus of* Tzav *is the instruction that a portion of each sacrifice belongs to the priesthood and becomes the core of their sacred meals, eaten within the walls of the sanctuary.*

Tzav *begins with a discussion of the* kodesh kodashim *(the most sacred offerings), which are four: the* Olah *(burnt offering) and the* Mincha *(grain offering), since both are part of the public ritual; and the* Hattat *(sin) offering and the* Asham *(guilt offering), the latter which are not part of the routine public ritual but result from an individual's private penitence.*

Afterward, the Torah describes the kodashim kallim, *offerings of lesser sanctity. These include the* zevah ha-shelamim, *peace or whole offering. This was used in private worship, except for the* Shelamim of Shavuot.

With chapter 8, the Torah moves on to the Hakhel *(gathering) of the entire community and the ordination and consecration of the altar and the priests over the course of seven days. The ordination includes sacrifice, and also the ritual of Moses taking some of the sacrificial blood and smearing it on Aaron's right earlobe, his right thumb, and his right big toe.*

Parashat Tzav/Command
Take 1

Ears, Thumbs, and Toes

Traditionally, the Book of *Va-Yikra* was known as *Torat Kohanim,* Teachings of the Priests. Its contents are directed to those ministering in the Temple in Jerusalem, and its topics pertain to priestly sacrifice, ritual, and purity.

Yet our tradition also holds that the eternal task of the Jewish People is to mold ourselves into a *nation* of priests, a holy people. In doing so, the standards that apply to a *kohen* in the *Beit Ha-Mikdash,* the Temple, are essential tools for elevating our own spiritual and ritual status as well. The same guidance that the Torah provided the *kohen* at his task can ennoble and uplift the serious Jew of today as well. In seeking to fulfill our divine mission, we turn to the very book that trained God's servants in antiquity as well.

At the outset of our commitment to become a nation of priests, we can look with special benefit to the ordination of the *kohanim* into their sacred service.

That installation took place amidst elaborate ceremony. The *kohanim* washed themselves to become ritually pure, and then donned special clothing to demarcate themselves for their activity in the Temple. Anointed with a special oil, the *kohanim* made a "sin offering" to atone for their own shortcomings and errors before attempting to intercede for the atonement of the people. After sacrificing the ram of burnt offering, Moses took some blood from the ram of ordination, and "put it on the ridge of Aaron's right ear, and on the thumb of his right hand, and on the big toe of his right foot." He then repeated the same ritual for each of Aaron's' sons. Finally, the remains of the animal were boiled and consumed by the newly ordained *kohanim.* That same ritual was repeated throughout seven complete days of celebration.

Why was blood applied to those particular extremities—the right thumb, toe, and ear?

An ancient commentator, Philo, perceived that "the fully consecrated must be pure in words and actions and in life; for words are judged by hearing, the hand is the symbol of action, and the foot, of the pilgrimage of life."

Thus, Philo reads specific meaning into each of the three body parts by analyzing the special function of each part in terms of their human use. Our words, actions, and life all must cultivate our highest potential of growth, expression, and humanity.

Rabbi Abraham ibn Ezra argues, on the other hand, that the ear "symbolizes that one must attend to what has been commanded" and the thumb "is the origin of all activity." Unlike Philo, ibn Ezra sees the two pivotal points as obedience to God's *mitzvot* and a commitment to a life of sacred deeds.

While ibn Ezra provides different reasons than Philo, both agree in reading metaphoric meaning into the details of the ritual. However, both sages ignore the requirement of spilling blood, and both fail to explain the entire ritual as an interrelated unit.

Building on their insights, we can extend their vision by utilizing the methods and findings of the modern study of religion as well.

Blood is an ambivalent symbol. A symbol of life (recall the emblem of the Red Cross) and of death (think of the devil's pitchfork), it is a simultaneous expression of both life and death that blood becomes such a prominent symbol for moments and places of transition. At a child's birth with *brit milah* (circumcision), at the first Passover when blood was smeared on the lintels of Jewish homes, blood marks the moment or the place as a transition between death and renewed life.

Here, too, by placing sacrificial blood on the priest's extremities, the Torah indicates that the newly ordained *kohen* has passed through a transitional moment from being a private citizen to becoming a representative of God and a public leader. Ear, hand, and foot—an abbreviated code for his entire body—emphasize that service to one's highest ideals, to one's people, or to one's God must be total.

Through his induction into the Temple ritual, the *kohen* entered a higher state of purity, devotion, and service. To become a *nation* of priests requires of us no less.

On Sacrifices and Repentance

Ever since the great Rambam, Jewish apologists have argued that the Temple ritual was superseded by the "service of the heart."

According to this opinion, after the destruction of the Temple, the "external" service of sacrifice and incense was replaced by the more "spiritual" service of prayer and *teshuvah* (repentance). Sacrifices, after all, were bloody, primitive, and crude. Newly liberated slaves, enmeshed in the pagan culture of Egypt, assumed that all worship required magic and death. Wanderers leaving Mesopotamia would harbor those same assumptions. Indeed, in ancient pagan cultures, human beings were often the prize object of sacrifice. While establishing the Temple might serve a useful pedagogical role to wean the slaves from pagan practice, its pervasive bloodiness and physicality would repel the sensitive soul. Naturally, God got rid of those practices as soon as possible.

This argument makes an implicit assumption that the opposite of sacrifice is spirituality, and that one must choose between *teshuvah* and ritual.

Such a dichotomy, however supported by a partial reading of the Rambam, is foreign to biblical and rabbinic perspectives. It also ignores a great deal of contemporary religions around the world.

For those who would relegate the notion of blood and sacrifice to the distant past, one need merely consider contemporary Christianity, based as it is on the blood sacrifice of an itinerant Jew from Nazareth. Or consider the tremendous emotional power of *brit milah,* circumcision, which derives no small part of its power from the requirement of the spilling of blood.

But the forced dichotomy, requiring opposition between some internal *teshuvah* and an allegedly external ritual, rails even according to the evidence of the Torah itself.

The Torah speaks of several kinds of sacrifices: the *Olah* (burnt offering), *Minha* (grain offering), and *Zevah Shelamim* (offering of well-being or peace). These three offerings are purely voluntary—they do not "atone" for any sin, and they are not coerced by any external authority. Jews brought them to the Temple simply because they wanted to do so.

Rather than excluding an inner feeling, these sacrifices were the result, and consequences, of an exalted spirituality.

The *Hattat* (sin offering) was for an individual who erroneously committed a prohibited deed, such as eating forbidden foods without knowing it. This offering, too, is not the result of external coercion. When an individual realized that a mistake was made, the *Hattat* provided a way to resolve feelings of guilt or sinfulness.

Finally, the *Asham* (guilt offering) was to atone for robbery or fraud.

Surely this is an external offering! As if one could atone for a grievance against another human being by slaughtering an animal! Isn't this an example of a primitive, externalized, and hollow rite?

No. According to the Torah, this offering can only be made *after* a person has repaid the victim. This notion of compensation only recently entered American law, but the Torah already speaks of the requirement of compensating victims beyond the financial loss incurred by the theft.

Every type of sacrifice in the Torah came after, not before, *teshuvah*. Only the individual, looking into the human heart, could decide whether or not to bring an offering. Only that individual could recognize that he or she could have done better in the past.

The issue of biblical sacrifice is not an argument between inner conviction and external performance. All of the sacrifices in the Torah are dependent on, and follow after, an inner realization and turning.

The real question is whether an inner feeling is enough. Aren't there times when the validity of an inner feeling is proven by its ability to inspire action?

Such are the moments of sacrifice.

✦

Parashat Tzav/Command
Take 3

A Word of Thanksgiving

For the second week in a row, our Torah presents a detailed account of the sacrifices offered first in the *Mishkan* in the wilderness and later in the Temple of Jerusalem. Sin offerings, guilt offerings, burnt offerings, and thanksgiving offerings, each with its own regulations and procedures, claim Jewish attention as the central means for biblical Jews to atone for wrongdoing and to renew themselves as children of God.

After realizing that they had committed a sin, Jews in the biblical period would offer a sacrifice as a way to acknowledge their own imperfection and their resolution to do better in the future. With one exception, the sacrifices we read about this week respond to human violations of the covenant with God.

But the *Korban Todah,* the thanksgiving offering, was different at its core. Rather than an expression of human shortcomings, this offering was meant as a response to the abundant goodness of God. Whereas the other sacrifices attempt to compensate for human imperfection or even evil, the *Korban Todah* is a celebration of life and its wonder.

The rabbis of antiquity were so enamored of the *Korban Todah* that they declared "in the coming time, all sacrifices will be annulled except for the thanksgiving sacrifice. And all prayers will be annulled except for prayers of thanksgiving." In the language of a messianic future, this passage from *Midrash Va-Yikra Rabbah* asserts that suffering and failure to live up to our own highest potential is not an inevitable part of human identity. Instead, our shortcomings are products of the disappointments and pain that life entails. Human evil and violence is circumstantial—the harvest of preexistent suffering. Hence, in the future, the need for sacrifices meant to atone for wrongdoing will disappear.

But goodness and gratitude are everlasting, at the very center of what it means to be a human being. According to this Talmudic view, long after human suffering has ended, long after the world has attained its full messianic promise, people will still feel a need to sing, to celebrate, and to thank.

The task of the Jew is to start the singing early. In the midst of a world at war, a world of illness, poverty and ignorance, we can light up the world with the fires of our thanksgiving.

Too often, we let the sufferings of life overwhelm our appreciation for its beauty. Sorrow may be the inevitable price we pay for love, but who would abandon love simply to lessen pain? Life summons us to rejoice at the bonds we can form with one another, moments of special kindness or creativity, and pleasure, a wonderful day, a flourishing tree.

The *Midrash* tells a story of a king who received callers. As each person offered the king a gift, the king would inquire who that person was. When informed that the person was one of his tenants, or a member of the court, the king would instruct his servants to take the offering and that would be the end of it.

But when someone appeared before the king who was neither a member of his entourage nor a tenant on his land, the king would be so moved by this spontaneous gift that he would have a special chair brought for this thoughtful citizen. "Likewise [with sacrifices]: a sin-offering is brought for a sin, a guilt-offering is brought for a sin; but a thanksgiving-offering is not brought for a sin [and therefore the Torah records]: 'If it be for a thanksgiving, God will bring him near.'"

We can all sincerely regret our own failures. We most often do so when the price for our selfishness or insensitivity is more than we are willing to pay. Then, though, our expressions of regret also have the reek of self-interest.

But gratitude and celebration have little to do with self-interest, and everything to do with appreciation for the sheer miracle of our lives. We open our eyes to the loveliness of the world; our ears, to the symphony of life within and around us. Despite the difficulties of life, we offer thanksgiving to the Holy Blessing One and by doing so, enhance the gift of joy in the world.

May our prayer of thanksgiving never be annulled.

SH'MINI/Eighth

Leviticus 9:1–10:47

Parashat Sh'mini *begins with the first celebration of sacrifice after the seven days of ordination. This sacrifice on the eighth day marks the first time that the altar is used for a sacrifice on behalf of the people Israel. Moses underscores the purpose of sacrifice when he says, "This is what the Lord has commanded that you do, that the Presence of the Lord may appear to you." Aaron and his sons follow the instructions of Moses, and perform the sacrifices exactly as God has commanded. Then Aaron lifts his hands and blesses the people. God's Presence appears to all the people, and a fire from God consumes the burnt offerings. The people respond by rejoicing and worshipping.*

Joy turns to tragedy as Aaron's sons offer alien fire, rather than performing the sacrifices in accordance with God's command. As a result, a fire from God consumes them and they both die instantly. Aaron is silent in the face of God's power and his sons' death, and Moses tells Aaron and his remaining sons not to engage in public displays of mourning. Instead, he instructs the entire community to mourn for the burning. Moses then instructs the priests to refrain from wine or other intoxicants when performing the sacred service. He lays out the role of the priesthood: "You must distinguish between the sacred and the profane, and between the unclean and the clean, and you must teach the Israelites all the laws which the Lord has imparted to them through Moses." The Torah then provides the laws of kashrut *(the dietary laws), reflecting the conviction that what and how one eats has spiritual consequence, creates strong communal bonds, and reinforces important religious insights.*

The first listed are permitted land animals: those with fully cleft hooves and who chew their cud. Other land animals are prohibited. Of water creatures, the permitted animals are those with both fins and scales. Prohibited birds are listed without any broad principle offered to explain the list. Most winged swarming creatures are prohibited, except for four types of permitted locusts. These form the core of the kashrut *system still observed by traditionally religious Jews today.*

The reason for these kosher laws is offered by the Torah: "For I the Lord am your God: you shall sanctify yourselves and be holy, for I am holy. For I the Lord am He who brought you up from the land of Egypt to be your God: you shall be holy for I am holy."

✦✦✦✦

Parashat Sh'mini/Eighth
Take 1

Kashrut After Refrigerators

Without attempting to justify the elaborate Jewish dietary laws, the Torah this week provides a lengthy list of which foods are kosher and which are not.

Animals with cloven hooves who chew their cuds are kosher. Fish with fins and scales are kosher. Birds able to fly, who eat grain and vegetables, are kosher. Insects, shellfish, and reptiles are not.

Since the earliest stages of our history, Jews have understood the patterns of *kashrut* to be at the heart of our heritage. Jews have even sacrificed their lives rather than desecrate themselves with *treif* food. From the biblical and into the rabbinical period, new guidelines and restrictions developed as Jews encountered different cuisines and aesthetic standards, yet the core of *kashrut* has remained unchanged over the millennia.

Some of our most stirring stories of Jewish martyrdom—of Jews who preferred to lay down their lives rather than abandon their Judaism—center around the laws of *kashrut*. Thus, as early as the time of the Maccabees in 167 B.C.E., we have stories of Jews forced to eat pork by the Syrian oppressors. In those tales, the Jews chose to die with their integrity intact, still obedient to the dictates of God and Torah. They could not conceive of a Judaism without *kashrut,* so central were the dietary laws to the entire rhythm of Jewish living.

Yet the Torah gives no justification for *kashrut*. Not surprisingly, then, Jews throughout history have struggled to understand the reasons underlying kosher eating.

Popularized by the Rambam, one explanation is found in *Sefer Ha-Hinnukh* (the Book of Education). For this school of thought, God is a cosmic doctor and *kashrut* is a medical plan to ensure the health of individual Jews. God prohibited foods that were harmful, thus ensuring that Jews would be vigorous and fit. God, they tell us, was the first health food nut, and *kashrut* was the macrobiotics of its time: "God knows that in all foods prohibited to the Chosen People, elements injurious to the body are found. For this reason, God removed us from them so that the souls can do their function."

One problem with such a viewpoint—that pigs cause trichinosis and were prohibited for that reason, for example—is that it implies that God doesn't care about the health of the rest of humanity. After all, *kashrut* applies only to the Jews. If God is the creator of all humankind, isn't it logical to expect God to care about everyone's health?

Another interpretation of *kashrut* is that it was an early compensation for unsanitary conditions. If the Jews of the Torah had invented refrigerators, they wouldn't have required *kashrut*; given modern technology, we don't need these archaic prohibitions. My grandmother was one of the most devoted exponents of that opinion. But no sacred text links the practice of the dietary laws to a fear of an epidemic, or to a need to avoid rotting meat.

If not health or physical well-being, then, what is the goal of the dietary laws? Why are they significant?

The answer is found in the Torah itself: "You shall sanctify yourselves and be holy, for I [the Lord] am holy."

Kashrut is a way of welcoming the holiness of Judaism into our daily lives. We rededicate ourselves to sacred living and behavior each time we sit down to eat. The intimate fabric of Jewish values—loving our neighbors, caring for the needy, affirming a connection to the Jewish People, and establishing justice and holiness on earth—gain strength and depth through the regular practice of *kashrut*.

Every form of effective pedagogy involves regular repetition and frequent exposure. Since we eat (at least!) three times each day, *kashrut* is the elementary school in which we remember that our lives are lived in covenant with God, and we make the values of our faith visible through our deeds and priorities.

Observing *kashrut* awakens us to a greater awareness and commitment to the values of Torah, to justice on earth, and to holiness in every aspect of life.

Parashat Sh'mini/Eighth
Take 2

Leadership: Where's the Beef?

This portion begins with the seven-day ordination ceremony that marks the investiture of Aaron and his children as priests in the *Mishkan,* the Tabernacle in the wilderness. As the ordination ends, Moses hands over the authority for making the required sacrifices to Aaron and the other *kohanim.* He tells them,

> Come forward to the altar and sacrifice your sin offering and your burnt offering, making expiation for yourself and for the people, and sacrifice the people's offering and make expiation for them, as the Lord has commanded.

The instructions seem simple: Aaron is to perform two sacrifices, the first for himself, and the second for the people. But the ancient rabbis, alert to nuances in the Torah, noticed an odd repetition. The first offering atones for *both* Aaron and for the people. Why, then, does Aaron have to offer a *second* offering for the people only?

The Rambam notes that the apparently redundant offering teaches a specific lesson: "Learn that [only] the innocent can atone for the guilty." In other words, when Aaron offers the first sacrifice, to expiate the sins of the people along with his own, he still needs expiation himself. Because he is not yet free of guilt, how can his offering be expected to assist those for whom he was supposed to offer sacrifices? Before he can truly atone for the sins of others, he must be freed of sin himself. In offering this interpretation, the Ramban is expressing another side of the insight of the Talmudic sage Resh Lakish, "First adorn yourself, then adorn others."

Rabbi Abraham ibn Ezra expanded on the Ramban's commentary: "No one can atone for another," he wrote, "until first cleansed of all personal sin."

Our rabbis are teaching us that the challenge of real leadership is in living up to the highest standards of the community's aspirations. A leader who fulfills the community's ideals encourages the rest of us to do the same. By making themselves living examples, leaders demonstrate that our values can indeed translate into a life ennobled and enriched.

So our portion this week reveals that true leadership requires even more than skill, insight, and experience. True leadership, says the Torah, involves remaking oneself in the light of one's ideals.

And who are the leaders of Judaism in our day? The answer is: each and every Jew. For the Torah teaches us, "You shall be My kingdom of priests, a holy people." Our heritage will flourish when each of us is a walking, living, breathing embodiment of the traditions, practices, and perspectives of Torah. We become living proof of how a vital Judaism can transform and elevate human existence. We demonstrate anew that all its paths are peace.

Aaron was the first model of a leader committed to embodying in his personal life the same values he taught. Can you make the same commitment?

✦✦✦✦

Parashat Sh'mini/Eighth
Take 3

We Are What We Eat

"Would you kill Flipper for a tuna sandwich?" a bumper sticker asked a few years ago.

The message asserted a connection between what we eat and who we are. Our community and our character are reflected in our choices of food. Vegetarians, macrobiotics, those who limit their cholesterol intake, those who won't eat red meat: All assert that we are what we eat.

For most animals, and for many people, eating is simply a response to a biological need, or at best an aesthetic pleasure. We satisfy our hunger without thinking at all about how eating is also an act of identification and of education. Particularly today, when our lives increasingly revolve around "instant" food, fast-food restaurants, and microwave ovens, we don't pay attention to the significance of what we consume.

This thoughtless approach to eating was not always the case, and need not be so now. Today's Torah portion establishes the core of Judaism's teaching that how we eat and what we feed ourselves are both sacred and communal matters that nurture identity, morality, and relationship, while simultaneously nourishing the body.

Kashrut summons us to transform eating from a biological response to an encounter with holiness; our kitchens and our dining room tables become sacred altars, our meals become occasions to experience our deepest values as Jews.

For thousands of years, the dietary laws served as a vehicle for strengthening Jewish identity, for connecting Jews with history and with one another, across the globe. Jewish meals can link family and friends into communities committed to a humane order on earth. Through the practice of *kashrut,* we learn that we can discipline ourselves, our drives, and our impulses, enjoying the pleasures of life while simultaneously affirming our richest humanity. Motivated at its core by a recognition of the holiness of every living creature, *kashrut* instills a sensitivity to the suffering of animals and to our responsibility to all forms of life.

Any undertaking that has the power to renew meaning and enrich a sense of community cannot come easily. The practice of dietary laws requires commitment, self-discipline, and striving. Yet look at what can result from the endeavor: an opportunity to become a fully conscious and caring person whose meals inculcate reverence for life rather than simply respond to hunger, one whose way of eating is an invitation to a noble sense of self and a continuing affirmation of sacred Jewish values.

Unlike book learning, *sh'mirat kashrut,* the observance of the dietary laws, is available to every Jew—young and old, adult and child, scholar and beginner. By integrating the Jewish dietary laws into our lives, we begin a spiritual practice that constantly evokes for us a knowledge of the preciousness of life.

We bring the world, and those we love, that much closer to redemption.

TAZRIA/Delivery
Leviticus 12:1–13:59

The next two parashiyot *detail issues of* tumah *(ritual impurity) and* tohorah *(ritual purity).*

A woman who bears a son is tamei *for seven days, and fourteen days for a daughter. The boy is to be ritually circumcised on the eighth day. There is a subsequent period of* tumah *for either boy or girl, and then the matter brings a sacrifice to restore her* tohorah.

Tzara'at is an eruption that affects human skin (and has often been confused with leprosy). It also affects fabrics, leather, and plastered building stones. The Torah speaks of four different categories regarding tzara'at: *(1) in humans, (2) in fabrics and leather, (3) a ritual to restore the purity of a person healed of* tzara'at, *and (4)* tzara'at *in plastered or mud-covered building stones. The role of the* kohen *is strikingly non-magical: He doesn't "cure" anyone of the illness; he merely diagnoses it and, when it is already cured, restores the person's ritual wholeness. In cases of acute* tzara'at, *the sufferer was banished from the camp for the duration of the illness, often for life.*

METZORA/The Leper

Leviticus 14:1–15:33

Metzora *continues the discussion of the ritual response to* tzara'at, *and is often read together with the preceding* parashah *during synagogue Torah-readings.*

The parashah *opens with the rites for restoring the* tohorah *of a person who suffered from acute* tzara'at. *These elaborate rituals were similar to those for a person who comes into contact with a corpse. Like the ordination of the priests, this ritual takes a full seven days plus one (marking a new creation or rebirth of the individual). Also like the ordination of priests, the person has sacrificial blood smeared on his right earlobe, right thumb, and right big toe.*

Within Eretz Yisrael, *this plague also affects homes. The home is then cleared prior to the priestly inspection. If it is indeed infected, the home is shut up for seven days. At the end of this period, the priest inspects again, and the affected stones are removed from the home (and from the town). The plaster inside the home is scraped off, and new plaster is applied. If* tzara'at *breaks out again, the home is demolished. The ritual for purging a "healed" home is almost the same as for a healed individual.*

The parashah *now moves to consider discharges from sexual organs, male or female. These discharges result from illness or infection, not from menstruation or normal seminal emissions. As with much of Leviticus, illness is subsumed under the category of* tumah *(ritual impurity), making illness a religious concern and equating healing with* tohorah *(ritual purity). Abnormal male and female discharges are both referred to by the same term:* zav. *The philosophy underlying this religious attention is expressed at the end of the* parashah: *"You shall put the Israelites on guard against their uncleanness, lest they die through their uncleanness by defiling My Tabernacle, which is among them."*

Parashat Tazria/Metzora/Delivery/The Leper
Take 1

Toward Healing

Like others in the ancient Near East, our people suffered from frequent eruptions of skin diseases, called *tzara'at*. Many of these "leprosies" were severe and in all the cultures of the ancient world they bore a severe social stigma. Countless stories in the Bible and the Talmud attest to the dreaded consequences of these diseases and the devastation they could bring in the lives of individuals, families, and communities.

According to the biblical view of how the world works, *tzara'at*—like all illness—was a divine punishment. If everything comes from the One God, then illness, too, must have its origin in divine will. The logical assumption was that people became diseased because they deserved it. The only question was which illness resulted from which deed. According to the *Midrash Va-Yikra Rabbah,* God inflicted "leprosies" as punishment for libel, bloodshed, vain oaths, sexual crimes, robbery, and the refusal to offer *tzedakah.*

It would follow that if God punishes through illness, anyone who tries to heal the sick is the equivalent of one who helps a murderer escape from prison. Logically, a physician who heals a leper or anyone else whose illness is understood to come from God is violating God's plan, rebelling against the way God rules the universe.

Logical, yes. But also cruel. Such a viewpoint requires blaming an individual for being sick—as if we could "earn" cancer or heart disease, as if the wrong thoughts are enough to merit pain and death. Such a viewpoint treats a victim like a criminal, ultimately withholding sympathy, company, or care.

Judaism has always valued the mind. "Talmudic" is often a synonym for "logical" and has been throughout the ages. Yet logic was not permitted to restrain compassion. According to rabbinic tradition, the overriding obligation of humanity is to become God's partner in creation—actively applying our learning and our skill to intervening and improving on the world as we find it.

Where Jews find illness, they are commanded to heal.

Where Jews find hunger, they are commanded to feed.

Where Jews find suffering, they are commanded to empathize with the sufferer and to alleviate the pain.

According to *Midrash Temurah,* the psalmist compares people to grass because "just as the tree, if not weeded, fertilized, and trimmed, will not grow and bring forth its fruits, so with the human body. The fertilizer is the medicine and the means of healing, and the tiller of the earth is the physician."

The Talmud understands the biblical injunction "not to stand (idly) by the blood of your brother" as mandating medical care. The Ramban sees that obligation in the verse "Let your brother live with you" and in "love your neighbor as yourself" (Leviticus 19:18).

Judaism's rejection of the "logical" position reflects its notion of how God and people are to relate. Rather than viewing God as an unchanging monarch and humanity as the passive recipient of whatever happens, the Jewish view of God and people is like that of mutual lovers. The lovers yearn for and work on a deepened relationship. In caring for one another, we express our love, both of God and of God's creatures.

※

Parashat *Tazria/Metzora*/Delivery/The Leper
Take 2

Of Leprosy and Lips

With today's Torah portion, we learn a great deal about the ritual function of the *kohanim* in helping people cope with infectious illness. *Tzara'at,* leprosy, becomes the focus of sustained attention, presumably because it was a common one in the ancient Near East.

Basing their ideas on a story found in the Book of Numbers, the rabbis of the *Midrash* viewed leprosy as an external sign of internal decay. Illness became a symbol for corruption, immorality, and callousness. This link between illness and a lapse of ethics arises from the story of Miriam's criticism of Moses's wife for being a Cushite. Clearly, Miriam uses her sister-in-law's ethnicity as a pretext for attacking her brother.

In a condemnation that neatly parallels Miriam's criticism that Moses's wife is too black, Miriam is stricken with an illness that leaves her skin a flaky white. Since her *tzara'at* resulted from her critical words, the rabbis naturally associated the two. Thus, the biblical laws on infectious disease became an extended metaphor for self-centeredness, critical or slanderous speech, and hateful deeds.

Midrash Va-Yikra understands the law of leprosy as an allusion to seven traits the Lord hates:

> haughty eyes, a lying tongue, hands that shed innocent blood, a heart that devises wicked thoughts, feet that run eagerly toward evil, a false witness, and one who sows discord among people.

How many of these violations pertain to an irresponsible use of language! Speaking and thinking ill of another person, construing their actions in the worst possible way, gossiping, and spreading rumors that harm the reputation of another person—these activities are so familiar to us that they may scarcely attract our notice at all. Yet they strike at the core of the kind of world Judaism is trying to establish. They provoke a cynical disregard of human decency; they cultivate our suspicion of each other and our anxiety that others are speaking ill of us behind our backs just as we are of them. In Hebrew, such speech is called *l'shon ha-ra* (literally, "an evil tongue").

L'shon ha-ra is the practice of speaking *about* other people negatively rather than speaking to them. It involves transforming a living, complex human being into a caricature—an object of evil, sloth, or competition. In speaking ill of others, we participate in their dehumanization, initiating a process the end of which is uncontainable. In the words of the rabbis, "A loose tongue is like an arrow. Once it is shot, there is no holding it back."

The *Midrash* notes that five times, the word *torah,* teaching, is used to refer to *tzara'at.* From this superfluous repetition, the sages derive that "one who utters evil reports is considered in violation of the entire five books of the Torah."

A marvelous tale is told of a wandering merchant who came into a town square, offering to sell the elixir of life. Large crowds surrounded him, each person eager to purchase eternal youth. When pressed, the merchant would bring out the Book of Psalms, and read them the verse "Who desires life? Keep your tongue from evil and your lips from guile."

We all need to commit ourselves to a language of responsibility, kindness, and compassion. Rather than spreading rumors to make others look bad, we need to use our empathic imaginations to understand why someone might have acted in a disappointing way. Rather than speaking *about* other people behind their backs, we need to speak *to* them and *with* them, creating a shared community together.

A trusting community rooted in goodwill and integrity is what establishing "God's rule on earth" actually means.

❀

*Parashat Tazria/Metzora/*Delivery/The Leper
Take 3

All That You Can Be

Today's Torah portion opens with the ritual implications of childbirth: "When a woman gives birth . . . " The miracle of birth is itself a significant religious event, often the closest a person comes to feeling God's presence in an immediate and overwhelming way.

Posed on the border between life and death, divine and human, the miracle of birth make us question the basic assumptions of what it means to be human. What does it mean to be a man or a woman?

In the world of scholarship, a debate rages over whether the emotional and temperamental differences between men and women are culturally induced, the result of years of social conditioning, or instead the natural expression of innate distinctions. Persuasive scholars support opposite positions with passion and with extensive documentation and eloquence.

Some insist than men and women are different at core; that, due to hormonal and biological traits, women are more gentle, caring, nurturing, and private, whereas men are naturally aggressive, competitive, and playful. Women automatically translate feelings into words, and rely on lengthy discussions of feelings, moods, and perceptions to cultivate a sense of intimacy and closeness. Men, on the contrary, don't discuss their feelings, preferring instead to show feelings through deeds and moods. Women get together to talk; men gather together to play.

While not denying the reality of many of these differences, those who argue in favor of the impact of society on behavior insist that we don't really know what differences are natural because all children are raised with gender expectations. Even if gender differences are innate, we cannot possibly identify what *is* innate because the social construction of gender begins at such an early age.

Jewish tradition provides an interesting meditation on this issue. Looking at the verse on childbirth, *Midrash Va-Yikra Rabbah* records the thought of Rabbi Samuel ben Nahman, "when the Holy Blessing One created the first human, God created a hermaphrodite, fully male and female."

Rabbi Levi expands on his colleague's insight; "When the *adam*, the first person, was created, God made *adam* with two body-fronts, and then sawed the creature in two, so that two bodies resulted, one for the male and one for the female."

According to this provocative *midrash,* the original state of the human being was both male and female, fully at home as both masculine and feminine. What a remarkable idea! In the beginning not only of the world, but also at the beginning of every human life we are potentially both male and female. Only in the course of our development, as a species and as a fetus, do we gradually assume the distinct and exclusive identification with a particular gender. In fact, the process of gender identification continues throughout one's lifetime, as the notions of what is "male" and what is "female" shift and alter across the years.

But this *midrash* also hints at something more profound than simply recapitulating our origins. It alludes to the notion that in our ideal state all human beings are not merely one gender or the other, but in important ways are still both. We have room to express the fullest range of human responses and emotions, both the nurturing which we define as "feminine" and the drive we consider "masculine"; both the reliance on words to communicate feelings, and the ability to savor silence in a loved one's company.

By adhering rigidly to either a masculine or a feminine self-definition, we chop ourselves in half—denying a significant part of our own longings, development, and possibilities.

Rather than struggling to reduce our souls to the severed half which remains, we might direct our energy, as Judaism does in so many other areas, to hastening the advent of the messianic utopia. In the realm of social justice, that means restoring the primal harmony symbolized by the Garden of Eden. In the depths of personal expression and gender identity, it means reclaiming our severed halves—learning from the men and women with whom we share our lives how to allow our souls to blossom and be infused by the full range of human potential.

AHAREI MOT/After the Death

Leviticus 16:1-18:30

Picking up the narrative after the death of Aaron's sons Nadav and Avihu, who had offered alien fire and died in the process, God tells Moses to tell Aaron that he and his sons are to enter the shrine only when performing the sacrifices in a fashion commanded by God.

The rituals for Yom Ha-Kippur (the Day of Atonement) receive the attention of chapter 16. The purpose of these rituals is to remove the tumah of the Israelites, the priests, and the altar, transferring them onto the goat of Azazel (the scapegoat), who is then driven into the wilderness. The biblical purpose of the Day of Atonement is to purify the sanctuary, allowing God to dwell in the midst of the Jewish People and maintaining the efficacy of the Temple ritual. Later Jewish thought shifts the focus from restoring the sanctuary to atoning for the people. This shift is reflected in the Torah in the words, "On this day atonement shall be made for you to cleanse you of all your sins; you shall be clean before the Lord."

The unit from Leviticus 17:26 is known as the Holiness Code because its dominant theme is the holiness of the people Israel. The constant refrain "You shall be holy, for I, the Lord your God am holy" becomes the vocation of each individual and of the entire Israelite people. As a result, the laws of this section pertain to all Israel, not just to Moses or the priesthood. Like the two other great biblical collections of laws (the Book of the Covenant—Exodus 20:19–23:33, and the Book of Deuteronomy) it begins with a prologue that outlines the proper mode of worship and concludes with an epilogue consisting of blessings and curses.

After the prologue, the Holiness Code moves on to the commandments pertaining to forbidden sexual practices, which are designated as to'evah (abominations) inconsistent with priestly purity. The overarching principle of this section (and the following sections) is God's injunction: "My rules alone shall you observe, and faithfully follow My laws: I am the Lord your God. You shall keep My laws and rules, by the pursuit of which a person shall live: I am the Lord."

KEDOSHIM/Holiness
Leviticus 19:1–20:27

Kedoshim contains a distillation of the essence of Torah/instruction. Chapter 19 lays out the duties of the people Israel, and presents representative teachings from the broad range of the mitzvot. This was already recognized in antiquity, as Midrash Va-Yikra Rabbah records: "Most of the essential laws of the Torah can be derived from it." A list of imperatives ("you shall") and prohibitions ("you shall not"), this chapter blends what we would call ritual requirements with ethical mandates in a way that is utterly characteristic of the Torah's genius.

These commandments are explicitly directed toward the entire community, beginning with the peroration, "You shall be holy, for I, the Lord your God, am holy." Note that these laws often echo those of the Ten Commandments in content and in form, and lay out an agenda of ritual profundity, ethical sensitivity and rigor, and a passion for social justice.

Chapter 20 moves into a reformulation of laws on the subject of incest and forbidden sexual activity. Whereas chapter 18 is in apodictic form ("Do not" or "You shall") without listing any penalty, chapter 20 is casual ("If . . . , then . . ." or "When . . . , then . . ."). Both chapters assume a connection between pagan religion and sexual immorality, and both recognize that nexus as a cause of exile.

The penalties in chapter 20 deal with capital offenses and with those that carry the penalty of karet (banishment from the community). The goal of these laws is that "you shall possess the land, for I will give it to you to possess, a land flowing with milk and honey. I the Lord am your God who has set you apart from other peoples, so you shall set apart the clean from the unclean . . . . You shall be holy to Me, for I the Lord am holy, and I have set you apart from other peoples to be Mine."

Parashat Aharei Mot/Kedoshim/After the Death/Holiness
Take 1
And You Shall Live by Them

With today's Torah portion, *Aharei Mot,* we begin one of the distinct law collections of the Torah: the Holiness Code. Chapters 17–26 in the Book of Leviticus explain how the members of the Jewish People are to attain a level of holiness and integrity that will allow us to reach our maximum potential as a covenanted people and as individuals in the service of God.

At the very outset, such an enterprise provokes an important question: Do these laws and rules represent a goal in and of themselves, or does their importance derive from some encompassing, extralegal values that inform their pedagogy and provide the *mitzvot* with direction and guidance?

Do we observe the rules of the Torah simply because they are rules, or is the Torah authoritative because it directs us on how to attain a sacred and meaningful Jewish life?

One productive area to explore in response to that question is the case in which a *mitzvah* pertaining to ritual conflicts with a requirement of health: If the rules are ultimately important as goals in themselves, no health concern should override their proscriptions and requirements. However, if the *mitzvot* are meant as commanding *because* they mold a community of sacred seekers and direct them in their journeys, we would expect a ritual *mitzvah* to recede in the face of considerations of life and death, or even of health.

One verse from the beginning of the Holiness Code relates that: "You shall keep My laws and My rules, by which man shall live; I am the Lord." Those two Hebrew words, *va-chai bahem,* "by which you shall live," reverberate through the ages as a witness both to the central function of Torah, and to the nature of its centrality as a path toward a sacred goal, rather than as that goal itself.

The rabbis of the Talmud consider, for example, whether a sick person should fast on Yom Kippur. Remarkable for its courage, their answer is that one who is sick, and who must eat to maintain health, is forbidden to fast. For such a person, it becomes a *mitzvah* to eat! Why? Because, in the words of the Rabbi Leo Baeck, "the great commandment is to live."

Living itself is a *mitzvah*. Without life, no other *mitzvot* and no other holiness is possible.

Therefore, the *mitzvot* should be understood as practices along the path toward the sublime, not themselves the summit. They are irreplaceable, yes, even obligatory and sacred. But the *mitzvot* are not the same as the goal; they are the *means* toward attaining the goal.

Choosing not to rely only on their own authority, the rabbis of the Talmud remark that the Torah itself tells us that the purpose of the *mitzvot* is to help us to live, not to put life at risk. "You shall live by them," says the Torah, not die by them.

And in that distinction, our tradition mediates a complex and dynamic balance. The *mitzvot* are commanded, for without them we will be unable to find our way back to the Source of holiness and oneness. Without them we cannot hope to repair our characters, our people, and our world.

Yet for all their tremendous value and their indispensability, the *mitzvot* themselves are but lights to guide us in our walk.

Our destination is a rich inner life, a pulsating love for the Jewish people and all humanity, and a sense of responsibility for our planet and its denizens, so that out of that rich spirituality, loyalty, love, and connection will emerge that most precious of all Jewish figures: a true sacred servant.

Such a person—open to the Divine, respectful of other seekers yet true to the path of Judaism, able to learn from others and to share with all—witnesses through deed and word the oneness of the universe and the wisdom and the love of its Source.

Va-chai bahem.

Parashat Aharei Mot/Kedoshim/After the Death/Holiness
Take 2

What Does It Mean to Belong?

In the movie *Zelig,* Woody Allen portrays a man who rises to the pinnacle of success repeatedly through his uncanny ability to become identical to those in power. Time after time, Zelig is able to transform himself into the image of people around him, who in turn reward his ability by offering him influence, prominence, and prestige. The audience sees Zelig in photographs with Indian chieftains, Nazi generals, and capitalist millionaires. In each case, he has become more like them than they are themselves. Always in the center, always a passionate advocate, Zelig's zeal bears the mark of his insecurity, his very passion revealing his anxiousness to belong.

Zelig indeed is a portrait of the Jews throughout history. We, too, have managed to adopt the look and the rhythm of the cultures in which we dwell. We take it as a matter of pride that we become better guardians of the dominant culture than are its biological children. Always under suspicion of being outsiders, we seek to prove our right to belong through our zeal and our ingenuity.

Assimilation, the drive to become like the people among whom we live, has long been a Jewish passion. It is certainly one of our consummate talents. American Jews talk, dress, vacation, and work in the same ways as all other Americans. With a few exceptions, our habits and lifestyles reflect the priorities of American culture. It is no coincidence that "I'm a Yankee Doodle Dandy" was written by a Jew, or that "You're a Grand Old Flag" was sung by one.

Our Torah portion this week addresses this issue in clear terms: "You shall not copy the practices of the land of Egypt where you dwelt, or of the land of Canaan to which I am taking you . . . You shall keep My laws and My rules, by the pursuit of which man shall live."

God is thus denouncing the practice of assimilation. The guiding assumption of this passage is, of course, that there is a need to speak out against this all too natural impulse, because we are obviously so tempted to become like those we behold.

Why does God denounce assimilation? Because we cannot blindly adopt the standards of other people and simultaneously remain true to the values of the Torah and rabbinic traditions. We cannot serve two masters.

Or can we? Is the condemnation of assimilation really that sweeping? Isn't it possible to learn from the accumulating wisdom of human experience, science, and insight?

Two medieval interpreters do read the verse in a more restricted light. Rashi understands this as applying *only* to the Egyptians and Canaanites, who were "more corrupt than all other nations." Abraham ibn Ezra explains that this stricture applies to "the Egyptian legal system."

Both of these sages perceive that there is much to be learned from the wisdom of non-Jews. Not only in the realm of science, but also in human relations, Jewish traditions have been open to insights from other peoples.

The key, both to this Torah verse and to later interpretations, lies in the final phrase. Those non-Jewish practices and insights which strengthen Jewish survival, which sensitize us as a people, which teach us how to be loving, caring, and sensitive, which increase our understanding of Judaism and prompt us to practice it fully, pose no threat to our Jewishness. On the contrary, we benefit from their inclusion. An openness to learn, however, should not be mistaken for the blind adoption of all Gentile standards.

Torah and later Jewish traditions stand as the ultimate counterculture —opposing all that would cheapen human life or reduce our consciousness of the holy.

Much in modern life deserves our opposition. But insights that strengthen Torah, that make Jewish identity vibrant and central, deserve our study and our adoption.

In cultivating those insights, we harvest a growing Torah. By adding to the riches of our heritage, we assure its continued greatness.

Parashat Aharei Mot/Kedoshim/After the Death/Holiness
Take 3

Holiness at the Center

In any five-book anthology, the third book always forms the center. So it is that *Va-Yikra,* Leviticus, is the center of the Torah. At the center of *Va-Yikra* is *Kedoshim,* the Holiness Code. Not coincidentally, a pinnacle of spirit and morality, the Holiness Code embodies the high-water mark of all religious writing of any period.

What makes *Kedoshim* uniquely magnificent is its insistence on a maximal Judaism—one which demands much, teaches even more, and which creates a completely new orientation in the hearts of those who try to take it seriously.

Kedoshim does not tailor Judaism to fit the personalities or ideologies of any particular group of Jews. Instead, it posits a lofty set of standards and then challenges the Jews of every age to rise up to match its high ideals. It asks all of us to grow beyond our own comfortable conventions, our own sleepy standards, to confront our evasion of excellence.

There are some Jews for whom Judaism is primarily a set of behaviors. What matters is whether a Jew performs the required ritual in the proper manner. Such people measure "religious Jews" by the number of homes they won't eat in or by their punctilious performance of ritual deeds.

Yet another group of Jews see Judaism exclusively as a form of social action. Ethics, for them, is the sum and total of any "living" Judaism. Marching against injustice, petitioning Congress, and writing letters to the editor—this forms the entirety of what is important in being Jewish.

Neither of these approaches fully captures the totality of *Kedoshim,* however. At core, this week's reading demonstrates the *indivisibility* of ritual and ethics. For the Torah speaks about paying a laborer his wages promptly, observing *Shabbat,* honoring parents, not making idols, the proper mode of sacrifice, and leaving food for the poor—all at the same time. In its purposeful jumble of ritual and ethical injunctions, the Torah offers only a single justification: "You shall be holy, for I, the Lord your God, am holy."

What a staggering claim! A maximal Jew practices rituals that are rooted in ethics, and acts on an ethical system that finds expression and reinforcement through ritual.

Ethical rigor and ritual profundity—that is the Jewish definition of holiness. By blending those two strands, we create a tapestry stronger and more enduring than either individual thread alone.

Ritual requires ethics to root it in the human condition, to force it to express human needs and to channel urges, to serve human growth and to foster insight.

Ethics requires ritual to lend substance to its ideals, to remind one on a regular basis, of ethical commitments already made, and to create a community of shared values and high standards.

Ritual without ethics becomes cruel. Ethics without ritual becomes hollow.

One of Judaism's central insights is to fuse ritual and ethics into a single blazing light—the *mitzvah*—and then to reorient that new composite creation, holiness, to reflect the very nature of God. Our standard is no longer tailored to concede our own imperfections or to cater to our mendacity.

Ethics alone makes man the measure of all things. Ritual alone surrenders the intellect to the power of unregulated passion. As many people have perished from emotion unleashed as from an unfeeling mind. The two need each other to teach restraint, balance, and compassion. By blending ritual and ethics, we shift the focus from our perspective to God's.

"You shall be holy, for I, the Lord your God, am holy."

EMOR/Speak
Leviticus 21:1–24:23

The beginning chapters of Emor deal with laws of the priesthood, including laws of purity and priestly contact with the dead, marital restrictions for the priests, bodily wholeness, and participating in the sacrifices as food. Just as the priests must be physically without blemish, so, too, the animals used as sacrifice are required to be physically free of defect.

The end of chapter 22 deals with rules pertaining to the sacrifices offered by Israelites: The sacrificed animals must be whole of limb, without mum (blemish), and they may not be sacrificed when they are younger than eight days old nor on the same day as their mothers. Finally, the Torah lays out the regulations for a Todah (thanksgiving offering).

The Torah flows naturally from a consideration of the sacrifices of the Temple to the calendar of sacred times—holy days and festivals—which mark the key moments in the history of God's covenant with the people Israel. "These are the fixed times, the fixed times of the Lord, which you shall proclaim as sacred occasions."

First in order is the holiest day: the Sabbath. The Torah repeats the prohibition on work during the entire period of the Sabbath. Then the Torah proceeds to the other sacred occasions of the year: Passover and the Feast of Unleavened Bread, Sefirat Ha-Omer (counting the new barley grains each night for forty-nine nights), Shavuot (the Festival of Weeks), the first day of the seventh month (now celebrated as Rosh Ha-Shanah—the New Year), the Day of Atonement, Sukkot (the Festival of Booths).

The parashah concludes with a collection of miscellaneous laws pertaining to lighting the menorah and the showbread in the sanctuary, and a tale of a son of an Israelite woman who blasphemed against God's name. He is imprisoned while Moses speaks with God to determine what to do, and God commands his execution. Afterward, the general law prohibiting both blasphemy and murder is explained, along with the famous "eye for an eye." Finally, the parashah concludes with the remarkable assertion, yet to be attained in our own time: "You shall have one standard for stranger and citizen alike: for I the Lord am your God."

Sacrifice and a Broken Heart

As modern people accustomed to worship through prayer, study, and the performance of loving deeds, we are repelled and shocked by the notion of serving God by killing animals. Yet most people throughout the ancient world, and in many contemporary communities as well, worshiped by providing offerings of animal or human flesh, as though God would eat.

With the destruction of the Second Temple by the Romans in the year 70, the practice of animal sacrifice was indefinitely suspended. Kosher sacrifice had been permitted only on the Temple altar in Jerusalem and nowhere else. Synagogues, houses of prayer, study, and *mitzvot* replaced the Temple, a place of animal sacrifice and the chanting of psalms.

Early rabbinic literature reflects that transitional relationship toward sacrifice which has characterized traditional Judaism ever since. Judaism recognizes the value that animal sacrifice possessed for our distant ancestors, and anticipates some future idyllic age in which the Temple will be rebuilt—signifying a more intimate relationship between God and humanity than is possible at present. In the meantime, we struggle with an imperfect world, one in which people face grave disappointments and crushing tragedy, one in which we and our loved ones will grow old and infirm, and will ultimately die.

Rabbinic Judaism is a religion which helps us cope in the real and difficult world of the present, while also recalling a holistic past and affirming the messianic possibilities of a better future. Precisely because of that insistence on facing reality directly—even the unpleasant aspects of reality—rabbinic Judaism retains the notion of animal sacrifice as a practice to read about and to study.

One striking lesson that emerges from a careful examination of today's Torah portion is that the animal victim strongly resembles the human slaughterer. The Torah records God's instruction to Aaron: "No man of your offspring throughout the ages who has a defect shall be qualified to offer the food of his God." The defects which follow— blindness, scurvy, a broken limb, a boil or scar, a limb too long or too short, crushed testes, or an abnormal growth in the eye—are precisely the same defects which render an animal impure for sacrifice.

That the same defects disqualify both the person and the animal involved in the sacrifice caught the attention of ancient and medieval Jewish commentators as well. *Midrash Va-Yikra Rabbah* asks, "How do we know concerning one who has repented that it is considered as if that person had gone up to Jerusalem, rebuilt the House of the Sanctuary, built the altar, and offered on it all the sacrifices that are specified in the Torah?" The *midrash* derives the answer from the Book of Psalms: "The sacrifice acceptable to God is a broken spirit."

In other words, it is the human heart itself that is the ultimate sacrifice. We humans are the ultimate version of what the sacrificial animal could only approximate.

Similarly, *Sefer Ha-Hinnukh* notes, "There are disfigurements that disqualify a *kohen* from serving, and if they are in an animal, they disqualify it from being brought as an offering."

The shocking parallel between the slaughtered and the slaughterer, between the animal and the *kohen,* highlights a disturbing truth implicit in sacrifice. The sacrificial animal *does* resemble a suffering and terrified human being, as anyone who has witnessed the slaughter of a cow, sheep, goat, or pig can attest. The terror in its eyes, and the panic in its throat, is a visible reminder of our own frailty and our own mortality.

Like the sacrificed animal, we, too, shall die someday. Like that powerless creature, we, too, lack ultimate control over our own lives. By slaughtering an animal in the sacred confines of the Temple, our ancestors were able to look death in the face and to respond to it through the rituals and context provided by Judaism.

Where can we turn to cope with the reality of death? Here, too, the wisdom of the rabbis provides guidance: Our tradition teaches that reading about the sacrifices "counts" as the actual performance. By imagining the rituals of death and of slaughter, we too engage in a controlled encounter with violence and dying. In the safety of the synagogue and its ritual, we, too, can explore and respond to the realities of life.

And in that response, the insight of tradition and the company of community can provide the real bridge to the sacred and the eternal, a link to the God who assures eternal life.

Parashat Emor/Speak
Take 2

The Pursuit of (Group) Happiness

Our culture glories in individuality and autonomy. The foundation documents of the United States affirm the right of each individual to "life, liberty, and the pursuit of happiness." Pilgrims fled England and Europe, so we are told, to practice religious liberty and to find individual freedom as well. Justly proud of our national ideals of personal liberty and freedom, we cherish the ability to pursue happiness each in our own way.

Even those Americans who came later were in search of economic freedom and personal expression. The ability to move wherever one chose, to work in any field one could, to rise as one's talents could propel a career, speaks still to the core of our ideals as Americans.

While there is certainly merit to that perspective, it reflects a different priority than that of traditional Judaism. Where American law speaks primarily of individual rights, Jewish law emphasizes duties to others. America understands *freedom* as an absence of restraints; Judaism perceives *freedom* as the ability to be fully caring, involved, and responsive.

The syntax of this week's Torah portion reflects that interdependent notion of human connection. In describing the anonymous man who blasphemes against God, the Torah informs us that "his mother's name was Sh'lomit, the daughter of Dibri of the tribe of Dan."

Why do we need such a lengthy presentation of this anonymous punk's family and kin? Alone, he provoked a fight, and he cursed God alone, so why involve his innocent mother, grandfather, and tribe? The rabbis of antiquity assumed that the Torah would not waste words on unnecessary information. If the name of the mother and the tribe are there, the Torah must have meant to teach us something. What would that be?

In this unexpected list, Rashi recognizes a message about human responsibility and belonging: "The wicked bring shame on themselves, their parents, and on their tribe." Similarly, the righteous earn "praise for themselves, praise for their parents, and for their tribe."

In other words, our deeds implicate those who love us and those who are connected to us through family or through culture. We may think we act alone, but we touch more lives than we know, and our deeds have the power to taint or adorn the lives of those who love us.

Each of us affects the reputation of all. In the words of the *Midrash Va-Yikra Rabbah,* "Why is Israel compared to a sheep? Just as if you strike a sheep on its head, or on one of its limbs, all its limbs feel it, so if one Jew sins, all Jews feel it."

All Jews have a stake in one another. Our deeds, our behavior, and our character alter the way other people perceive us as a people. Indeed, the behavior of one Jew can even influence how other Jews perceive Judaism!

- When Jews engage in fraud, we shame the values cultivated by our tradition.

- When Jews express contempt against other Jews—either through word or deed—we betray our common ancestry and endanger our shared future.

- When Jews ignore the suffering of other people—in our own communities and around the world—we implicate the Source of our humanity.

Identifying as Jews, we agree implicitly to preserve the Jewish people as a "light to the nations." How we act will affect how non-Jews think of us all. How we act will mold how *we* think of ourselves as well. Jewish self-hatred is often absorbed from the attitudes or behavior of our fellow Jews. And one courageous, pious, or decent Jew can inspire a score of us to emulate those same precious ideals.

The *kippah* on your head, the *mezzuzah* near your door, or the Star of David around your neck is a pledge to reflect the highest standards of Jewish morality.

We are one.

Parashat Emor/Speak
Take 3

Blemished People, Unblemished Tools

For several years now, our society has been discussing the countless ways in which we have made life difficult for people who are lame, blind, deaf, mute, or who suffer from one of the many physical impediments that can restrict living. Over the centuries, most of humanity responded to handicaps in others by turning their backs to them, preferring to blame them for their disabilities rather than strengthen the human connection that binds each to all.

The mentally ill, schizophrenics, and others were isolated in institutions—more often to shield the members of society from the reality of such people and their suffering than to provide any real assistance to them. Only of late are efforts being made to communicate with and to educate people whom in ages past would have been consigned to a life of silent degradation and exclusion.

The Torah also speaks about disabilities, reflecting a complex balance of values, priorities, and perceptions. On the one hand, many of the biblical leaders themselves suffered from physical handicaps. Jacob limped, Moses was a stutterer, Miriam suffered from leprosy, and Isaac was blind. Saul had bouts of insanity and severe depression. These leaders, and many others in the *Tanakh* and rabbinic literature, were able to surmount their disabilities and to lead the Jewish people in exemplary fashion.

Yet the Torah clearly prefers "wholeness." In describing what disqualifies a *kohen* from offering sacrifices in the Temple, today's Torah portion states, "No man of your offspring throughout the ages who has a defect shall be qualified to offer the food of his God." The Torah then goes on to specify what those defects entail: those who are blind or lame; those with a limb too short or too long or a broken arm or leg; those who are hunchbacks or dwarves; those who have a growth in the eye, a boil, a scar, scurvy, or crushed testes—all who suffer from these afflictions are prohibited from offering a sacrifice in the Temple.

Certainly this passage, and others like it, lent biblical weight to the dehumanization of the disabled. Legislation in rabbinics confirmed that the blind, deaf-mute, and developmentally disabled were not allowed to participate as full members of Jewish society, either by functioning as acceptable witnesses in legal proceedings or as members of the *minyan* in religious services. While those prohibitions may have been reasonable in a time when no one could figure out how to educate or communicate with the disabled, the legacy those rules leave remains a tragedy in our day.

But there is another way to understand this verse as well. As we noted earlier, medieval commentators realized that precisely those traits that disqualify a *kohen* from performing his duties also disqualified an animal from being a sacrificial offering. Both the sacrifice and the one performing the sacrifice could not suffer from any *mum* (defect). At the same time, anyone, regardless of health, was certainly welcome to bring a sacrifice to the Temple, and that sacrifice would be accepted by the *kohanim* and work to bring atonement between the individual and God.

In other words, both *kohen* and animal functioned not as representatives of human values and ideals, but rather as instruments in the Temple ritual. Just as you wouldn't use a broken hammer to build a house, the Torah insists that only *kohanim* whose bodies can represent the typical Israelite (by virtue of the lack of any singular or distinctive traits) are a fitting implements for repairing God's relationship with Jewish individuals.

Midrash Va-Yikra Rabbah picks up on this essential insight, and makes explicit that no one is disbarred from offering a sacrifice, regardless of his or her disability or handicap. To the contrary, God cherishes those who wrestle with their handicaps and have to make a greater effort to live their lives:

> Said Rabbi Abba bar Yudan, "Whatever blemishes God declared invalid in the case of a beast was declared valid in the case of a person." Just as God declared invalid in the case of a beast "one that was blind or broken," so God declared the same valid in the case of a person: "a broken and contrite heart, O God, you will not despise."

In a very real sense, we are all handicapped, all of us disabled. Each of us balances personal weaknesses, inabilities, and injuries, working to compensate for them so they don't prevent us from living our lives to our fullest. In this regard, the *midrash* and even this Torah portion remind us that only implements—like hammers, *kohanim*, and sacrifices—lack blemishes. And only in them is a blemish a disqualification. For the rest of us, struggling to be decent, loving, and good, blemishes and disabilities are the catalysts that force us to wrestle with our own fears and inadequacies, and to grow.

BE-HAR/On the Mountain
Leviticus 25:1–26:2

Be-Har *begins with an entire chapter dealing with use and ownership of land, the rights and obligations of landowners, and the process of selling and mortgaging real estate. It also contains laws both about indebtedness and becoming an indentured servant as a way of repaying debts through work. The chapter also establishes the remarkable practice of* Shemittah *(sabbatical year), allowing the land to lie fallow every seven years, and the* Yovel *(Jubilee year), adding an additional cycle of rest every half century.*

Providing coherence to these practices is God's assertion that "the land is Mine; you are but strangers resident with Me." Since God is the land's only true owner, our task is to maintain the land on behalf of its true owner. As a sign of God's dominion, the people are commanded to "proclaim liberty throughout the land, and to all the inhabitants thereof."

BE-HUKKOTAI/In My Statutes
Leviticus 26:3–27:34

This parashah *constitutes an epilogue to the Holiness Code, hence to the entire Book of Leviticus. Composed of neither legal nor ritual language, instead* Be-Hukkotai *expands on the blessings that are experienced by the community that adheres to the teachings just concluded, the curses which emerge for those who violate these teachings, and a final conclusion.*

The blessings for the observant community include peace and prosperity, a bountiful population, and victory over the nation's enemies. The blessings conclude with an affirmation of the covenant binding God and the Jews, and the eternity of that covenant: "I will establish my abode in your midst, and I will not spurn you. I will be ever present in your midst: I will be your God, and you shall be My people."

The curses follow, an escalating outpouring of ever more dire consequences. Each cycle of disobedience unleashes a heightened cycle of consequences-military defeat, disease, ravages of wild beasts, famine, death, and exile. At its height, however, the cycle is broken by hope and love: "Yet, even then, when they are in the land of their enemies, I will not reject them or spurn them so as to destroy them, annulling My covenant with them: for I the Lord am their God."

After this powerful conclusion, chapter 27 appears like an appendix, dealing with the important (from a priestly perspective) issue of funding the sanctuary, its services, and its clergy.

The book ends with an affirmation: "These are the commandments that the Lord gave Moses for the Israelite people on Mount Sinai."

Parashat Be-Har/Be-Hukkotai/On the Mountain/
In My Statutes
Take 1

Redeeming a Land

One of the central paradoxes of Jewish history is that the Jewish People were landless through most of our history, yet we were always profoundly aware of our link to *Eretz Yisrael*. Perhaps because we did not live in a place we could call our own, the intense love between Jews and our homeland permeated our prayers, our Torah, and our hearts.

Today's Torah portion speaks directly to the centrality of *Eretz Yisrael* in Jewish thought and deed. God instructs the Jewish People, "You must provide for the *ge'ulah*, redemption, of the land."

What does it mean to bring *redemption* to a land? It might make sense to use tangible terms—*irrigate* the land, *fertilize* the land, even *cultivate* the land. Those are terms a farmer can act on and recognize. But how does one redeem a land?

According to most biblical commentators, this verse is understood as mandating a loving Jewish presence in *Eretz Yisrael*. The Land is referred to as an *ahuzzah*, a holding—given to the Jewish People as God's part of our *brit,* our covenantal relationship. Our ancestors agreed to serve only God, and God agreed to maintain a unique relationship with the Jewish People. That relationship was given form in the detailed legislation of the Torah and the Talmud as a way of shaping and cultivating the reciprocal obligations between God and the Jews.

The one place in the world where the Jewish People could act on every part of our *brit* was within the Land of Israel. Only there could all the laws and practices of Judaism receive their full articulation, because, in the words of Rabbi Ovadiah Sforno, "outside of the Land [of Israel] there is no sabbatical year, nor a jubilee year." The many agricultural *mitzvot*—of leaving gleanings for the poor, of offering first fruits, and others—were operative only within the Land of Israel.

There, in *Eretz Yisrael,* the Jew could most directly encounter God and sanctity.

What was true in the past is true today as well. There is a special quality to *Eretz Yisrael* that, for Jews, exists nowhere else in the world. In the words of the Talmud, "the air of the Land of Israel makes one wise."

Our generation is uniquely blessed. While Jews have prayed facing Jerusalem for thousands of years, while our ancestors longed for the messianic future as a time when Jews could freely live as Jews in our homeland, we have seen the establishment of a Jewish state—a thriving democracy and a world center for Jews and Jewish expression—in our own time.

Unlike our great-grandparents, we can travel to Israel's holy sites any time we choose. Unlike the Jews of the past, we can learn our sacred language, Hebrew, from people who speak it on a daily basis. We can contribute to the liberation of Jewish people who have left lands of oppression and suffering to be reunited with our people and our history.

We can redeem the land. In our day, that might mean bringing our own growing ecological awareness to the renewal of Israel's streams and rivers and forests, spreading the word of the value of recycling to a crowded nation still delighting in the proliferation of plastic bags. It might mean aiding our fellow Jews in Israel in their quest for social justice and religious freedom for all, regardless of ethnicity, skin color, gender, or denomination. It might mean doing what we can to work for a just and enduring peace.

Provide for the redemption of the land. Why not begin to provide for that redemption today?

Proclaim Liberty, but What Kind?

Puritans and colonial Americans viewed themselves as the modern embodiment of ancient Israel. Like the Israelites, they saw themselves as fleeing from an oppressive Pharaoh, journeying into the wilderness in pursuit of freedom and the establishment of a religious and democratic society. It's no coincidence, then, that on the Liberty Bell in Philadelphia, the Hebrew Bible proclaims its ancient ideal: "Proclaim liberty throughout the land, and to all the inhabitants thereof." Like the ancient Jews, the colonial Americans saw their mission as one of proclaiming liberty.

What kind of liberty did the colonists spread, and what kind of liberty does the biblical passage intend?

Various cultures understand freedom differently; in the former Soviet Union, freedom theoretically implied relief from unemployment and homelessness. In America, those basic human needs are not considered freedoms at all, but rather privileges that too many Americans don't get to enjoy. On the other hand, Americans theoretically believe that freedom permits uninhibited expression of personal opinion and the right to practice one's religion unchallenged. In China, those values do not comprise freedom; instead they are considered subversive.

Within Jewish traditions, Rashi understands freedom to imply the ability to reside anywhere. He adds that freedom precludes living under the authority of others.

One cannot, he claims, be truly free unless one is able to choose where to live. Do the homeless in our major cities have that freedom? Can they choose where to live? What of recent college graduates, so saddled with untenable debts that they are unable to purchase a home? What about members of racial or ethnic minorities who are victimized in certain neighborhoods? What of the freedom of gay men and lesbians to live freely where they choose without fear of intimidation or assault?

Our elderly refrain from leaving their homes at night. Women are frequently the victims of rape or robbery on American streets and college campuses. Is a society where so many must worry about where they live truly free?

Rashi's second standard is equally intriguing: freedom from subjugation to the authority of others. This standard is necessarily more subjective: Whether we identify with those in power is a question of personal judgment. Do our politicians act based on our needs? Are we represented by the corporations that make boardroom decisions establishing the contours of our lives? Or by the press? Or by the scholars who advise those in power or who mold the thought and culture of the rest of us?

Clearly, no society is completely free. Our dual birthright—as Jews and as Americans—encourages us to struggle to increase our freedoms, so that a previous generation's aspirations advances the next generation's rights.

As Jews, our call to freedom emerges naturally from our relationship to God. Freed from human bondage in Egypt, we recognize that freedom is the corollary to divine service. In the words of the Talmud, we are *God*'s "servants, and therefore not the servants of servants."

In a world of social justice and spiritual depth, Jewish notions of freedom can thrive, the freedom to assume our rightful place in a world sanctified and at peace.

Parashat Be-Har/Be-Hukkotai/On the Mountain/ In My Statutes
Take 3

Between a Mountain and a Field

At its outset, today's Torah portion states, "The Lord spoke to Moses on Mount Sinai" and then commences a detailed exposition of the laws of the *Shemittah,* the seventh year, in which the land must lie fallow as testimony to God's exclusive ownership of all.

Since this is the climax of all priestly rules for the conduct of Jewish worship in the biblical period, we would expect something a little more ethereal, a little grander and loftier as a summary of all that came before. After all, this is God's timeless message to the Jewish people. Is the most important part of that message really to leave our fields alone once in a while?

That same question occurred to the rabbis of antiquity. In the *Midrash Sifra,* an ancient commentary to the Book of Leviticus, the rabbis open by asking, "What is the connection between Sinai and *Shemittah?*" Consider all the commandments given at Sinai, not just this one. So why does *Shemittah* merit the honor of its position as conclusion of all the priestly rules? What's so special about *Shemittah?*

The *Sifra* responds to its own question by asserting that the juxtaposition of *Shemittah* here teaches that "all commandments originated at Sinai." Rashi and the Ramban both concur with that judgment.

But it is possible to go beyond that reading, to see something more essential in *Shemittah* that singles it out for this place of honor. After all, any other commandment could have demonstrated the same point, that all *mitzvot* originate in the meeting of God and the Jewish people, in the sacred dialogue that unfolded in the Torah and the Talmud and in our own day as well. So if any *mitzvah* could have demonstrated that point, what is so special about *Shemittah?* What is the unique link between *Shemittah* and Sinai, between a vacant field and a mountain?

To respond to that question, we must first look at the function of the sabbatical year. The Israelite farmer planted and worked the field in accordance with the practices of Judaism; for example, by leaving the corners of the field for the poor to glean, and bringing tithes to Jerusalem. As idyllic as a people at home in their land might be, there was a danger as well. Jews living freely in their own homeland could well begin to think of the land as theirs by right. It would be a small step to assert that since the land responds to human labor, it is ultimately a tool for humans to use as they see fit.

Once every seven years, the *mitzvah* of *Shemittah* arrives to remind us that while we may cultivate the earth, ultimately the land is not to be owned by any human being. We may borrow land as we borrow utensils and material things, but ultimately we must return all to the cycles of nature. We as a species are part of that natural cycle, and thus are permanently linked to the limitations and rules imposed on the world. Through the institution of *Shemittah,* the Torah records God's sacred truth that "the land is Mine; you are but strangers resident with Me."

The Ramban clarifies that verse by paraphrasing it as "don't think that you are so essential." The world is not a plaything for human beings, and the vast array of organic and living things serves a purpose higher than that of human whim. Together with humanity, the rest of the cosmos is a living, interlocking symphony to our Creator. We are the tenants, but God is the only *baal ha-bayit*.

Distracted by the brilliance of human achievement, and deafened by the clatter of our own insolent self-absorption, we can too easily forget that we are part of an order we neither made nor sustain. A little lower than the angels, yes, but still a long way from being masters of the universe, human beings are trapped in illusion if we consider ourselves or our species to be the measure of all things.

Only by linking our own destiny to the transcendent, by aligning ourselves to a divine living force, by shaping our deeds into a song of praise and gratitude, can human beings escape the despair of our mortality and fallibility. Focusing on our own needs and desires, we will always be disappointed in the world and ourselves. But if we lift our eyes to a higher vision, if we set our feet on a more tested path, we can soar above our plight, as on eagles' wings.

In the words of the *Sifra,* "it is enough for the servant to be like the Master." By making ourselves godly, we partake of God's fullness: "When it is God's, then it is ours."

NUMBERS

BE-MIDBAR/In the Desert
Numbers 1:1–4:20

The Book of Numbers begins in the wilderness of Sinai (Be-Midbar means "wilderness"). The people are organized into a military camp, which requires taking a census to know their precise number. Moses, Aaron, and the chiefs of the tribes register all the men over the age of twenty. The total comes to a little over 600,000. The Levites are not included in the census with the other Israelites.

Once Moses has ascertained their numbers, each Israelite is told to camp in military divisions with his own tribe, with each tribe assuming an assigned position around the Tabernacle. The Levites are assigned to be attendants to the priests, and the priests are given sole responsibility for performing the rituals of the sanctuary. All of this takes place around the foot of Mount Sinai.

In the wilderness near the mountain, God tells Moses to perform a census of the Levite males from the age of one month. Their total was 22,000. In lieu of God possessing the firstborn among the Israelites, the Levites are now pledged to divine service. There follows a second census of the Levites, this time numbering those between the ages of thirty and fifty, for the purpose of determining the workforce available to transport the Tabernacle through the wilderness.

Parashat Be-Midbar/In the Desert
Take 1

My Nephews, My Sons

One of the greatest *mitzvot* in the Torah, the very first command given to humanity, is that of bearing children. "Be fruitful and multiply" is the necessary underpinning of Jewish life, since without new generations of Jews, there can be no Torah, nor, of course, any Judaism either.

But parenting is more than simple biology. Any animal can spawn, and most animals have the necessary instincts to guide their young through a relatively brief infancy before the new generation takes off on its own, guided by its own internal barometer. Humans are distinctive in the extraordinary length of our infancy and youth, the extreme degree of dependence of our young, and our lack of instincts to fall back on to guide us in raising our children.

Instead of instinctual imperatives, we rely on social norms and religious values to guide our parenting and to mold our children. Our friends, our parents, books, rabbis, magazines, and popular psychologists all instruct us about how to raise our children and what standards and expectations we can rightly apply to them.

Human parenting, then, is executed within a network of other adults, and is guided by the cumulative experience of our own communities.

Anthropologists speak of the transmission of a traditional culture in similar terms. A culture is normally passed from one generation to another, from knowledgeable adult to learning child. Since the adult has absorbed the norms and practices of the culture from older acculturated adults, this transmission is often simply through exposure and example, the stuff that memories are made of: watching Bubbe lighting *Shabbos* candles, sitting next to Zeyde at a Seder.

The Torah records that point clearly in today's reading. The *parashah* opens by noting, "This is the line of Aaron and Moses at the time that the Lord spoke with Moses on Mount Sinai. These were the names of Aaron's sons. . . ." What follows is a list of Aaron's children and grandchildren.

This strange juxtaposition of *Moses*'s name with Aaron's children raises an obvious question. In the words of the *Midrash Ba-Midbar Rabbah*: "Surely 'the line of Moses' is not required here! Why, then, is it stated?"

The answer provided by the *midrash* is that Moses's name is listed alongside that of the natural father, Aaron, "out of respect for Moses, in order not to diminish any of his dignity." Yet we still must ask, what did Moses do to deserve being listed as parent to Aaron's children?

The answer is found in the commentary of Rashi. Rashi tells us that Aaron's children "are called the line of Moses because he taught them the Torah. This teaches that whoever teaches Torah to the child of a friend . . . is accounted as the bearer of the child."

Moses becomes the equivalent of his nephews' parent by teaching them who they are and where they belong. As the children watched

Moses fast on Yom Kippur, study Torah, build a *sukkah,* care for widows and orphans, eat *matzah* on *Pesah,* keep kosher, dispense justice, and observe the Sabbath, they absorbed the meaning of Jewish identity without even knowing it. By teaching them the Hebrew alphabet and how to pray, study, and live as Jews, Moses assured the continuity of Judaism and the Jewish People. Isn't that precisely the role of the Jewish parent throughout time?

Today, far too many of us live without the ability to be Jewish parents to our children. Instead of teaching Judaism to them, we hope to pick up fragments of what they themselves gleaned from religious school. In many homes, parents are unable to parent their children in this most important area of the child's identity. How can we change that?

Every synagogue in existence is really an empowerment center, dedicated to providing Jews with the ability and knowledge to create Jewish homes and to teach their children Jewish ways and Jewish values. Putting parenting back in the hands of Jewish mothers and fathers is precisely what rabbis, educators, and adult education programs are eager to do. So, reach out to them—go and learn!

❧

*Parashat Be-Midbar/*In the Desert
Take 2

Who Counts in the Book of Numbers?

The Book of Numbers, *Sefer Be-Midbar,* begins with a series of census counts to establish the number of adult males, the number of Levites, and the number of *kohanim* among the people of Israel. The endless list of random names can bore you to tears. Rabbis have been frustrated trying to find some hook to make these lengthy Torah passages seem worthwhile. Columns of numbers may interest accountants, but the rest of us may strain to experience either spiritual or moral resolve in a census of who was who in ancient Israel.

Yet we return to these verses every year. Surely there must be a reason why the Torah includes them. Normally terse and laconic, the Torah must have a rationale for the recitation of this tedium. Why this attention to numbers? Rashi has a moving explanation. The concern for counting each individual, he says, reflects God's intense love for each member of the Jewish People: "Because they are cherished before God, they are counted at every occasion." Each and every one is counted, for in God's light, each and every individual is unique and precious.

But in this enumeration of the people of Israel, there is a surprising omission. As the rabbis of the Talmud point out, neither Aaron nor Moses is included at all. They are not in the general census, since Levites are excluded from that numbering. Nor are they counted when the Levites are polled separately.

If being counted is a sign of being loved, why weren't Moses and Aaron—both of whom God clearly loved—included in the census?

Perhaps their omission teaches us a lesson about human love.

The love of humanity is a virtue found throughout Jewish literature, where it is called *ahavat ha-briyot*. Indeed, most cultures value the love of humanity, a love mentioned so often, as well, by politicians, poets, and philosophers of all opinions and persuasions.

But such a love is also too often ignored when it comes to specific groups of human beings. In the words of a character from the late Charles Shultz's cartoon strip, "Peanuts," "I love humanity, it's people I can't stand!"

But there is no generic humanity: Everybody is a particular kind of person. Is it really possible to claim to love humanity and at the same time to despise or discriminate against particular *kinds* of people—Jews who are different from us, human beings of another ethnic or racial group, gays or lesbians, anyone at all?

The Torah addresses this very point. After reading the census of the twelve biblical tribes, followed by the census of the Levites, we rightly expect to see a census that will include Moses and Aaron. When no such count is forthcoming, we are shocked into dissent. If the Torah can't include Moses and Aaron, then surely the census is fatally flawed.

And so it is with us as well. If we cannot learn to love *all* groups of human beings, which is distinct from necessarily loving everything that they do, we cannot claim to love humanity.

Humanity is made in God's image; an inability to love all groups of people thus constitutes hatred of an aspect of God as well. For the sake of our human future, there is no time to lose. May we resolve to cultivate our own ability to love precisely where we find love most difficult.

Parashat Be-Midbar/In the Desert
Take 3
Operation Desert Insight

One confusion about being a Jew is understanding the concept of "chosenness." One mistaken interpretation is that chosenness implies Jewish superiority to the rest of humanity or even that God cares only for Jews. So uncomfortable is such an idea that some Jews have rejected chosenness altogether despite its centrality in both the Torah and the Talmud. Fearing the dangers of triumphalism and religious bigotry, they cannot see a way of understanding chosenness that would be compatible with a broader love of humanity.

Today's Torah portion helps us to understand what chosenness is all about. The beginning of the fourth book of the Torah, *Be-Midbar,* Numbers, opens with the report that "the Lord spoke to Moses in the wilderness at Sinai."

Apparently, during the first year following the liberation of the Israelite slaves from *Mitzraym,* they had journeyed to and camped around Mount Sinai. Now, they began to move into the wilderness. They will spend the next thirty-eight years here, continuing their travels and the intimate dialogue with God that will form the root and essence of our Torah.

For the generation of liberation and wandering, most of life was spent in the wilderness. Why? What is so significant about the wilderness? According to *Midrash Be-Midbar Rabbah,* "Our sages inferred from this that the Torah was given to the accompaniment of three things: fire, water, and wilderness." Why "fire, water, and wilderness"? Because, the *midrash* goes on to comment, just as fire, water, and wilderness belong freely to all humanity, so also are "the words of Torah free, as it is said, 'All who are thirsty, come for water' " (Isaiah 55:1).

The wilderness, for the sages, is that territory belonging to no single person and no single people. So, too, God's love, loyalty, and concern are not the prerogative of a single people. To claim a monopoly on them is to diminish the grandeur of the Holy One, an expression of human arrogance, even blasphemy.

Why was the Torah given in the wilderness? To warn Jews not to mistake this precious gift for favoritism nor imagine that possessing the Torah makes us more worthwhile, more valuable, or better than others.

On the contrary, our tradition views our relationship with God as distinct because it bestows on us particular responsibilities. Time and time again, the Torah summons us to fulfill our responsibilities to all humankind, to be a nation of priests and a holy people, facilitating the relationship between God and all people everywhere through our fidelity to Jewish living, study, and observance.

The wilderness has yet another significance. A wilderness, says the *midrash,* is open on all sides; similarly, one who "does not throw himself open to all . . . cannot acquire wisdom and Torah." In the words of Rabbi ibn Gabirol, wisdom can come only through "a willingness to accept truth from any source." To be a spiritual seeker means becoming as the wilderness our ancestors wandered; taking in travelers from all directions, willing to listen to and learn from all.

God spoke from the wilderness of Sinai to remind us of the need for humility; to urge us to be open to all sources of wisdom and knowledge, and, finally, to remind us that we must ultimately serve all of humanity and work for the redemption of the entire world.

What, then, of chosenness? Being chosen means maintaining our distinct peoplehood, learning from all without losing our own character and identity. God delights in variety, rather than sameness, but in the symphony of humankind, in which each group plays its own notes and melodies to create a music more profound and lovely than any one part could possibly produce by itself.

We are chosen to be Jews and to embody the ways of Judaism in our daily lives. And in so doing, we deepen our connection with all human beings, all chosen, each in its own way, to contribute to creating the harmony of life.

NASO/Take

Numbers 4:21–7:89

Parashat Naso *begins in the middle of the description of the duties of the Levitical clans, focusing on the duties of the Gershonites and the Merarites.*

The next two chapters, 5 and 6, interrupt the preparation to march through the wilderness to lay out several laws designed to preserve the ritual purity, and to remove any impurity, from the Israelite camp, thus allowing God to remain in the midst of the people and their camp.

The first instruction is to remove any person with a bodily discharge, or who has been in contact with a corpse, and is thus ritually impure. The Torah then lays out the laws for an Asham *(guilt offering for one who has made a false oath).*

If a husband suspects his wife of committing adultery, but there is no proof, he may bring her before a priest. The priest makes her drink a mixture of sacred water, dust from the sanctuary, and parchment containing a curse that mentions God's name. If her body becomes distended, then she's guilty. If not, she is innocent.

In biblical Israel, there was no way for an ordinary person to live a life of full-time religion. The remedy for this was to provide for the Nazirite. The Israelite (man or woman) makes a vow for a finite period of time, to abstain from intoxicants or any grape products, to grow the hair long, and to avoid contact with a corpse. During this Nazirite period, the individual serves in the sanctuary in consecration to God.

One of the duties of the priest is to bless the people Israel. The Torah here lays out the words of that blessing, the well-known priestly benediction. This benediction is still recited by kohanim *in traditional congregations during the Days of Awe and Festivals, and often by parents to their children on Friday night as* Shabbat *candles are kindled.*

The interruption now concluded, the finishing touches make the Tabernacle ready for use. The chiefs of the tribes supply gifts, the menorah is completed and lit, and the Levites are placed in service. At the end of this elaborate preparation, the sanctuary can function as the site where God and humanity meet. "When Moses went into the Tent of

*Meeting to speak with God, he would hear the voice addressing him
from above the cover that was on top of the Ark of the Covenant between
the two cherubs. Thus God spoke to him."*

⊷⊷⊷

Parashat Naso/Take
Take 1

From a Small Silver Plaque to You

How do you approach a classic within a classic?

The Bible as a whole embodies a pinnacle of literary, moral, and spiritual accomplishment. Translated into every language of the globe, the Bible is the all-time best-seller for humanity. Particular passages echo through the ages, so resonant are they with meaning and depth.

One such passage is the *Birkat Kohanim,* the priestly benediction, found in this week's Torah portion. God instructs Moses to speak to Aaron and his sons:

> Thus shall you bless the people of Israel. Say to them:
>
> The Lord bless you and protect you!
>
> The Lord deal kindly and graciously with you!
>
> The Lord bestow favor upon you and grant you peace!
>
> Thus shall they link My name with the people of Israel, and I will bless them.

This is one of only *two* prescribed blessings within the entire Torah; the other forms the core of the Passover *Haggadah.*

How carefully crafted this gem is becomes particularly evident in Hebrew. We see an increasing pattern of words on each line (three, five, seven), and an increasing pattern of both consonants (fifteen, twenty, twenty-five), and syllables (twelve, fourteen, sixteen). The very wording thus contributes to a sense of order, climax, and completion.

What is ultimately apparent is that the *kohen* serves a vital but limited role. Unlike a magician who himself generates the magic, the *kohen* is only the channel for the blessing to pass through on its way from the

Holy One to the Jewish People. For that reason, each line begins by mentioning God as the active agent, and the last line explicitly states, "I will bless them."

We are thus made to realize that no human being is conceived of as holy in a way that is different from the holiness of any other human being. At the same time, the priestly blessing reminds us of the sanctity of all humanity, and the awesome otherness of the God of Israel.

The blessing also links us moderns to the antiquity of our people and to God's own need to love and be loved.

Several years ago, I went to the Israel Museum in Jerusalem to see the latest archaeological finds. Among the digs displayed was the excavation of a burial plot (*Ketef Hinnom*) from the end of the First Temple Period (1000–586 B.C.E.), complete with jewelry, pottery, and glass. Of all the artifacts, a small silver plaque, the size of a thumb, caught my breath. On this thin sheet of silver the *Birkat Kohanim* was inscribed in the Hebrew script of the seventh century B.C.E.—the oldest biblical text then in modern possession!

According to the description of the archaeologist, Professor Gabriel Barkay, this silver sheet had been rolled up and worn around the neck of some pious Jew over 2,600 years ago. That same prayer which observant Jews recite each morning as part of the *Shaharit,* morning service, which *kohanim* use to this day to bless the congregation on Yom Kippur, *Rosh Ha-Shanah,* and the Three Festivals, that same prayer was cherished by our ancestors so many centuries ago.

As I stood in the Israel Museum in Jerusalem, capital of the Third Jewish Commonwealth, I started to cry.

I cried because of the privilege we Jews enjoy in a spiritual continuity extending back to the very beginnings of our people. What an extraordinary blessing to share the same prayers as our most distant ancestors, to be moved by these words that have echoed through countless generations, and to pass them on to my own children today.

Much in human history changes; our customs, styles, and cultures swell and shift throughout the ages. But there are three constants: The human heart retains the same needs, urges, and concerns across time; the God of Israel has not changed or altered despite our shifting perceptions and understanding of the Divine; and the bridge between the human heart and the God of Israel—Judaism—is still the encapsulation of the *brit,* the covenant, which binds the Jewish People to each other throughout time, and to the Holy One, Who transcends time.

Parashat Naso/Take
Take 2

Gilligan, God, and the Sotah

The "moral position" has often been considered the one that adheres to an objective standard of right and wrong. Someone who evaluates an action in the light of immutable values is viewed as demonstrating a higher level of moral development than a person who uses more situational standards.

The roots of this perspective lie in ancient Greek thought, which associated the true with the eternal: What was perfect never changed. Similarly, the highest level of morality would be immutable. The Greek mind sought out laws of nature which functioned in the realm of human morality no less than in the realm of astronomy.

Modern psychologists of moral development—primarily students of the late Lawrence Kohlberg—looked to those Greek suppositions and found confirmation in the moral development of boys and men. Apparently, the highest level of moral development among males involves recourse to external rules of ethical standards that are considered to be always true and always definitive.

A challenge to this notion of moral objectivity emerged in the work of Carol Gilligan, who argued that girls and women base moral decisions not on objective or immutable standards, but rather on how the decision will affect human relationships. Gilligan argued that women govern their moral lives by weighing the cost for different human beings. Consequently, their view of morality is situational and relative.

The Torah thinks more like Gilligan's women, for it also holds that ethics ought to be dynamic and intersubjective, whether between one person and another, or between a person and God.

For example, examine the way the Torah considers a jealous husband who accuses his wife of committing adultery. She appears before the *kohen* in the Temple and drinks a mixture of bitter water, "*Sotah* water," dust from the Temple floor, and a charcoal curse containing God's name, which is melted into the water potion.

If her body begins to deteriorate after drinking the water, the court and the entire people consider her guilty. But if nothing happens (which is much more likely because, after all, all she did was drink dirty water), her innocence is established beyond doubt.

The ritual of the *Sotah* thus provides a method for vindicating an innocent wife in the face of a paranoid husband.

What caught the rabbis' attention as they studied this passage was God's role in the process: God allows erasing the divine name—mixing it in the waters—to confirm the wife's innocence.

This act of divine self-effacement becomes all the more striking if you recall Judaism's insistence that God's name is too sacred to be pronounced out loud. Books containing God's name can never be thrown out; instead, they are buried with full funeral rites or stored forever. Such is the reverence traditional Jews have always accorded God's name.

Yet here *in the Torah itself* a ritual requires God's name to be erased publicly!

Why? Because, according to *Midrash Ba-Midbar Rabbah,* "in the case of the Holy Name, inscribed in sanctity, Scripture orders that it is to be blotted out in water to bring about peace between a man and his wife." What God's example teaches is that preserving a relationship is often more important than dignity or honor. God is willing to forego the normally mandated honor in the service of harmony between people.

What we come to realize is that God demonstrates the same situational ethics that Dr. Gilligan attributes to women. Rather than referring to some unchanging rule (for example, "never desecrate God's name") mandating ethics that are inflexible and absolute, God's moral imperative is to preserve the relationship between husband and wife. Toward that end, God mandates what is normally prohibited.

As portrayed in the Torah and in later Jewish traditions, the Divine One is passionately involved in relationships—with the Jewish People and with all humanity. The lesson for us is that at its best, morality is in the service of compassionate and caring human living. Morality, at its core, is about relating.

The Passionate Faith of the Nazir

One of the most striking institutions in biblical Israel was that of the Nazirite, a person who took a vow to abstain from grapes or grape products such as wine, from cutting the hair on the head, and from contact with the dead. The vow would cover a specific period of time (according to the Talmud, at least thirty days) and was applicable only in the Land of Israel.

Today's Torah portion provides the framework for the Nazirite, including the proper procedures in case the Nazirite became ritually tainted and the appropriate method to restore cultic cleanliness. While there is abundant evidence for this religious practice in the biblical period—both Samson and Samuel were Nazirites—and even in the Talmudic age, the custom of swearing to become a Nazirite seems to have ended somewhere during the Middle Ages, as there is no further mention of Nazirites after the close of the Talmud.

What was the significance of this stringent order? And what are we to make of such a group, who forswore the pleasures of wine, who refused to come into contact with the dead, and whose lengthy curls were an emblem of their special status?

In the Torah, there is a threefold division of the people, a hierarchy of holiness, corresponding to *Kohen, Levi*, and *Yisrael*. Elaborate procedures specify the spiritual duties of the *kohen,* how to administer in the *Mishkan,* the Tabernacle, and how to offer sacrifices that would be pleasing to God. Similarly, the Torah provides a function for the *Levi'im* that allowed them a unique role in the service of God.

But what of *Yisrael*? How, in the biblical period, could an average Jew who was motivated by burning piety find a way to express that devotion and faith? Granted, the festivals were available to all, and the pilgrimages they fostered were high points every year. But many of the rules of the Torah pertain only to judges and to the administration of the sacrifices by the *Kohanim*. What of the Jews who wanted to do more, who wanted to make of their lives an offering of love to God, a symphony of holy deeds in praise of the sacred?

For such a holy one, a *tzaddik,* the Torah provides the institution of the *Nazir*. Noted scholars have commented on the parallels between the *kohen* and the *Nazir,* how both cannot touch alcohol during their moments of *kedushah,* holiness, how both are described as "holy to the Lord." Neither can expose themselves to the remains of the dead, and in both instances, the head is the focus of sanctity.

Perhaps, then, what the Torah is telling us is that clergy do not have a monopoly on holiness. The privileges of being a rabbi or a cantor are many—the right to lead the service, to select the sermon topic, to organize the community, and to spend every waking moment in the service of God and the Jewish People. For many laypeople, it is enough to leave that all-consuming Judaism in the hands of rabbi or *hazzan,* enough that it is there when they need it for celebration or for comfort in times of sorrow.

But for other Jews, it is not enough. Proud heirs of the prophets and sages, Jews are members of a people in covenant with God. That covenant was not made merely with Moses and Aaron, but with every Jew, past and present. Each one of us is summoned to a unique relationship with God, one that can become as all embracing as we allow it to be.

The *Nazir* was the path for the biblical Jew who wanted to make that relationship central and public. But what of our own age? What of the Jews who have those same deep spiritual needs, the same burning desire to make their Judaism a priority?

Those people need look no further than their own synagogues. Every rabbi is eager to respond to Jews who are ready to take steps to reclaim their heritage. Every cantor is eager to teach the methods and melodies of the sacred prayers and Torah chanting. Learning opportunities abound throughout our communities, often inspired by the request of a seeking congregant who was looking for something that did not yet exist.

The challenge of participating with a full heart in the pageant and drama of Jewish living is still before us. Not as Nazirites, but as enthusiastic participants in learning and in worship services, as practitioners of the *mitzvot,* each one of us can claim a unique place as a servant of the living God.

BE-HA'ALOTEKHA/
In Your Lighting
Numbers 8:1–12:16

Once God speaks to Moses from the Holy of-Holies, Moses receives the final instructions about the menorah and its operation.

The parashah then discusses the purification of the Levites, who are charged with building and dismantling the Tabernacle, but must be in a state of tohorah (purity) to do so. Those Levites older than age thirty were inducted into this sacred labor. An additional task given to the Levites is to serve Aaron and his sons. Finally, the Book of Numbers establishes an age limit of fifty for active duty, after which the Levite may still perform guard duty.

Two years after their departure from Egypt, the Israelites prepare to move on from the wilderness of Sinai. Once again, they offer the Pesah sacrifice, but some of the men were in a state of tumah (ritual impurity), and could not participate. God authorizes a second Passover offering, one month later, for those who were tamei (impure) during the first one. Non-Israelites are explicitly permitted to offer a paschal sacrifice.

Once the Tabernacle is built, a cloud hovers over it by day, and it looks like fire by night. It moves as a sign that God wants the Israelites to proceed, so they march whenever the cloud moves forward, and they camp whenever the cloud settles down.

God then instructs Moses about the trumpets, final preparations before the Israelites march. They are to be used to mobilize the people for marching, to call out the soldiers in defense of Israel, "that you may be remembered before the Lord your God and be delivered from your enemies." And the trumpets blow for Israel's festivals and new moons, as "a reminder of you before your God."

The Israelites now resume their march, from Sinai toward Jordan. Moses invites his father-in-law (here referred to as Hobab) to join them as their guide through the wilderness. The ark guides them as they journey.

Unfortunately, the people begin to complain, first at Taberah, where a fire breaks out amidst the people, then at Kibroth-Hattaavah, where *they cry out for meat. God is furious with them, and Moses feels the full burden of his leadership, so God agrees to divide his load among seventy elders. God also agrees to provide the people with meat, although Moses expresses doubt that God will be able to feed so many. God's spirit rests on the seventy elders, who speak in ecstasy whenever God's spirit rests on them, even on Eldad and Medad, who aren't physically near the other elders. Moses is delighted. "Would that all the Lord's people were prophets, that the Lord put His spirit upon them!" God provides the people with quail until they feel sick. The* parashah *closes with Miriam and Aaron complaining about Moses because he married a Cushite woman. They claim that God also speaks through them, and God gathers them together and asserts the uniqueness of Moses. Miriam is afflicted with white scales, and Moses offers the Bible's shortest prayer on her behalf: "El na refana lah, God, please heal her." After seven days Miriam is restored, and the people set out from Hazerot to the wilderness of Paran.*

✦

Parashat Be-Ha'alotekha/In Your Lighting
Take 1

For Whom the Menorah Shines

Welcome to the world of medieval Jewish debate. The subject: the purpose of the *mitzvot,* the commanded deeds of holiness that constitute Judaism. At the core of the discussion: To whom is religion directed? Should Judaism exist to meet the needs of human beings, or should it exist to meet the needs of God?

Many Jews whose piety is a point of pride and the object of devoted cultivation often claim that our efforts should be directed toward meeting divine needs. For such people, Judaism exists to assist God. When other Jews ask what they can "get out" of Judaism or Jewish practice, they are seen as expressing a self-centeredness that is corrosive to true religiosity. If we are the center, then we displace God to the periphery. Only by directing our spiritual life to *God's* concern, only by satisfying *God's* loneliness, can our Judaism possess the balance, power, and ability to lift us beyond our own limited perspectives.

There is much to be said for this viewpoint. Many of us often fail to take God seriously—we prefer to believe in God without the consequences of believing in God. With God as a cosmic "Big Buddy" we can tailor our Judaism to make us comfortable wherever we are now. If we were to recognize God as a commanding presence, Judaism would become a demanding faith, compelling us to struggle toward deeper levels of insight, caring, community, and response.

The other extreme, of maintaining a religion that is always affirmative, always accepting, and always condoning, also has many advocates. Viewing religion as a response to human needs, these Jews argue that each individual can best set the parameters for his or her own Judaism, and that the central institutions of Judaism should facilitate those choices rather than impose fixed standards.

This approach, too, has much to commend it. Religions tend toward a certain insularity and self-satisfaction. By emphasizing the legitimacy of human needs and the reality of contemporary perceptions, this view of Judaism restores the imperative of caring for God's children. The difficulty arises because this viewpoint regards individual desire as the ultimate criterion of right and wrong, thus often confirming a person's laziness or ambivalence when clear guidance and more exacting standards might have been more helpful.

Both extremes—placing God at the center or seeing each person's perspective as the pinnacle—have a valid insight, and both go too far in their exclusivity. The balance of traditional Judaism, the balance of the living traditions of Torah, Talmud, and later rabbinic commentaries, insists on the two positions as complementary, creating a richer synthesis than would have been possible without their interplay.

Today's Torah portion contains an instance of that call for balance. The *parashah* opens with God's instructions to Aaron: "When you light the lamps [of the menorah], let the seven lamps give light at the front of the lamp stand." Aaron promptly fulfilled God's decree. The *Midrash Ba-Midbar Rabbah* notes that the way the menorah was set up would mean that its light was shed on the worshipers and their service. In answer to the question "Who needs the light?" the *midrash* responds that God ordained the lighting of the menorah wicks to provide for human growth, rather than to meet a divine need:

> The Holy Blessing One said to Moses, "It is not because I require lamps that I have reminded you about them, but only in order that Israel may acquire merit." . . . God is all light and does not need

Israel's light. Why then did God command you to kindle lamps? In order to enable you to acquire merit.

This *midrash* rejects two extreme possibilities—that we light the menorah simply to satisfy a divine need or that we light the menorah simply to benefit ourselves. By accepting the importance of both perspectives, the human *and* the divine, the *midrash* provides a fuller impulse that underlies Jewish observance.

Jewish observance rejects bifurcation: We act in order to respond to God's command *and* to meet the psychological and spiritual needs of Jewish individuals.

The *mitzvot* harmonize two otherwise conflicting agendas; through the performance of sacred deeds, Jews care for themselves while also loving God. We grow to meet the standards that Judaism provides us, and in the process, we make of ourselves better people, more rooted in our Judaism and better followers of the living God.

Parashat Be-Ha'alotekha/In Your Lighting
Take 2

In Diversity, There Is Strength

If asked, most Jews might assert that leadership in the Torah is almost exclusively the prerogative of two primary figures, God and Moses. Repeatedly, God instructs Moses, who in turn relays the new standards to the entire people. Ritual, ethical, and social instruction all proceed from God through Moses to the Jewish People.

That exclusive possession of power shifts during the second year following the Exodus from *Mitzraym,* after a year of revelation at the foot of Mount Sinai, when the Jewish People resume their wanderings through the wilderness. Sinai represents the pinnacle in more than one regard: Not only is it the peak of God's intimacy with the Jews, but it is also the high-water mark of Moses's authority. His stature shines so brightly it blinds those who see him. Alone on that mountaintop, Moses doesn't share his glory or his power with any other human being. As the synagogue hymn *Yigdal* puts it, "there never was another prophet like Moses."

Simultaneously with their renewed wanderings, the people also resume their complaints, their stubbornness, and their disagreements. Moses, now exhausted by leading these contentious people alone, pleads with God for additional assistance. Recognizing his own limits, Moses's modesty is a lesson for all aspiring greats—greatness comes in what you can give to others, not in being the center of all things at all times.

God accedes to Moses's request, instructing him to "gather for Me seventy of Israel's elders . . . and I will draw upon the spirit that is on you and put it upon them: They will share the burden of the people with you."

The medieval commentator the Ramban notes that the number seventy has special significance in Judaism. It represents the total number of nations in the world and the total number of sacrifices offered during the holiday of *Sukkot*, as well as the total number of those Jews who originally went down to Egypt.

Seventy is a number representing completion. The Ramban explains that the choice of seventy elders is not fortuitous, since "this number includes all opinions (that are possible in a given case)."

Through the authorization of seventy sages, God establishes diversity as a Jewish virtue. By providing the leadership, the prototype of the Second Temple, and the rabbinic *Sanhedrin* with dissenting opinions, God assures that every possible view will be articulated and considered.

Diversity, then, is not a threat. Instead, the Torah presents diverse viewpoints as a source of richness, stability, and vitality for Judaism; indeed, the Ramban suggests that this pluralism of viewpoint is at the very center of Jewish law, from the time of Moses to our own day.

The ability to incorporate dissenting viewpoints within the same religion is the great innovation of rabbinic Judaism. Every page of the Talmud records rabbis arguing with each other. Their commitment to Judaism includes a willingness to disagree with each other while still respecting each other, a recognition that there can be such a thing as "a dispute for the sake of Heaven" in which many viewpoints, although they may contradict one another, reflect the "words of the living God."

Our own age is sorely in need of this rabbinic insight, rooted, as we see, in Moses's appointment of the seventy elders. What threatens the vitality and strength of Judaism today is not pluralism and an array of different ways to be Jewish. What threatens Judaism is indifference, an all-too-common attitude Jews have toward their heritage; and an artificially imposed uniformity, which would deprive the Jewish People of the insights and flexibility which are the crowning virtues of rabbinic Judaism.

Instead, each of us can contribute to the continuing health and development of Jewish law, theology, and culture. By developing our own understandings, by engaging other Jews in study, discussion, and growth, we cultivate the resources of a richer Judaism.

In the process of expressing commitment to Judaism through a celebration of Jewish diversity we affirm the traditional Jewish characteristic of unity without uniformity, a goal established so long ago in the wilderness of Sinai.

❧❀❧

Parashat Be-Ha'alotekha/In Your Lighting
Take 3

Trying to Remember the Reason I Forgot

The human brain presents us with both a marvel and a mystery. Capable of mastering a remarkable range of complex tasks, of remembering obscure experiences or facts, that same organ will also forget an important appointment, an acquaintance's name, or the contents of this morning's breakfast.

Though able to outperform a computer in our supple manipulation of data into concepts, each of us also faces the unpleasant reality that we continually forget information we desperately desire or need. Anyone who has reviewed notes taken in college or remarks scribbled in the margins of books read years ago has admitted to the enormity of what is routinely forgotten. It is not uncommon for authors to report rereading their own writing after several years with the uncomfortable sense that they are no longer the masters of what those essays or books contain.

Today's Torah portion hints at this problem, and the rabbinic tradition suggests a remarkable reason for such frustrating lapses of memory. In our portion, Moses "told the people of Israel that they should keep the Passover." Nothing surprising here; Moses often tells the Jewish People what they should or should not be doing. But the *Midrash Sifrei Ba-Midbar* objects that, in this case, the information he conveys is redundant. Didn't the Torah already relate in the Book of Leviticus that "Moses declared the festival seasons of the Lord to the people of Israel"? So why does he have to repeat himself now?

Sifrei goes on by answering its own question: "This teaches that he heard the passage of the festival seasons at Sinai and stated it to Israel, and then went and repeated it to them when the time had actually arrived to keep the rules . . . He recited to the people the laws for Passover at Passover, the laws for *Shavuot* at *Shavuot,* and the laws for *Sukkot* at that season."

Why does Moses repeat the same injunction twice? Because he knows just how forgetful people can be. Recognizing that even the most intelligent, learned, and scholarly people forget much of what they learn, Moses knew that the Jews would have to be reminded of the appropriate *mitzvot* just before the time of their observance. A keen student of the human heart, Moses knew that learning is either renewed, or lost.

Learning is not a possession, something to *have*. It is a process of growth and unfolding that is a permanent accompaniment to human life. Mistakenly viewing learning as a form of conquest leads to the gradual loss of competence in a professional field—that is why so many professions require continuing education to be able to remain active, why professors and rabbis need regular opportunities to renew themselves through study, even sabbaticals. Knowledge and wisdom do not merely grow stale; they dissipate if not freshened each day.

Midrash Kohelet Rabbah understood that point, insisting, "It is for our own good that we learn Torah and forget it; because if we studied Torah and never forgot it, the people would struggle with learning it for two or three years, resume ordinary work, and never pay further attention to it. But since we study Torah and forget it, we don't abandon its study."

Here the rabbis make a virtue out of what might otherwise seem like a universal shortcoming of human life. Even what we cherish, even what we spend hours poring over, trickles through the sieves of our minds, ultimately lost to us.

The corollary of this forgetfulness is the imperative to make learning a lifelong process. Keeping a Jewish book by the side of the bed; enrolling in a study program at the synagogue, community center, or university; learning Hebrew through cassettes, courses, and books—all of these are ways not only of keeping our minds supple and our knowledge growing, but, in fact, of providing the only possible antidote to the pervasive forgetfulness around us.

One of the laws of thermodynamics is the principle of entropy—that everything returns to chaos eventually. In the world of biology and physics, only the investment of new energy can counter the inevitable spread of disorder.

This is true of the world of spirit as well. Judaism has made a cardinal *mitzvah* out of *Talmud Torah*, Jewish learning. Jews studying together, the *Mishnah* teaches us, experience in the process the presence of God.

So go ahead; learn a little.

SH'LAH-LEKHA/Send
Numbers 13:1–15:41

One of the most significant sins committed by the generation in the wilderness involves the spies sent to scout out Canaan.

God commands Moses to send spies, one from each of the tribes, and to report back on the land and the people there. The spies find grapes so large that a single cluster requires two men to carry it, and they name the location Eshcol in honor of the enormous bounty. After forty days of scouting, they return, reporting that the land "does indeed flow with milk and honey." But they also report that the land is fortified; the Canaanites, strong. In fact, the spies insist that they are too strong, that Israel will not be able to conquer the land. Only Caleb affirms faith in God's promise of the land.

Hearing the spies' evaluation, the people burst into tears, saying it would have been better to remain slaves. Joshua and Caleb continue to insist that God can bring about the gift of the land, but the people try to stone them, and only the appearance of God's presence saves them. God threatens to destroy the people, and to make a new chosen nation out of Moses and his descendants. Moses manages to dissuade God, pleading for pardon on their behalf. God insists that none of the naysayers (nor the Israelites of that generation) will live to enter Eretz Yisrael. God then redirects their steps by way of the Sea of Reeds (the Red Sea). Frantic, and too late, the Israelites gear up and attack the Amalekites (against the instructions of God and of Moses), and they are routed at Hormah.

A chapter that provides some laws that will take effect when the children of the wilderness generation enter the land now interrupts the narrative. These laws include the libation accompanying meat sacrifices, the hallah (dough) offering, expiation for unintentional error (either by individuals or the group), the punishment for a man who gathered wood on Shabbat, and the commandment to wear tzitzit (fringes) with a thread of tekhelet (a special blue dye) on the corners of their garments.

Parashat Sh'lah-Lekha/Send
Take 1

A Land Still of Milk and Honey

Parashat Sh'lah-Lekha contains a justly famous description of the Land of Israel as a "land flowing with milk and honey." The riches of *Eretz Yisrael* have endowed our people with a sense of home and of promise since our people's earliest days. But why should a contemporary Jew, at home in America and comfortable with English, care about Israel? What has Israel done for us lately?

Any visitor to Israel cannot help but be moved by the archaeological testimony of the Jewish past—David's city; the steps leading up to Solomon's Temple; Massada, site of the Jewish resistance against Rome; the tomb of Maimonides; the synagogues of the fourth and fifth centuries; the synagogues of the medieval mystics of Safed. Each age of Jewish civilization has left its mark in *Eretz Yisrael,* and the great treasures which have come to light due to the careful studies and exploration of Israel's archaeologists—the most notable of which are the Dead Sea Scrolls—enrich our sense of belonging and of peoplehood for Jews everywhere.

For too long, Jews were reputed to be weak, passive, and incapable of productive work. Hidden inside dimly lit houses of study, Jewish pedants supposedly would mull over obscure and archaic books, while Jews lived in fear, poverty, and ignorance.

While that characterization is not an accurate reflection of Jewish history, many Jews share it as well. The Zionist movement and, later, the State of Israel deliberately encouraged a new self-image for the Jew. No longer a figure of weakness or passivity, Zionist women and men were pioneers—transforming the desert into bounteous farmland, restoring ruined cities to prosperity and habitation. Israel's ability to defend itself against hostile and implacable neighbors, Israel's vibrant if often chaotic democratic system, and Israel's first-rate system of schools and universities have restored an image of Jewish self-worth that had been denied for too long.

While it is certainly true that many Jewish artists, writers, and thinkers adorn Jewish communities of the Diaspora, it is no less true that Israel has had a tremendous impact on Jewish culture throughout the world.

Think, for a moment, about how many synagogues and Jewish centers offer Hebrew classes. Now recall that until this century, Hebrew was not a spoken language. Like classical Greek or Latin, Hebrew was a language that only scholars read. But Hebrew hadn't been used as a living language for two thousand years, until Zionism restored it to life.

Israel is a living laboratory for Jewish expression in the modern world. In Israel, Jews must resolve questions of power, violence, government, and of being a majority in ways that Jews elsewhere only ponder. As a consequence, Israel's writers and thinkers exert an influence out of proportion to their numbers. Writers such as Amos Oz, Shulamith Hareven, and A. B. Yehoshua; poets like Yehudah Amichai and Dahlia Ravikovitch; and philosophers such as David Hartman, Emil Fackenheim, and Eliezer Schweid have profoundly shaped Jewish thinking and Jewish culture.

During the *Shoah,* every nation in the world closed its borders to fleeing Jews. Countless millions might have survived if the Western democracies would have welcomed them. During World War II, Jews had nowhere to go. With the establishment of the State of Israel, all Jews acquired a second home. Israel has taken in hundreds of thousands of refugees from Egypt, Yemen, Syria, Iraq, Iran, Eastern Europe, the former Soviet Union, Ethiopia, and elsewhere. Oppressed Jews are no longer abandoned; they now have a haven in Israel.

That concern for the abandoned extends even beyond a concern for Jews alone. When the "boat people" of Southeast Asia were drowning at sea, Israel opened its arms to them. In fact, Israel took in more Indochinese refugees than any other country except the United States. When Arabs in neighboring countries need advanced medical help, they utilize the free medical expertise of Israeli hospitals. Israeli experts flew to the Ukraine to save lives following the catastrophic nuclear accident at Chernobyl, to Africa to heal victims of famine, to Eastern Europe during recent murderous wars.

For all of these reasons—biblical memory, rabbinic longing and love, unity of the Jewish People, a renewed Jewish culture, pride, and character, and a haven for oppressed Jews—Israel is still the land of milk and honey, still our eternal homeland, regardless of where we hang our *kippot.*

Parashat Sh'lah-Lekha/Send
Take 2

The Power of Perception

Moses instructs twelve spies, one for each of Israel's tribes, to investigate the characteristics of the land the people are about to enter. They travel throughout the Land of Israel during the course of forty days, and they return to the camp bearing an enormous load of the fruit of the land.

Yet when they return, their testimony is contradictory. On one hand, they assert that the land is one which "flows with milk and honey," a land bounteous and fertile. On the other hand, they also insist that the people in the land are giants—*nefillim*—who cause the hearts of those who see them to collapse.

Based on the perceived strength of the inhabitants, the spies urge Israel *not* to occupy the land, despite the assurances of God and Moses that they would do so successfully.

Alone among the spies, Caleb and Joshua assert with complete faith that Israel *should* enter and take the land immediately.

What is striking about the spies' report is the central role of their subjectivity. What mattered to them was not a simple compilation of facts, but rather an internal sense of what those facts mean: "We looked like grasshoppers to ourselves," they said, "and so we must have looked to them."

Faced with the sight of fortified cities and armed soldiers, the spies look at each other, and what they imagined they saw revealed their own lack of imagination and failure of vision. Rather than experiencing themselves as carried by God's promise, sustained by the covenant of Israel, they became overwhelmed by the facts as they appeared on the surface.

Caleb, on the other hand, saw the same facts and refused to bow before them. Infused with passion, conviction, and Torah, he intended to shape reality to conform to his vision.

And his vision was one of a faithful Israel, led by a loving God, occupying the land of its promise.

The facts looked glum—they demonstrated just how unlikely Israel's occupation of the land would be. Yet Caleb, with his idealism and his energy, proved to be correct.

The history of the Jewish People is the continuing saga of the power of ideas to alter statistics. One hundred years ago, no one expected traditional forms of Judaism to survive and today they are flourishing. In twelfth-century Egypt, the time of Maimonides, people wrote of the demise of Judaism, only to have their predictions ignored. When the Temple of Solomon was destroyed and the Jews were exiled, few expected the survival of our people. Yet here we are; still thriving, some 2,500 years later.

We have witnessed the rise and fall of Egyptians, Hittites, Babylonians, Assyrians, Greeks, Romans, the Holy Roman Empire, the British Empire, and the Ottoman Empire, just to name a few. They rose and fell, and we remain. As Psalm 20, exults: "They stumble and fall, but we rise and stand firm."

That there are still Jews who care about Judaism is a statistical impossibility. Yet we are still here, still passionate and still Jewish. The secret of our survival is our continuing excitement and fascination with our ideas. Passionate about our relationship with God, thrilled with the challenge of doing *mitzvot,* energized by the values and ethics that form the core of our rich inheritance, we make ourselves eternal by linking our identity to the One who is eternal. As the psalmist explains, "some trust in chariots, others in horses, but we honor the name of the Lord our God."

Through passion and convictions, we mold mere reality to match our vaunted dream.

Parashat Sh'lah-Lekha/Send
Take 3

The High Price of Silence

It is virtually impossible to read through the morning newspaper, or to listen to the daily news on the radio, without confronting a series of atrocities that shock and appall. Demagogues who murder, rape, and torture are now a daily expectation. Gangs destroying the neighborhoods of our cities, robbing our teenagers of the end of their childhood and much of their future, and schools no longer able to impart either knowledge or values, speak to a futility in trying to aim for a better tomorrow. Each day, we read of a new leader assassinated, of a new war or epidemic or famine that has wiped out the hopes or lives of thousands of people. And behind these episodes of catastrophe lurk the ever-present shadows of environmental poisoning.

How easy to respond to this overwhelming (and incomplete) list of disasters by developing a callousness that ignores reality in favor of a more pleasant fantasy. The world is simply too much of a mess, the level of human suffering too staggering for us to comprehend, let alone try to repair.

Facing the choice of feeding the hungry child or of turning the page, how many of us have opted to turn the page? Most of us don't even stop to think that we made a choice when we did so. Unable to feel *everything,* we shut down our hearts, choosing instead to feel *nothing.*

And so we remain silent in the face of the unspeakable. We surrender our common humanity, our ability to care, in the interests of preserving our sanity and our sense of purpose. Looking steadily into the abyss is impossible, so we shut our eyes and stop our ears. We become deaf and blind to the needs of our fellow human beings, willfully ignorant of the consequences of our own lifestyles and economy on the health and survival of the planet itself.

We are not the first generation to make this choice. Today's Torah portion relates the tale of the twelve spies, sent by Moses to scout out the Land of Israel and to report back on its habitability for the tribes of Israel. Of the twelve who see the land and its produce, its storehouses and its people, ten become adamant that they do not want to move there, that the inhabitants are giants who will obliterate the Israelites. Only two of the spies argue on behalf of trusting God's promise and entering the land.

And most of the people say nothing. In silence they listen to the arguments back and forth, and in silence they refuse to take a stand. In anger, God sentences the entire community, every single adult, to die in the wilderness. Their silence condemned them.

Is that fair? After all, it might have been that they were intimidated by the volubility of the ten spies in opposition. Perhaps they secretly agreed with the two who wanted to move in, but they simply lacked the will to speak out. Or they chose not to do so, since no one wanted to draw attention to himself.

Despite their silent neutrality, God appears to judge them as acting *de facto* on the side of the opposition party. The rabbinic tradition affirms that *sh'tika ke-hodayyah*: Silence is assent. By refusing to speak out on God's behalf, they made themselves into active opponents of the sacred path before them.

Many years later in sixteenth-century Bohemia, the great Rabbi Judah Loew, the Maharal of Prague, wrote,

> Individual good will pale in the face of the sin of not protesting against an emerging communal evil. Not only will such good not avert the impending evil, but such a person will be accountable for having been able to prevent it and not doing so. Such is a communal wrong that it prevails over individual merit.

One can lead a personally pious and decent life, caring for one's neighbors and family, and still be accountable for the misery in the world. By remaining silent in the face of that evil, by refusing to take an active and public stance on behalf of justice and the good, the decent acts of our private life become trivial and powerless in the face of the massive injustices and dangers which form such a public and overwhelming threat to human health and potential.

Each of us is called to "hate evil and to love good" on two levels. On the personal level, we struggle to remake ourselves as fitting role models, as personal embodiments of the virtues of a *ben* or *bat Torah*: modest, diligent, studious, loving, and forgiving. But at the same time, we must also become *rod'fei tzedek* and *rod'fei shalom,* pursuers of justice and peace.

For in the redemption of the world, the individual can find a haven.

KORAH/Korah
Numbers 16:1–18:32

The theme uniting Parashat Korah is the question "Who is allowed to approach the altar and perform sacrifices there?" Beginning with the rebellion of Korah against Aaron's priesthood, the parashah establishes that only kohanim descended from Aaron may offer the sacrifices, but that when they do, other Israelites may safely participate in the worship. The parashah ends by listing the benefits the kohanim and Levites receive for assuming the risk of guarding and tending the altar and the Mishkan (Tabernacle).

Korah, a Levite, along with Datan and Aviram, rebels against Moses, as do 250 chieftains. Moses responds by asserting that God will clarify who is to speak on God's behalf, and who has access to God's altar. Each is instructed to take their fire pans and put incense in them. Aaron did the same. Then, in front of the Tent of Meeting, God's presence appears, threatening to wipe out the entire fickle community. The community pleads with God to punish only the guilty, and God agrees. Moses instructs the people to withdraw away from the abodes of the rebel leaders, Korah, Datan, and Aviram, and the earth opens and swallows them alive. Then a fire issues from God and consumes the 250 rebel chieftains as well.

The rebellion now suppressed, God tells Moses to hammer the fire pans into plating for the altar, as an eternal reminder. The community is infuriated at Moses and Aaron, and threatens to kill them. The two leaders repair to the Tent of Meeting, and Moses notes that a plague from God has already begun to strike down the stiff-necked Israelites. He tells his brother to take his fire pan and bring incense among the people to make expiation for them. Aaron is able to stop the plague in this way, although many people die.

Next, God has each chieftain inscribe his name on a staff, instructing Aaron to do the same for the tribe of Levi. All leave their staffs before the Ark of the Covenant, and the next morning, Aaron's has blossomed and borne almonds. His staff is to be displayed as a permanent reminder.

Finally, God instructs Aaron and his sons about their exclusive role as priests, establishing that they will be maintained from the sacrifices and offerings that the Israelites bring to the Mishkan (Tabernacle).

✦✦✦

Parashat Korah/Korah
Take 1

Different as Day and Night

The rebellion of Korah against Moses and Aaron is painful to most Jews who read it, precisely because it is so complex and so timeless. While we are trained to sympathize with Moses and his supporters by our upbringing and by Jewish tradition, it is difficult for anyone passionate about democracy not to be stirred by Korah's powerful message. Our Jewish loyalty seems pitted against our democratic commitments. That conflict hurts.

Moses and Aaron have successfully led the tribes out of slavery in Egypt and through the dangers of the wilderness, and they are now relatively secure and comfortable. God regularly speaks through Moses to the people, and the families live out their lives waiting to move into the Promised Land.

In the midst of this idyllic serenity, Korah rebels. He resents having to follow Moses in all matters, and challenges him with the moving line, "All the community is holy, all of them, and the Lord is in their midst. Why then do you raise yourselves above the Lord's congregation?"

Korah's challenge strikes at the heart of the democratic values so cherished by both our Jewish *and* our American traditions: If all people are created equal, then why should any one person have any authority over another? Why should one person ever have access to power, wealth, or prestige in a way that another person does not?

Korah's challenge echoes in the words of the prophets Samuel and Amos, as well as in those of Thomas Jefferson and Abraham Lincoln, Karl Marx, and Leon Trotsky. Great leaders in every age have fought for the assertion that each person has intrinsic worth, that all people have equal value.

Few in America would challenge this claim. But what does equality mean? All people are indeed equal in light of the infinite God who created us, but we are not all the same. To be equal in worth does not mean we all have the same God-given abilities.

Korah's flaw was to confuse equal worth with equal skills.

People are *not* the same. The most rudimentary glance around a crowded room reveals differing degrees of intelligence and strength, various personalities and states of health. Great athletes are different than the rest of us, and Nobel laureates do, in the words of the Wizard of Oz, "think deep thoughts with no more brains than you have." There *is* a difference. Korah was threatened by diversity, by specialization, by distinction.

Yet Judaism is based precisely on the celebration of diversity, the importance of distinction. One can be different and still be equal.

Midrash Ba-Midbar Rabbah articulates that insight when it says, "God divided the light from the darkness in order that it might be of service to the world." Korah's position would be to try to fuse the two, to resist the difference between darkness and light. Korah would fail to perceive—would even be threatened by—the distinct contribution of each to the maintenance of the world.

But we need night *and* day. Each one's unique integrity is vital for life to continue.

Similarly, the *midrash* continues, "just as God distinguished the light from the darkness in order that it might be of service to the world, so God made Israel distinct from the other nations . . . and in the same manner distinguished Aaron (and Moses)."

For Jews to be able to contribute to the world—by living the values and practices that make for a society of sacred learning, divine service, and deeds of love—we must remain distinct.

Not better, not isolated, but *distinct*.

Just as we needed Moses to function as a leader—a part of the people, yet distinct from them—so the world needs Jews and Judaism; with a distinct role to play in the participatory drama of human life.

Parashat Korah/Korah
Take 2

Leadership of Compassion

Korah challenges—but how does Moses react? Faced with the most threatening rebellion of his entire leadership, Moses could well be expected to respond with tremendous passion and force, lashing out ruthlessly to crush his rebellious underling.

But the God that Moses celebrates is *El Rahum ve'Hanun*: the God of compassion and mercy. Thus, Moses first reacts to the insubordination by repeatedly expressing concern for the rebels themselves. Rather than punishing them immediately, he engages in a series of maneuvers to postpone the inevitable clash, hoping all the while that Korah and his followers will back down.

Initially, Moses summons two of the leaders of the revolt, Datan and Aviram, in the hope that their obedience to his call would demonstrate a willingness to renew their loyalty to Moses and to God. When they refuse to come, Moses again postpones the public contest, saying only, "Come morning, the Lord will make known who is His."

The Torah records that when first faced with the rebels, Moses "fell upon his face." Rashi understands this to mean that he was dismayed that they would yet again rebel against God. He notes that this is the fourth rebellion, following the Golden Calf, the murmurings, and the recalcitrant spies. Three times Moses intervened with God to overlook the rebellion, but now, at the rebellion of Korah, his hands sank down. This may be compared to a prince who sinned against his father, and the councillor conciliated his father for him once, twice, and three times. But when he offended the fourth time, there sank down the hands of the councillor, for he said, "How long can I impose upon the king? Perhaps he will no longer accept advocacy from me!"

Rashi's *midrash,* taken from *Midrash Tanhuma,* illustrates a powerful mode of leadership not often accepted by our contemporaries. Rather than lash out, Moses demonstrates sufficient confidence in his own leadership to try to reestablish a connection with his enemies. Rather than simply use force to impose his will, Moses makes the effort to persuade, discuss, and negotiate.

In our own time, when some leaders are praised for their ability to impose their will and "get things done," and others are condemned for being too emotional, the compassionate efforts of Moses can encourage us to consider a higher level of interpersonal accommodation and understanding.

Power can be more than the ability to use force, the might to impose will. Perhaps the ultimate power, as our rabbis understood so well, was the ability to control our own inner drives, to hold them in check, and to occasionally rise above them. In the world of international politics, as in the world of friendship, family, and love, taking the time to persuade, explain, and educate can produce results the depth and degree of which can far surpass a begrudging acquiescence to force.

Wouldn't that make this planet a more peaceful place to live?

◈◈◈◈

Parashat Korah/Korah
Take 3

Serving Through Rebellion

Less patient than Moses in the face of Korah's rebellion, God is infuriated. God's wrath is so great that the Holy One is prepared to destroy all Israel out of rage and desperation. God tells Moses and Aaron, "Stand back from this community, that I may annihilate them in an instant!"

But Moses and Aaron do not obey. Instead, they demonstrate remarkable courage and leadership, simultaneously recognizing God's sovereignty while also contesting God's will. "They fell on their faces and said, 'O God, Source of the breath of all flesh! When one man sins, will You be wrathful with the whole community?' "

Moses and Aaron recognize that God has the power, even the legitimate authority, to wipe out an entire people. By referring to God as the "Source of the breath of all flesh," they acknowledge that God gave breath and can therefore take it away. But then they turn that idea around: Since God is unique in being the author of life and death, God's anger can discriminate between the guilty and the innocent.

Midrash Bamidbar Rabbah contrasts this Divine ability with that of a mortal king. Filling in the Torah's terse report of the words of Moses and Aaron, the *midrash* quotes them as saying:

> Sovereign of the Universe! In the case of a mortal king, if a province rebels against him and rises and curses the king or his deputies, even if only ten or twenty of them have done so, he sends his legions there and carries out a massacre, slaying the good with the bad, because he cannot tell which of them has cursed them. You, however, know the thoughts of people and what their hearts and minds counsel. You discern the inclinations of your creatures and know which person has sinned and which has not, who has rebelled and who has not. You know the spirit of each and every one.

Because of that Divine ability to know the human heart, God doesn't have to act with the blindness of a human despot, wiping out countless innocents in order to guarantee that the guilty are punished as well. God can distinguish between the good and the bad, between the rebel and the innocent, Moses and Aaron imply, and thus God must do so.

No less amazing than their courage to stand up and argue with God is God's response to them both. In a sense, their words to God constitute no less a rebellion against Divine will than did the incendiary actions of Korah. They too speak against what God decreed. Yet God welcomes their words, instantly altering the consequences to accord with Moses and Aaron's view of justice.

God is willing to learn from them. Why?

Perhaps rebellion against God isn't always opposing the literal presentation of Divine will. Perhaps sometimes God wants us to search our souls, to ask, "But is that right?" When we stand up for the values and teachings that form the essence of Jewish belief and morality, even if we do so in opposition to established practice, God may actually be pleased by our intransigence.

Certainly, in this instance, Torah law is itself amended: God rejects the notion of collective punishment, in which an entire people pays the price for the misdeeds of a few in their midst. Instead, in response to the unshakable dual loyalty of Moses and Aaron—loyalty to God and loyalty to the Jewish People—a new principle is established: Only the straying individual is responsible for his or her own evil deed.

Korah and those who rebel pay a terrible price for their arrogance and jealousy. But those who did not support the rebellion are spared punishment. Even though they are associated with Korah by blood or proximity, they bear responsibility only for their own actions.

Because our leaders felt a religious obligation to dissent from Divine will in the service of loyalty to God and Torah, a great ideal became a firm principle of Jewish law, and later, of Western jurisprudence as well.

Dare we do less?

HUKKAT/This Is the Statute

Numbers 19:1–22:1

Hukkat *begins with one of the most complex and puzzling rituals in the Torah: that of the red heifer. This cow must be completely red, and its ashes are used to remove the most severe degree of* tumah *(impurity), that of contact with a corpse.*

The Israelites resume their journey, this time to the wilderness of Zin, at Kadesh. There, the prophet Miriam dies and is buried. At that time, there is a drought, and the people begin to rebel against Moses and Aaron once again. God instructs Moses and Aaron to take the rod, gather the people, and order the rock to produce water, as a miraculous sign of God's providence. Instead of doing as God instructs, Moses strikes the rock, twice. Water gushes from the rock, and the people drink and water their animals. God, however, is angry with Moses for lacking sufficient faith to simply speak to the rock, and therefore ordains that Moses will not enter Eretz Yisrael. *The place receives the name Meribah, meaning quarrel.*

Moses contacts the king of Edom, requesting permission to pass through his land, but the king refuses his request. Edom sends out an army to attack the Israelites, so they turn away, seeking another route toward their goal.

At Mount Hor, Aaron dies, and is mourned by the entire people. His son, Eleazar, becomes the new Kohen Gadol *(high priest).*

The king of Arad attacks the Israelites in the Negev, near Atarim. Israel emerges victorious, and renames the place Hormah, meaning "destruction."

As they continue on their march, the people again start to complain about God and Moses. As punishment, God sends serpents, which bite and kill many of the people. The people plead with Moses to intercede, and God tells him to construct a copper snake statue, called Nehushtan. When people look on it, they are immediately healed.

The march continues to the border of Moab on the east, to Be'er, where there was a famous spring of water, and finally to Pisgah. Moses sends messengers to Sihon, the king of the Amorites, requesting permis-

sion to pass through. Instead of acceding, Sihon launches an attack, and he is routed. The lands of the Amorites, and the town of Heshbon, are now occupied by the Israelites. A similar encounter with Og, king of Bashan, leads to a second Israelite victory. The parashah ends with the Israelites victorious and encamped on the very borders of the Promised Land, across the Jordan River from the city of Jericho.

Parashat Hukkat/This Is the Statute
Take 1

Miriam: Water Under the Bridge?

Careers of public figures take on a life of their own, ebbing and flowing with shifts in public opinion and contemporary values. One Jewish figure whose popularity is at an all-time high is the prophet Miriam, the sister of Moses and Aaron.

Though featured prominently in the Torah, Miriam's claim to fame traditionally paled in the face of her more visible brothers. After all, Aaron was the first *Kohen Gadol,* the link between the Jewish People and their religion, and Moses was the intimate friend of God, transmitting sacred teachings to the people. Compared to those two leaders, Miriam seemed to fade into the background. True, we celebrate her powerful song at the shores of the Red Sea, but even that is overshadowed in the Torah by Moses's far-lengthier song.

The celebration of Miriam in our own day is rooted in our more liberated culture's determination to honor historically unrecognized women. Our own tradition, however, also celebrated her. The medieval commentator Rashi noticed the strange juxtaposition in the description of the prophet's death in today's *parashah:* "Miriam died there and was buried there, and the community was without water." From that juxtaposition, said Rashi, "we learn that all forty years they had a well because of the merit of Miriam."

Miriam's well entered the realm of *midrash* as evidence of her greatness. As the ancient Hebrews wandered through the wilderness, Miriam's wisdom, integrity, and nourishing power was such that God provided in response a miraculous well of water, one which moved with the people throughout their wanderings until the prophet died. Without

Miriam, the well disappeared. The role of Miriam and her well in Jewish legend points to two lessons we can carry with us through our own personal wildernesses.

While most of our prophets emphasize the power of words and the centrality of rules of conduct, sanctity, and justice, Miriam's prophecy was one of deed. Rather than offering stirring speeches or administering justice, Miriam taught her people to sing in moments of triumph, and she sustained them during times of exposure and fragility. Miriam's example is one of action, the performance of deeds of love and support. Without Miriam's actions, who could have listened to the words of Moses? Who could have studied God's Torah?

Notice also that, until after she died, there is no comment on her well. In that regard, this prophet of Israel can be seen to foreshadow the tragic reality of the women who came after her. How much recognition has been given to the generations of women who have raised children, taught students, tended the sick, or performed the countless other difficult, tedious tasks that have long sustained and made human life possible? While public honors historically accompanied the splashier achievements of men, many women labored for years without public attention or commendation. Only when they are no longer able to serve are their services noticed, and then only because they are missed.

Why wasn't Miriam's well noticed while she was still alive?

It is time for our generation to reexamine its own values and its heroes today. Do we honor those whose contribution is support of others? Do we still relegate such vital care to others, or have we all yet sought to become not only disciples of Aaron, not only children of Moses, but also personifications of Miriam—using our hands and hearts, just as she did, to enable the lives of our people and of all people to flourish?

***

*Parashat Hukkat/*This Is the Statute
Take 2

When Moses Lost His Temper

In the sweltering heat of the summer sun, Israelite tribes wander in the wilderness. Fatigued, stripped of hope, after the death of Miriam they again complain to their leader, Moses.

Whining that they would have preferred to die in Egypt, where at least they had certain minimal comforts, they bemoan the absence of water to drink or at least leeks to eat. By comparison, the old slave days in Egypt seemed pretty good. At least there they had a regular place to sleep.

In response to their litany of complaints, Moses and Aaron speak to God, who tells them to take their rod and speak to the rock, out of which water will flow. In the face of yet another popular rebellion, God's patience seems endless. Moses and Aaron follow God's command: They take up their rods and stand before the rock. All the people gather around them, hushed and expectant.

Moses lifts up his rod, and twice he strikes the rock with great force. At the end of the second blow, the rock erupts with an enormous flow of fresh, cool water. The problem seems solved.

One would expect that God would be pleased with Moses. After all, Moses publicly affirmed his loyalty to God, and he assured the continuing loyalty of the tribes of Israel to their God. The Jews get their water, and Moses gets a more docile and satisfied populace. Everyone wins.

Yet immediately after the water flows from the rock, God tells Moses and Aaron that they cannot enter the Land of Israel, "because you did not trust Me enough to affirm My sanctity in the sight of the . . . people."

Rashi correctly understands that "but for this sin alone, they would have entered the Land." To what sin is he referring? Didn't Moses do as God had instructed?

A close look at the words of the Torah reveals that while God told Moses to *speak* to the rock, Moses instead *hit* it. And not once, but twice.

Moses's sin was to resort to force when words would have been enough. He needed only to speak to the rock and water would have flowed forth. There was no justification for the needless striking.

The *midrash* goes even further, saying that Moses's sin was not just the physical act, but the fact that he lost control; he lost his temper in the face of Israel's stubborn rebellion.

According to *Midrash Ba-Midbar Rabbah,* "Moses had been guarding himself during all those forty years of wandering against losing his temper with them." The sin here was that "he instantly lost his temper and struck the rock."

Anger is not always sinful; there are times when anger is a righteous and appropriate response, as Moses demonstrated against the Egyptian taskmaster or against the Jewish rebel, Korah. What made *this* outburst of anger sinful was that it blinded Moses to the real possibilities that dialogue would have offered. He was so angry that all he could see were his own grievances and his rage. All he could remember was the long list of abuses suffered at the hands of the tribes.

Lashing out against a painful past, Moses misread the present. The challenge, then as now, is to know when anger and force are appropriate responses and when, instead, they are inappropriate and destructive. How often do we become so blinded by the hurts and wounds of the past that we carry them into our present, precluding the possibility of ever transcending the very wounds that hurt us? In a very real way, we become our own torturers, making certain that old injuries continue to harm us, that old cuts continue to sting.

In our day, no less than during our ancestors' wanderings, what we need is the ability to turn ourselves to God, to tap into God's patience, forbearance, and magnanimity. By reaching out to that reservoir of strength, compassion, and insight, we gain the inner power to let the past recede and read the present for what it is.

By misjudging the present as the past, Moses lost his claim to the future, and was forbidden to enter the Promised Land.

Based on a sermon by Rabbi Simon Greenberg, vice-chancellor of the Jewish Theological Seminary of America, and founding president of the University of Judaism.

Parashat Hukkat/This Is the Statute
Take 3

Lipstick, Ties, and a Red Cow

How often do we ask why we Americans do things as we do? How often do we question our own assumptions about the "American way of life" or subject our familiar customs to scrutiny? Fireworks and barbecues on the Fourth of July? Of course!

Not so with our Judaism. At best an adopted stepcousin, Jewish traditions and writings are mostly unfamiliar to us, and most of us are far less observant of Jewish practice than we are of proper etiquette at a ball game. As a result, we constantly ask, "Why do that?" or "What's the reason for that?" We notice Jewish customs because they are not familiar. We are not equally the products of two civilizations.

Our own Jewish community is, of course, not the first in history to be sometimes bewildered by the reason for some Jewish practices. In today's Torah portion, we read about one of the strangest rituals in the Bible, that of the red cow (*parah adumah*). According to the Torah, anyone who suffers ritual impurity (*tumah*) because of exposure to a human corpse can be made pure again by being sprinkled with the ashes of a perfectly red cow.

What is the connection between ritual purification and the ashes of a cow? Why does a red cow restore purity after exposure to corpses?

Pesikta de-Rav Kahana, a *midrash* on the annual Torah-reading cycle, reports that a pagan questioned Rabban Yohanan ben Zakkai about this strange ritual, insisting that it was a form of sorcery. Rabban Yohanan was able to appease him by comparing it to a similar medical practice of the day. Once the pagan walked away, however, the rabbis' students berated him for offering such a shallow rationale. What, they wondered, is the true reason for the rite of the red cow? Rabban Yohanan answered, "The truth is that the purifying power of the red cow is a decree of the Holy One. The Holy One said, 'I have set it down as a statute, I have issued it as a decree. You are not permitted to transgress My decree.' "

In other words, Rabban Yohanan doesn't provide a reason either. He simply asserts that we are Jews and it's a *mitzvah,* so we do it without justification. Doing the *mitzvah* identifies us as Jews; links us with the values, teachings, and wisdom of Judaism; and provides a way to respond to the presence of God in our lives.

Think for a moment about American culture. Why should a male executive have to hang a thin piece of silk around his neck every day? That cloth makes it hard to breathe, gets messy at meals, and is uncomfortable. There is no rational reason for a tie. Or consider a woman doctor. Why should she have to smear colored paint in a small circle just under her nose? What if she would rather make that same circle with the same paint, but do it about five inches higher, on her forehead? There is no rational justification for lipstick either.

So many of the things we do without question as Americans make no sense on the specific level, but contribute to our identification as participants in a certain part of American culture. The tie lets us know something about a man's values, community, income, education, and work. A woman's lipstick does the same. These things gain their value not from the particular practice, but from the context that such practices creates.

So, too, with the *hukkim,* the unexplainable *mitzvot* in the Torah and in rabbinic literature. Any living culture requires distinct customs and practices to maintain its own special identity, to affirm the loyalty of its members and its continuity across generations. Judaism has those same needs.

But Judaism posits an additional reason as well. The ultimate justification of parental instruction is always, "Because I said so, that's why." Judaism claims to preserve the loving *brit* between God and the Jewish people.

Just as close-knit families develop special customs to maintain their closeness, just as nations develop unique foods or holidays to heighten the loyalty of their members, so God and the Jewish People developed the *hukkim* in the context of creating deeds that cement the loyalty among Jews and with God.

BALAK/Balak
Numbers 22:2–25:9

Balak, the king of Moab, seeks to hire Balaam, a soothsayer of great repute, to curse the Israelites so he can defeat them. When the elders offer this invitation to Balaam, he tells them to wait so he can inquire as to God's wishes. God tells him not to go with the Moabites, nor to curse the Israelites, since they are a blessed people. The dignitaries return to Balak, who sends another delegation. Once more, Balaam inquires of God, and God permits Balaam to go with them, but insists that "whatever I command you, that you shall do."

Balaam saddles his donkey, and proceeds. But God is furious at Balaam and sends an angel with a drawn sword. The donkey sees the angel and swerves from the path, but Balaam beats it to force it to return. This happens again and again, until God causes the donkey to speak, berating Balaam for his lack of gratitude or vision. Then God allows him to see the threatening angel.

When Balaam arrives, he tells Balak, "I can utter only the words that God puts into my mouth." They make a sacrifice, and then Balak leads Balaam to a place where he can see some of the Israelite encampment. Balaam builds seven altars and offers seven bulls and rams. God tells Balaam what to say. This is a blessing that includes the famous description of the Jews: "There is a people that dwells apart, Not reckoned among the nations. . . . May I die the death of the upright, May my fate be like theirs!"

Balak is distraught that the seer he hoped would curse the Israelites blessed them instead, so he tries again from another locale. A similar message emerges: "The Lord their God is with them, and their King's acclaim in their midst."

Balak attempts a third oracle, which offers the blessing, "How fair are your tents, O Jacob, Your dwellings, O Israel!" At this final blessing, Balak sends Balaam back to his home. Before leaving, Balaam offers a fourth oracle, unrequested, predicting Israel's victory against the enemy nations that surround it. He then returns home.

While encamped at Shittim, the Israelite men are enticed by Moabite women to participate in the idolatrous cult of Baal-Peor. As a result, a plague erupts among the Israelites, and God commands Moses to impale the leaders of the rebellion. Before he has a chance to carry out God's grim decree, however, the priest Pinhas finds an Israelite man and a Moabite woman copulating near the sanctuary. Zealous on God's behalf, he impales the two with a spear during their copulation, and his action stops the plague.

Parashat Balak/Balak
Take 1
Balaam: Gentility and Compassion

With great anguish, the Holocaust taught the Jewish People that we ourselves must be the guardians of our own survival and our own needs. The vaunted "civilization" of the West, at whose altar post-Enlightenment assimilated Jews worshiped, revealed itself to have moral and religious shortcomings for which Jews paid with their lives.

The tragedies of our past taught us that our own identity as Jews, the sacred traditions of Judaism, and our people's *brit* with God merit another look, a renewed allegiance, and greater fidelity.

But we can also go too far if we look only inward and reject the claim of universal values. Today's Torah portion about the Gentile prophet Balaam is about balancing those extremes. The Torah describes Balaam as speaking directly with God. Time and time again, following God's instruction, Balaam blesses the Jews, praising their beauty as a people, and reminding us of the legitimacy of our distinctiveness: "There is a people that dwells apart, not reckoned among the nations." Coming from the mouth of a prophet from another nation, these words force us also to look at the larger human context that transcends the particularity of our identity.

Midrash Ba-Midbar Rabbah comments on how striking it was that God should speak through a Gentile prophet. The rabbis then ask why, if in the biblical period, it was possible for prophecy to transpire through non-Jews, why was that no longer true? The answer, according to the *Midrash,* was that Balaam eventually lost compassion for the Jewish

People since they weren't his own nation: "The reason the section of Balaam was recorded was to make it known why the Holy Blessing One removed the holy spirit from the idolaters, for this man rose from their midst, and see what he did!"

Not so the prophets of Israel. According to these same rabbis, "all the prophets retained a compassionate attitude toward both Israel and the idolaters." That compassion for others was what marked the prophets of Israel as worthy of transmitting God's voice to the world.

What was true then is no less true today. Our concern with explicitly Jewish issues—our sense of identity, life in Israel, religious observance, our spiritual lives as Jews—is a vital part of who we are. But it is only *part* of who we are. If we turn our back on social and humanitarian involvements with the larger world, we betray what was distinctive about our prophets of old, and what was beautiful about an earlier vision of what Judaism should be.

As we plumb the depths of our sacred traditions, becoming increasingly at home with Torah, Talmud, and *midrash,* as we learn to pray and to converse in Hebrew, as we grow in observance of the *mitzvot,* may we always remember that we are descendants of those prophets who knew that God's revelation to our ancestors was based on love and compassion for all peoples.

Parashat Balak/Balak
Take 2

Who's Really the Ass?

Our relationship with animals is ambivalent, yet strong. On the one hand, we allow animals into our homes, our bedrooms, and our most intimate moments, lavishing our affection on them during the quiet moments of our days. We love to go hiking to watch birds and see deer, rabbits, and other wild animals, reveling in our sense of union with the natural order. We admire animals for their beauty, grace, and the warmth they bring to our lives. At the same time, we also perceive ourselves as their superiors. After all, only people were made in God's image. Humanity seems never to have quite settled on what animals mean to us or how we should treat them.

In today's Torah portion, we see that same ambivalence, this time in the relationship between Balaam and his remarkable donkey. Balaam has been summoned by the king of Moab to curse the Israelites, making it easier for the Moabites to destroy their Jewish victims. Saddling up his animal companion, Balaam is infuriated when the donkey refuses to follow orders. Ironically, we know that the donkey is trying to protect her less-insightful human cargo. After enduring several blows, the animal finally speaks out, saying, "What have I done to you that you have beaten me these three times? . . . Look, I am the ass that you have been riding all along until this day! Have I been in the habit of doing thus to you?"

Against Balaam's thoughtless fury, the donkey answers calmly and with reason. The rabbis of *Midrash Ba-Midbar Rabbah* expand this observation. They ask, "Why is it that animals don't use speech?" And their answer is, "had they been able to speak, it would have been impossible to put them to the service of people or to stand one's ground against them. For here was this ass, the most stupid of all beasts, and there was the wisest of all the wise, yet as soon as she opened her mouth he could not stand his ground against her." Therefore, conclude the rabbis, "the Holy Blessing One has consideration for the embarrassment of people, and knowing their needs, shut the mouth of beasts."

The *midrash* raises this inescapable question: What might animals say if they could speak?

Our dogs might ask us why they are able to be so agreeable and loving all the time while we seem incapable of achieving that same love and loyalty among ourselves.

Our cats might inquire about our admiration for their cleanliness and the care they take of their own bodies while we destroy our own health through our refusal to exercise or to control our eating, drinking, smoking, and any number of other destructive habits.

Those same cats might also puzzle about why we admire their independence while it is so difficult for us to be alone. Are we afraid of our own thoughts, or our own company?

Our pet birds might ponder with confusion as we rave about their beautiful singing but devote no time at all to our own creativity and playfulness. For most of us, poetry, art, and drama are child's play.

Always able to find time to play or socialize, our pets might ask why we always complain about our lack of time but never take the steps necessary to reorganize our lives to care for our real needs.

But most of all, animals—wild and domestic—would wonder why we so pervert and cheapen our own noblest instincts. Dogs are able to play together and to live up to our expectations. Cats and birds also care for their own kind.

Almost solely in the world, human beings demonstrate a level of aggression and cruelty to their own kind that would be considered truly beastly—except that beasts don't do it.

Balaam's ass embarrassed Balaam because the prophet was less able to live up to his own expectations than was the donkey. Blessed and cursed by our gift of reason, we rely on our brains just enough to get ourselves in trouble, but not enough to resolve to live better, more thoughtful, and more reasonable lives.

Think of all the secrets our pets have seen. And imagine how embarrassing it would be if they could speak.

⧫⧫⧫

Parashat Balak/Balak
Take 3

Blessed, and a Source of Blessing

Every year that I read the remarkable story of the Gentile king, Balak, hiring the Gentile prophet to curse the Israelites, I am struck by how remarkable this story really is. After all, how often does the Torah concern itself with the internal affairs of other peoples? Understood as the love letters between God and the Jewish People, it is quite proper that the Torah's focus is on the relationship, the *brit* between God and Israel. Yet this story stars a non-Jew who is seen as a holy and a wise seer.

Balak demands that Balaam curse the Jews so that they will be easier to defeat in battle. Faithful to God, Balaam explain that he cannot curse or bless without first receiving divine authorization. When he asks God what to do, God tells him, "Do not curse the people, *ki varukh hu,* for it is blessed."

What is God really saying about us? In what way are the Jewish People *barukh,* blessed?

The medieval commentary *Lekah Tov* understands this phrase to mean that we are blessed because of the *zekhut avot,* the righteous deeds of the patriarchs and the matriarchs. Their goodness was such that God blessed us with an irrevocable blessing. We, their later descendants, benefit from their blessing to this day.

Another related way to understand this verse is to ask ourselves in what way are we blessed. It does sound like God is saying that there is some intrinsic blessing with which we are imbued. How are Jews blessed?

- We are blessed with a rich memory: As a people, we enjoy a continuous identity stretching back to the very earliest layers of human history. From Abraham and Sarah down to the youngest Jewish baby alive today, we know where we come from, and we know who we are. In an age of rootlessness, in a time of confusion about identity, we Jews have the luxury of knowing our beginnings and of identifying with our rich and varied history. As the Passover *Haggadah* urges, each generation understands the history of the Jews not merely as something from the past, but as something informing our own identity today: *We* were freed from Egypt, *we* fashioned the Talmud, *we* explored the depths of Jewish philosophy and Kabbalah, *we* enjoyed the modern fruits of emancipation and of Zionism.
- We are blessed with a wise and profound way of life: Not only do we have a history that is ancient and continuing, but we also have a way of life that is rich and rewarding. The cycle of Sabbaths, holy days, and festivals adds shape and texture to our weeks and years, allowing us to rejoice with our loved ones and to create precious occasions to cherish and to enjoy. The beauty of the holidays becomes part and parcel of our love for each other and our sense of community. Linked as they are to ethical values and religious expression, their beauty is enhanced by moral depth and by great insights to be learned anew.
- We are blessed with being the messengers of God's love and justice: Our religious tradition harnesses beautiful ritual for the sake of ethical rigor. By teaching us to care for the sick, to feed the hungry, to shelter the homeless, to care for the earth, our religion offers a message as vital now as it was when it was first articulated. No less revolutionary today, the notion that all people reflect God's Divine image and are worthy of respect and dignity contin-

ues to transform and elevate the world. Ours is the privilege of carrying that message and reiterating it, even when it seems that others may have forgotten it.

In these and other ways, we are indeed blessed to be Jews. But there is another way that we can understand Balaam's rejoinder. The Hebrew word *barukh* may be passive, meaning blessed. But it might also be an active adjective, like *hanun* or *rachum*. In that case, it means "source of blessing" or "bountiful." When we say a *berakhah,* then, we are saying that God is generous to us, and then specifying how God's bounty is manifest in that particular instance.

Using this understanding, we can say that Balaam is refusing to curse the Jews because we are a source of blessing.

In that reading, Balaam offers us a great challenge: Our mission as Jews is to be a source of blessing, not merely for ourselves, but for all humanity. As Balaam says, "Blessed are those you bless, and cursed are those you curse." Our task as Jews is to serve as God's representatives on earth: Just as God is known as a source of blessing for creation, so we are to be a source of blessing for all.

The way we live our lives, then, must be measured not only by our ritual observances, important as they are, but also by how we embody the ethical *mitzvot*. By shouldering the burdens that weigh others down, by conducting our business lives in an honorable and productive fashion, by embodying patience and compassion in all we do, we live up to Balaam's and God's high expectations.

Are we a blessing? Are you?

PINHAS/Pinhas

Numbers 25:10–30:1

God bestows on Pinhas an eternal covenant of peace as a reward for his zeal on God's behalf. The Israelite who was killed, Zimri, was the son of a chieftain from the tribe of Shimon. The woman was Cozbi, the daughter of a chieftain of the Midianites. God commands Moses and the Israelites to attack the Midianites because of their role in luring the Israelites into idolatrous worship and apostasy.

The parashah continues with the rise of a new generation and preparation for the conquest of Eretz Yisrael. This new generation, unlike the generation of the Exodus, is characterized by fidelity to God and Torah.

At the end of the plague, God mandates another census of men who are over twenty years of age. Unlike the earlier census, this one is by tribal clans, and the total number is over 600,000 males of fighting age. Once the number of people is established, God discusses allocating the Promised Land by lot and by the size of each tribe.

The census confirms that the generation of the Exodus has died, fulfilling God's dictate that those rebellious Jews would die in the wilderness and their children would reach the land of Israel. The daughters of Zelophedad raise an issue with the justice of the inheritance system. Why, they ask, should their father's land allotment go outside the family just because he had no sons? Moses consults with God, who affirms the wisdom of the daughters and grants them the right to inherit. God tells Moses to ascend to the heights of Mount Avarim to view the land the Israelites will enter, after which he, too, shall die. Still concerned for the well-being of the people, Moses asks God to appoint someone to lead in his stead, so that the Lord's community may not be like sheep that have no shepherd. God appoints Joshua, and Moses signifies the choice in a public ceremony involving Eleazar, the Kohen Gadol (high priest).

Once the apportionment of the land and the succession of leadership is resolved, God establishes the calendar of public sacrifices, the festivals and holy days of ancient Israel and contemporary Judaism. These occasions of public festivity mark the daily offering, Shabbat (Sabbath), Rosh Hodesh (the New Moon), Pesah (Passover), Shavuot (the Feast of

Weeks), Rosh Ha-Shanah *(the New Year)*, Yom Kippur *(the Day of Atonement)*, Sukkot *(the Feast of Tabernacles), and* Shemini Atzeret *(the Gathering of the Eighth Day)*.

Parashat Pinhas/Pinhas
Take 1

Turn the Other Cheek; Get Slapped Twice

It seems obvious that striking back at an enemy is a gratifying but more primitive response than forgiving the trespass in the first place. A person who is able to overlook having been wronged reveals a higher form of moral sensitivity, by setting priorities that preclude a need to get back at someone else.

That line of reasoning was given its classical formulation in the Christian Scripture, with the mandate to "turn the other cheek." If someone slaps you on one side of the face, rather than slapping back, simply offer your other cheek to be slapped. By doing so, you confront your enemy with the power of love and the depth of your own humanity.

Such morality has retained its popularity from the time of Jesus into our own century as well. Mahatma Gandhi was the preeminent exponent of responding to hostility with passive resistance. He urged Indians by the thousands to resist the violence of British officers and soldiers with equanimity, allowing the British soldiers to beat, maim, and often shoot Indian opponents of British colonialism without opposition. Through this massive passivity, Gandhi and his followers hoped to show the British and the world the power of love to overcome hatred and oppression.

In our own country, the great Reverend Martin Luther King Jr. employed this same passive resistance to the racism which pervaded America. His followers, like Gandhi's, were clubbed, attacked by guard dogs, and hosed without resistance; they attempted to awaken the slumbering moral conscience of the nation.

But what if a nation has no moral conscience? Isn't it possible that the policy of turning the other cheek can work only with a democratic government, one in which the public recoils from brutality and is forced to witness its own police and citizenry in unfettered reporting every day?

In other words, might it not be that turning the other cheek works when the citizenry or government is fundamentally moral and open? In imperial Rome, they butchered the people who turned the other cheek. In the Jim Crow South, men were lynched.

Such an approach disregards the enormity of evil in the world, ignoring the fact that there are people and organizations that knowingly destroy human lives and families, willfully and without apology. Adolf Hitler could not be shamed out of Auschwitz, and Joseph Stalin was not embarrassed by the Gulags.

In such instances, rather than representing a higher spirituality, turning the other cheek becomes simply a form of cooperating with evil.

Our Torah portion addresses the issue of that kind of evil. In speaking of the Midianites, a tribe which attacked the stragglers and weak among the Israelites, the Torah instructed our ancestors to "harass the Midianites . . . for they harass you." The Torah recognized the reality of human evil—a malignancy which goes beyond not recognizing the consequences of one's actions, or underestimating how much one's policies hurt others, but rather evidences the reality that some people delight in oppressing others and putting them down. Such people cannot be won over through appeals to conscience or by showing one's own weakness. Rather, they can only be opposed with a greater force than they would have used to impose their own will on others.

An ancient *midrash* teaches, "If a man comes to kill you, rise up and kill him first." No turning the other cheek here. Unadulterated evil can only be opposed with superior power. There are times when discussion fails, when persuasion is beside the point. At such times, as our rabbis taught, "who begins with kindness to the cruel winds up being cruel to the kind."

Most people are not evil. Many simply need to see firsthand, and over a long period of time, the consequences of their own bigotry, anger, or greed. But that predominance should not blind us to evil and its reality.

The example of the Midianites, and the Torah's insistence that evil must be exposed and opposed, is the natural consequence of a passion for justice. Mercy is important as a way to temper strict justice. But as a replacement for justice, mercy results in the suffering of the victim instead of the wicked.

Our Torah insists on balancing mercy and justice—each with its own appropriate sphere, each with its own important jurisdiction.

Justice, an insistence that actions have consequences, requires that we oppose evil with sufficient force to prevent the wicked from harming the innocent.

Gandhi and King notwithstanding, Jews do not turn the other cheek. We strike back hard enough to prevent any further aggression.

✦✦✦✦

Parashat Pinhas/Pinhas
Take 2
To See with the Heart

In a remarkable story, the Torah relates the courage and the integrity of five women, known collectively as the daughters of Zelophedad. What makes this story truly astonishing is not only that the heroes are women, itself a rarity in the biblical age, but also that it represents the earliest revision of biblical law. Here, within the Torah itself, God revises an earlier piece of Divine legislation because of an overriding moral imperative. What a magnificent precedent to set for later generations in their dealings with *halakhah* as well!

The tale is worth telling. According to a law already established in the wanderings in the wilderness, men alone were permitted to inherit their parents' property. At the time, no one had objected. Neither Moses nor any of the seventy elders saw a problem with that procedure for transmitting a parent's holding in the Land of Israel. After all, it was universal custom for men to own and inherit property, to handle finances, and to run the economy, both household and community. Women lived on the generosity of powerful men.

Alone among the children of Israel, the daughters of Zelophedad pointed out that they had no brothers. If the law were rigidly followed, their father's family would be completely dispossessed.

Responding to their complaint with characteristic modesty, Moses promised that he would ask God what the law should be. And God acts in a very Godly way, taking the side of those who have been wronged, those who have been overlooked. Our God is passionate about human dignity, and, as a result, intervenes and changes the law. The daughters of Zelophedad do, indeed, inherit their father's land.

Why hadn't Moses, or any of the other elders, been able to point out this legal injustice on their own? What special trait allowed the daughters of Zelophedad to notice an injustice and to speak out?

The medieval Bible commentator Rashi explains that the story teaches us that "their eyes saw what the eyes of Moses did not see."

In this regard, our own eyes often resemble those of Moses. So many of us go through the routines of our lives without truly seeing. Understandably wrapped up in prosaic issues of our own, we fail to take the time to see other people as human. Instead, we wind up treating them like objects—a butcher is a source of meat, a teacher provides our children with skills, and so on.

Remember, as a child, just how shocked you were to see a teacher or your rabbi in the supermarket? Suddenly it dawned on you that he had a life, too, that his existence served a larger purpose than simply his role in your life.

As another example from the supermarket, I recall my shock the first time I saw a sticker from PETA (People for the Ethical Treatment of Animals) affixed to a flank steak in the frozen foods section. It said, "Meat stinks!" Since then I've seen others that point out that what is immaculately wrapped inside that cellophane is the carcass of a dead animal. But it is wrapped so beautifully that we don't even think about the fact that our dinner is a dead cow, lamb, or chicken. Our eyes simply don't see this.

People, animals, and scenery too often enter our worldview in terms of the function they can perform for us, rather than as "others" with feelings and problems and dreams, as living creatures, or as magnificent natural treasures. Most of the time, we look but we don't really see.

The daughters of Zelophedad teach us an essential lesson for being fully human. They teach us the imperative of truly seeing—not only with our eyes, but with our minds and our hearts as well.

They teach us not to turn away from the homeless, the elderly, the disabled, or members of other minorities. Rather than looking at people as objects, the Torah shows us, by example, that the constant struggle to be fully human is really the struggle to see all humans as people.

This *Shabbat,* and in the future, let us take up the gift of the daughters of Zelophedad.

Let us teach ourselves to see.

Parashat Pinhas/Pinhas
Take 3

Walking in a Crowd, Standing Alone

Rabbinic tradition provides a lovely *berakhah* to recite when seeing a crowd of over 600,000 Jews: "Praised are You, Lord our God, Ruler of the Universe, wise in secrets." Why at such a moment would we praise God for knowing secrets? Isn't it the size and power of the crowd that is truly impressive? Or the fact that the traditional number of Jews standing around the foot of Mount Sinai was 600,000, so that such a crowd today is a reenactment of the revelation? Why focus on *secrets*?

When I began as a pulpit rabbi, my overwhelming impression surveying a sanctuary full of people was their beauty and warmth. I had not yet had the chance to get to know them as individuals, so all I could see was their identity as a group. Over the years, however, I participated in countless *s'mahot* (celebrations) of bar and bat mitzvah children, births, graduations, honors, luncheons, festivals, holy days, and Sabbaths. I was also with them through the hard times—difficult pregnancies, developmental disabilities, behavioral problems, marital issues, divorce, illness, separation, job loss, and death. That first *Rosh Ha-Shanah,* I saw simply a sea of faces. After several years, I saw hundreds of individuals standing together. And what struck me was how many stories of suffering, courage, patience, and sorrow each face masked.

I am only a human being, aware of my limits and my foibles. If I can become so aware of the bottomless well of personality, history, joy, and suffering that each person brings into the sanctuary, imagine the symphony of feelings and experiences that serenade God.

Perhaps what is most remarkable about God is that each person is able to relate to God in a slightly different way from her neighbor, in a manner that speaks most directly to her own needs, aspirations, and ability. If God is truly *Ein Sof,* beyond limit, then it is the ultimate Godlike ability to respond to each individual as singular and special.

Our Torah portion expresses that insight this week. Moses prepares to transfer leadership to a new generation. He is concerned on behalf of his people that the new leader honor the individuality of each member of the community and not impose a bland homogeneity on all. Moses insists that the legitimate claims of the community must accommodate and celebrate individual expression and difference.

In addressing God, Moses uses the term "Source of the breaths of all flesh." The rabbis of *Midrash Ba-Midbar Rabbah* notice that Moses uses the word *ruhot* (breaths) rather than *ru'ah* (breath). Why did he employ this awkward plural form?

The rabbis understood that even though a crowd of people may look alike, that similarity is only superficial. Just as their faces are not like each other, so are their temperaments not like each other, every individual having a temperament of her own. God, therefore, manifests differently "for the spirit of each individual being." The *midrash* understands Moses's brief phrase to mean "Sovereign of the Universe! The mind of every individual is revealed and known to You. The minds of Your children are not like each other. Now that I am taking leave of them, appoint over them, I pray, a leader who will bear with each one of them as their temperament requires."

We are commanded to imitate God's attributes of loving-kindness (after all, what else can it mean to "walk in God's ways"?). Just as God responds differently to each individual person, based on His particular mixture of desire, need, perception, and ability, so, too, should we. No two people are alike. Even if they dress similarly, work in similar fields, and enjoy similar lifestyles and incomes, those similarities mask the profound depths of human individuality. Every person is unique.

And that unique difference of each person makes sense, not only psychologically, but from the perspective of theology as well. The Torah reminds us that we are made *b'tzelem Elohim*, in the image of God. If God is infinite, every creature made in God's image will reflect a different finite aspect of that infinite Source of life. That each new person presents a new aspect of God's image is a consequence of God's creative energy.

Communities, families, friendships, and governments would do well to remember the truth that Moses hinted at and the rabbis of the *midrash* made explicit: Everyone is different, and those differences are to be cherished, nurtured, and cultivated. Rather than seeing individuality as a threat to society, a godly community will celebrate distinction as yet another mark of the abundant fullness of God's presence in our midst, infusing us and all with passion, energy, wonder, and life.

MATTOT/Tribes

Numbers 30:2–32:42

This parashah *begins with the issue of oaths and vows, establishing their binding nature for all men, and for women, provided that the fathers of minor daughters or husbands of married adults don't retract the vow when they first hear it. The vow of a widow or divorced woman is binding precisely as that of an adult man.*

The last task facing Moses is to seek vindication from the Midianites for having drawn the Israelites into the licentious idolatry of Baal-Peor. Moses musters a force using soldiers from each of the tribes, and they vanquish the Midianites without losing a single Israelite warrior. In addition to executing the five Midianite kings, they also slaughter Balaam.

The soldiers take booty from the Midianite settlements, including women and children, beasts, herds, and gold. Moses is outraged that the very women who led the Israelite men astray are spared, and he orders their prompt execution as well. Then he mandates that the soldiers undertake a seven-day period of purification prior to reentering the camp.

The booty that remains is divided equally among those who fought and the rest of the community, at God's command. The officers, grateful for the remarkable victory and lack of Israelite casualties, donate all their gold plunder to the sanctuary.

With the last battle of the wilderness behind them, Israel moves into a new phase: that of settlement. The two tribes of Reuben and Gad petition to settle on the eastern bank of the River Jordan, rather than on the western bank of the Jordan. At first, Moses resists this proposal, but once he is assured that the two tribes will continue to fight along with their fellow Israelites, he consents.

MASSEI/Itineraries
Numbers 33:1–36:13

The final parashah *of the Book of Numbers recounts each of the forty-two camps of the Israelites, from Rameses to Sinai, from Sinai to Kadesh, and from Kadesh to the steppes of Moab. This listing of encampments is both a joyous recollection of God's miracles along the way, and a sobering reminder of Israel's many rebellions against God and God's servant, Moses.*

At the border of Canaan, God mandates the conquest and apportionment of the land. While Moses isn't allowed to enter the land, at least he is permitted to draw up the plans for its settlement and growth. He lays out the regulations for the conquest, the precise boundaries of the new Israelite home, and the authority of the tribal chieftains who will establish forty-eight towns for the Levites and the six Levitical towns of asylum for involuntary manslaughter.

The parashah *and the entire book, end with a follow-up from the family of Zelophedad, concerned that the women who will inherit family land will then marry into other families and their land will be lost. To remedy this concern, God mandates that the women must marry within their own clan.*

The Book of Numbers closes with this observation: "These are the commandments and regulations that the Lord enjoined upon the Israelites, through Moses, on the steppes of Moab, at the Jordan near Jericho."

When Silence Speaks

Today's Torah portion speaks, in the language of its own age, to the timeless question of when to get involved.

Parashat Mattot addresses the legal issue of the nullification of vows. It records the ancient law that a woman's vow can be nullified by her husband, provided that he cancels her vow immediately on hearing it. If he delays in silence, her vow becomes irrevocably binding.

While many moderns are troubled by the power of men to override the vows of women, it is also striking that the Torah insists that the husband either use his power instantly, or lose it forever. Why? After all, if he has the authority to nullify her oath, they why can't he choose to exercise that power later?

The answer given by the Talmud is that "silence is like assent." Once the husband knows what his wife has sworn, he becomes a participant in her oath. At that point, he can either object immediately—dissociating himself from her words and thereby nullifying them—or he can remain silent, which effectively links the husband and the vow. Silence is assent.

How often do we face acts of injustice or callousness with silence? A derogatory joke in our presence, an act of selfishness or cruelty, or simply reading about political oppression in our newspapers—all of these instances summon us to choose a side. We can either verbalize our opposition immediately, or, through our silence, become allies of the act or words we abhor.

There is no neutrality. Silence is assent.

Our society is producing homeless people in record numbers. Unemployment among minority males and violence in some minority communities have shattered normal human living for many in our inner cities. Our schools produce illiterate children who grow up to become unskilled and poorly motivated adults. Women are still, according to the most recent statistics, unfairly burdened and inadequately compensated. Jews, gays, blacks, and others are frequent objects of bigotry and violence.

This ought to be a time of profound embarrassment to religious people. Far from agreeing to serve as God's partners in Creation, establishing

God's rule of justice and love, we have effectively turned our backs on the welfare of many of our fellow Americans and on the health of our planet.

How do we participate in these evils? By not opposing them in public, we allow our silence to speak instead of our words and our deeds. Rabbi Judah Loew, the great sixteenth-century Maharal of Prague, wrote:

> While a person may be individually pious, such good will pale in the face of the sin of not protesting against an emerging communal evil. Not only will such piety not avert the impending evil, but such a pious person will be accountable for having been able to prevent it and not doing so.

In the midst of the dark ages of his time, the Maharal understood that his obligation as a being in covenant with God was to represent God's light and God's passion despite the powerful forces mustered against them.

In the midst of the current dark age, we, too, need to remember our eternal calling—to sanctify God in the midst of the people. By feeding the hungry, clothing the naked, healing the sick, pursuing peace, and identifying with the weak, we move from silence to eloquence. We provide God with hands and a voice.

There is no neutrality. Silence is assent.

Parashat Mattot/Massei/Tribes/Itineraries
Take 2

The Importance of Intention

Today's Torah portion addresses the issue of unintentional manslaughter. What is the appropriate penalty for someone who kills another person unintentionally? Should there be any penalty at all?

The *parashah* discusses the establishment of six cities of refuge, *Ir Miklat,* set aside as a permanent asylum for anyone who unintentionally killed another person. Once within their walls, the manslayer was protected by law against any revenge or additional punishment.

In this way, the Torah insisted that killing another person is reprehensible, but it also asserted a distinction between murder (which is deliberate) and manslaughter (which is not). Contemporary American law makes a similar distinction, mandating a varying degree of severity to correspond to the different levels of responsibility due to intention and circumstance. Three thousand years earlier, the Torah instituted those same legal distinctions based on diverse intentions.

One way to understand the profundity of the Torah's insight is to contrast biblical law with other ancient standards.

Ancient Greece, Sumer, Phoenecia, and other cultures all articulated a notion of asylum. In those civilizations, a murderer could flee to a local shrine and gain protection at the altar of the local deity. Whether the death had been intended was irrelevant to the power of the shrine to protect the murderer. The pagan idol was no less holy, no less powerful, just because the murderer intended to kill his victim.

Not so the Torah's law. The Torah asserts emphatically that the six cities of refuge would only protect the unintentional manslayer. The willful murderer was to be evicted, tried, and punished. No matter how powerful the divinity whose altar provides shelter, the Torah mandates that religion cannot interpose itself between a murderer and justice. Religion is a way of life, not a shield for violence.

Also diverging from other ancient law codes, the Torah does not determine the severity of punishment based on the status of the victim. Murdering a free man, woman, child, slave, or foreigner all resulted in the same penalty. Since all human beings reflect God's image, all people deserve equal protection and possess equal worth.

The notion of a city of refuge is not unique to the Torah. Nor is the idea of making legal distinctions for the same action. Nonetheless, in the law of the cities of refuge the Torah presented something breathtakingly new and exciting.

The assertion that *inner intention* determines the meaning of an action was revolutionary. While all intentional murders are abhorrent, they are not the same as an accidental homicide; one who kills unintentionally is still guilty, but of a lesser offense. In fact, the Talmud in *Massekhet Makkot* expanded upon this insight to provide for the release without penalty of those involved in complete accidents. Intention matters.

Unique among ancient law codes, the Torah consistently maintains its emphasis on *kavvanah* (intention). Indeed, Judaism continues that distinction to this day.

Human beings represent something precious—the only permissible representation of God in the world. And what is most godly about us is our knowledge of good and evil. That awareness, and our ability to act on our own moral impulses, represents both an opportunity and a challenge. The challenge is to grow to reflect that Divine image to the fullest extent we can. The opportunity is to create, through moral integrity and *mitzvot,* an environment in which God's presence is readily apparent.

As this week's reading says, "I, the Lord, dwell in the midst of the children of Israel." To which Rashi adds, "you shall not cause Me to abide in uncleanness."

Our actions must reflect our intentions, as we strive to make our intentions correspond, ever more closely, to God's.

⊁⊰⊱⊁

*Parashat Mattot/Massei/*Tribes/Itineraries
Take 3

And If I Am for Myself Alone . . . ?

Occasionally, we hear of an act of self-sacrifice so sweeping and powerful that it commands the respect of all who encounter it: a mother and father who willingly undergo life-threatening surgery to try to save the life of a beloved child; rabbis, nuns, or ministers who work with people suffering from highly contagious diseases without regard to the threat to their own lives; brave men and women who volunteer to serve as soldiers in dangerous missions or wars because the cause is just; civil rights volunteers who stand up to the prejudice of their own society against racial minorities, women, gays and lesbians, or the disabled, and do so without regard to personal comfort or protection. The very length of such a list is a challenge to any complacency the rest of us may feel.

Does such sacrifice make sense? Even granting that only through that kind of self-denial can the world be made more just, compassionate, and kind, is it reasonable to give up the only life a person will ever have in order to try to help the lives of others? After all, once we lose an arm, it will never grow back. Once some bigot kills us, our lives are over. We won't benefit from the improvements to the world that may result from our nobility of vision. Or will we?

In today's Torah portion, we come across an example of just such selflessness. God commands Moses to "avenge the Israelite people on the Midianites; then you shall be gathered to your kin."

In the past, I've taken it for granted that Moses set out to fulfill the order the moment he received it. But I came to realize that God doesn't tell Moses that he must act immediately, and, in fact, Moses has every incentive to postpone acting on the issue of justice, for he knows that once he's done it, his life will end. To put off dealing with Midian for as long as possible would be the obvious way for Moses to delay his own death.

The rabbis of *Midrash Ba-Midbar Rabbah,* always attentive readers of Torah, noticed the choice that God had placed before Moses. Rabbi Judah remarked,

> If Moses had wanted to live many more years he could have, for the Holy Blessing One told him, "Avenge" and "then you shall be gathered," thereby making his death dependent on the punishment of Midian. But the Torah tells us of the excellence of Moses. He thought, "Shall Israel's vengeance be delayed merely that I may live?" Instantly, Moses spoke to the people, saying "Let men be picked out from among you for a campaign, and let them attack Midian."

In fact, the Bible offers a counterpoint to the selflessness of Moses. Joshua, Moses's attendant and successor, was supposed to live 120 years, but lived only for 110. Why? Because when God told him to fight promptly, he reasoned, according to the *Midrash,* " 'If I kill them at once, I shall die immediately, as Moses our Rabbi did.' What did he do? He began to dally in wars against them." In response, God diminished his life by ten years.

We may admire Moses's choice but know in our hearts that Joshua's is far more readily understandable. He enjoyed living, he knew little about death, and he realized that if he fulfilled his mission he risked dying younger than if he delayed. So he made a decision that reflected his own desire to survive. Wouldn't we do the same?

Moses didn't. Moses chose to value the will of God and the well-being of the people as a whole, more than his own life.

The only way such a choice is conceivable is to perceive oneself as extending beyond the well-being of one's own body and mind and soul. If our highest interest is only ourselves, then Moses's behavior and that of Martin Luther King Jr., Rabbi Leo Baeck, and Mother Teresa is the height of folly. There is never a rational basis for letting any value take primacy over survival and personal interest.

Yet that is not the only way, nor is it the way conducive to a life of meaning and contentment. Only when we see ourselves as participating in a greater life beyond our own self-interest can we become rooted in a transcendent purpose. Linking our ancestors with our descendants, we are drops in a stream of living waters; what matters most is the flow, of which we are but a part. To be one of the Jewish People, *Am Olam,* the Eternal People, is our taste of eternity and our source of purpose.

Ultimately, even the Jewish People are finite. What connects us with a purpose that will survive the end of life on earth and the extinction of the sun is our reflection of that which was there before earth and sun, the One who will be there after they are gone. By placing God's love and will at our core, by centering our identity on the *Adon Olam,* the Eternal Holy One, we become everlasting.

The paradox then, is that the only way to discover our eternal worth is to discard it—like Moses.

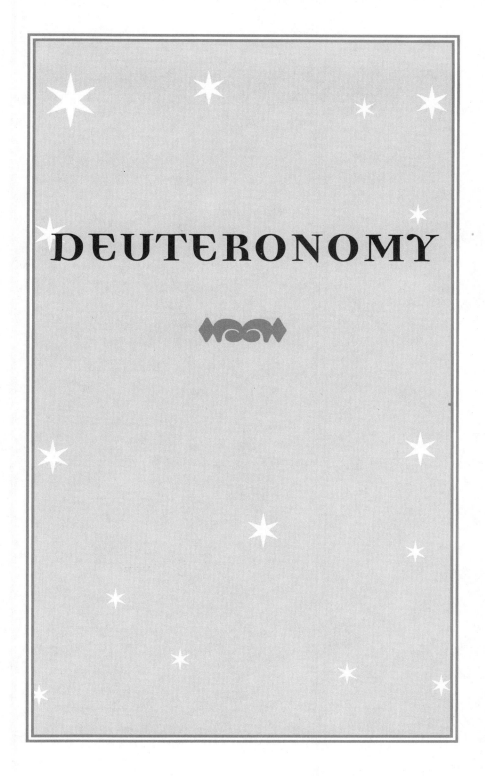

DEUTERONOMY

DEVARIM/Words
Deuteronomy 1:1–3:22

The fifth book of the Torah constitutes Moses's farewell address to the people Israel on the border of Eretz Yisrael. According to Jewish tradition, Moses's series of discourses took thirty-six days to deliver, beginning on the first of Shevat and ending on the sixth of Adar. Deuteronomy is portrayed as the time that "Moses undertook to expound this Teaching (ha-Torah ha-zot)." The purpose of this instruction is to convey law as well as teachings that must be studied and pondered, with the intention of molding character, establishing virtues, and making goodness and holiness habitual.

The first discourse describes the history of Israel from the liberation from Egyptian slavery up to this event some forty years later. The first section of the first speech offers a retrospective and culls important moral lessons for Israel to learn from its first half century. The theme of this section is neatly summarized: "Adonai your God has blessed you in all your undertakings. God has watched over your wanderings through this great wilderness. Adonai your God has been with you these past forty years: you have lacked nothing."

Moses uses this opportunity to remind the Israelites of key lessons they will need as they enter Israel: that a lack of trust in God and a lack of obedience to God's will results in calamity, and that, conversely, faith and obedience result in victory. God is the warrior who does battle on Israel's behalf. Moses relates how the disobedience and rebellion of the tribes led to their defeat by the Amorites and the condemnation of the first generation to death in the wilderness, and how the second generation's trust led to military victories over enemy rulers, King Sihon and King Og. The conclusion that Moses derives from Israel's liberation and early wanderings is this: "You have seen with your own eyes all that Adonai your God has done to these two kings; so shall Adonai do to all the kingdoms into which you shall cross over. Do not fear them, for it is Adonai your God who will battle for you."

Parashat Devarim/Words
Take 1

Jewish Unity—and Diversity

The oneness of God, for Jews, is a special aspect of God's glory, a distinct trait of divinity. From the recital of the *Sh'ma* in biblical times, through the rigorous philosophy of the medieval sages, the utter oneness of God has been a distinguishing trait of Judaism itself. In fascinating ways, the intuition that God is best conceived as a unity has been echoed by the search by contemporary physicists for a grand unified theory, as well as by the current study of ethics, which speaks of a single ground for goodness.

It's a short jump from the praise of God's oneness to the argument that such unity is also an ideal for human beings. If God's unity is a source of strength and continuity, Jewish homogeneity should provide powerful evidence of the oneness of the God who summoned our people into existence. The argument is that Jews should constitute one undifferentiated group, with one style of Judaism for all. "The more Torahs, the more blemishes."

From this perspective, diversity is a blemish. It suggests that we Jews are only guessing in the realm of religion, that our Torah is not a Torah of truth at all.

A second perspective argues that Jews have many different opinions because like all peoples, we encompass a range of personalities and characteristics. Particularly in a democratic society, no external force can impose an artificial unity on any group. Given this diversity of opinion, a choice of different forms of Judaism will actually strengthen the connection between Jews and our faith: The more forms of Judaism, the more each Jew will be able to find a voice within the larger Jewish community.

Today's Torah portion provides support for that second position, but it also institutes a Jewish standard for deciding when diversity is legitimate and when it degenerates into divisiveness.

In *Parashat Devarim,* the tribes of Israel prepare to cross the River Jordan and to enter *Eretz Yisrael.* Our national history is about to begin. At the river's edge, the tribes of Reuben and Gad remind Moses that he had agreed to permit them to remain east of the Jordan, where they would build towns and establish settlements for their families. Unlike the rest of Israel, their God-given inheritance was to be on the east side of the Jordan River.

This first assertion of Jewish diversity troubled Moses, but when he inquired of God, the Holy One confirmed that what Reuben and Gad proposed was permissible. The two tribes had particular needs that differed from those of the other tribes. Finding a way to meet their own needs was a healthy response to the richness of human variety.

Recognizing the distinct needs of Reuben and Gad, and not considering those needs as a threat to the larger group, required Divine revelation. God was able to see that human variety need not lead to anarchy or hostility.

Even while recognizing the value of diversity, God and Moses realize that diversity is not the only value. There are limits to how far diversity can go while still remaining a Jewish value. Moses instructs the two tribes that they may build settlements for the women and children, but the men must fight with the other ten tribes until all of Israel has received its inheritance:

> You must go as shock troops, warriors all, at the head of your Israelite kinsmen . . . until the Lord has granted your kinsmen a haven such as you have . . . Then you may return each to the homestead that I have assigned to him.

Diversity is legitimate so long as each Jewish group keeps the well-being of the entire Jewish People in mind. We are all limbs on one body. As the rabbis saw it, "all Israel are comrades."

So long as we understand that our Jewish self-interest requires us to care for, and to be involved in, the defense and love of all Jews, our particular understanding of how to be Jewish or what Judaism may mean can only enrich our larger Jewish community.

God is one. And, thank God, the Torah has many paths. As you walk along your path to God, remember to reach out a hand. That way, we'll all get there together.

Parashat Devarim/Words
Take 2

May I Have a Word with You?

The opening words of the fifth book of the Torah begin, simply enough, "These are the words that Moses spoke to all Israel."

The Torah had a choice here: It could use the word *amar,* for "spoke," or it could use the word *daber.* The rabbis of the ancient *Midrash Sifre Devarim* note that every place the *Tanakh* uses the verb *daber* indicates harshness or rebuke, whereas the Hebrew word *amar* conveys a sense of praise. In the opening lines of *Devarim,* the Torah uses the word *daber.* Why? Why did Moses speak harshly to the Hebrews as they gathered on the border of the Promised Land?

Because his final speech, the culmination of his long life of service to them and to God, consisted of chastisement, reminding them that they fell far short of the sacred standards embodied in the Torah and Jewish tradition.

And did the people resent Moses's apparent harshness, as most of us would? Did people say, "He never gives us a break," or note that even at the end he was still haranguing them instead of focusing, even for a moment, on their virtues and better natures?

Apparently not. The speech is, after all, dutifully recorded in the Torah and read every year in synagogues around the world. And when Moses concluded his words and then went off to die, the people mourned his loss, even as we still keenly feel his absence today.

Can you imagine what it would be like if, at a dinner honoring twenty-five years of service with a particular synagogue, rather than dwelling on warm memories, the rabbi enumerated all the flaws of the congregants as revealed during the past two and a half decades? Can you imagine how resentful and bitter most of them would feel?

Rabbi Tarfon, a great sage of the *Mishnah,* read this passage and sadly observed, "I doubt if there is anyone in this generation who is fit to rebuke others. For if one says to another, 'Remove the mote from between your eyes,' the reply invariably is, 'Remove the beam from between *your* eyes.' " No one in Rabbi Tarfon's time was exempt from the very faults they would point out in others; they were hardly role models capable of rebuking their neighbors with disinterest.

Rabbi Eleazar ben Azariah said, "I doubt if there is anyone in this generation who is able to *receive* rebuke." Rabbi Eleazar observed that people no longer accepted criticism as an act of love. Instead of listening openly to a description of how they had acted inappropriately and then seeking to change their behavior, the object of rebuke would respond defensively, ignoring or insulting the person who had pointed out the error.

Rabbi Gerson Cohen, past chancellor of the Jewish Theological Seminary, tells of the time he was a child at Camp Ramah in Wisconsin. As he and his friends were playing basketball, the game got a little rough, as sports often do. Without warning, one of the scholars in residence, a rabbi and professor of Talmud, intervened, scolding the boys, "There is a Jewish way to play basketball. And this is not the Jewish way." Rabbi Cohen remembers that they were stung by the remarks, and humbled. Instead of grumbling about it, however, they stopped their game and started a discussion about how they would try to play in the future. As the scholar was about to walk away, he said to the kids, "How wonderful, a group of boys able to receive rebuke."

Rabbi Akiva, a contemporary of Rabbi Tarfon, added a third portion of lament to those of his colleagues: "I doubt if there is anyone in this generation who knows *how* to rebuke." Pointing out someone's shortcoming or error should not be opportunity to feel superior, to humiliate, to gloat. Instead, offered with love and humility, a rebuke becomes an act of affirmation and faith: an affirmation that the person is worth the effort in the first place, and faith that he or she remains capable of improvement.

A rebuke is a gift and a challenge. Without our friends, colleagues, and families being willing to point out our own errors of judgment or action, we bind ourselves to our own faults. Their courage to articulate disappointment in our actions is an indispensable prerequisite to self-improvement and refinement.

We cannot afford to wait for the perfect, loving hero to inform us of our flaws. Instead, we rely on those around us to act as our early warning systems, pointing out moral failure and ethical obtuseness before it's too late to improve. And when they do, we must be able to really listen.

Are We Really Equal?

Every American child knows that our nation's founding document proclaims the equal worth of every human being: "We hold these truths to be self-evident: that all men are created equal." Our entire structure of government, our economy, and our approach to education is predicated on the notion that each person has precisely the same value as any other person, regardless of who that person is, what family they are part of, or how much money they own.

If different people possessed different value, then it would be ridiculous for each person's vote to have the same weight. Instead of the "one person—one vote" approach that we currently take, we might prefer to have a political scientist's vote count five times more than, say, a simple country rabbi's. After all, the political scientist is a highly trained scholar in the areas the vote is considering. Or, perhaps the president of Ford Motor Company should have a few more votes than one of the janitors from the same company.

We don't allow some individuals to have a weightier vote than others because of the American credo that all people possess equal worth.

But is that true? Are people really equal? Don't intelligence, reliability, integrity, and drive vary greatly from one person to another, so that some will work long hours to achieve real excellence, while others might accept mediocrity or failure? Some earn top grades in school while others barely make it through the system. Some perform acts of heroic caring while others commit violent crimes.

By any objective standard, people are not equal, whether in physical appearance, emotional temperament, or mental prowess. The only way in which people can claim equality is if we posit some other point of perspective from which to compare them to each other. That second point of perspective must be so radically superior to even the best human being that in comparison to it, all people are *relatively* equal. For the founders of the American republic, as for Judaism, that point of comparison is God, the Creator of all.

When contrasted to an all-knowing, all-powerful, all-good God, the distinctions among human beings level out to insignificance. Indeed, to insist on human equality requires the reality of God; otherwise, that assertion shrinks into a beautiful but unsupportable illusion.

Today's Torah portion raises a similar point. In instructing a judge how to handle a case between the prominent and the unknown, the Torah relates the instruction "You shall not be partial in judgment: hear out low and high alike. Fear no man, for judgment is God's."

Rashi explains this to mean "let a case involving a small coin be as dear to you as a case involving a hundred coins, that if the former came before you first, don't postpone it until the end."

Rashi's explanation recognizes the fact that a case involving little money is different than one involving a tremendous fortune and that a prominent person is not the same as an unknown. From the perspective of quantifiable facts—what can be measured, weighed, and tested—these are as objectively unequal as two different human beings.

Yet, says Rashi, what the Torah's message teaches is that the source of human worth is not based on any facts. The infinite worth of each human being springs from our equality in the sight of God. That perspective alone—of an external position from which all humans appear to be functionally equal—mandates a system of justice that accords equal worth to otherwise unequal people.

Our entire democratic enterprise, then, is based on a spiritual truth; that in the sight of God, all people are equal and deserving of dignity, respect, and justice. Precisely because the cosmos is a creation of the God of the Universe, precisely because each human being is a unique reflection of God's image, every one of us can lay claim to the same portion of infinite value that, ultimately, adheres to God alone.

All of us, the great and the small alike, are equal not because of our skills, our strength, or our insight. Our equality is not a function of what we do. It is a function of what we are: children of the living God.

VA-ET'HANAN/I Besought
Deuteronomy 3:23–7:11

With the opening of chapter 4, Moses moves into the second section of his address, exhorting the people to obey God's laws so that they might dwell securely in the Promised Land. In a sense, chapter 4 introduces what follows: general themes that Moses will repeat throughout the book. Here Deuteronomy highlights relying on Israel's experiences of deliverance and wandering, of the threat of exile, and of God's forgiveness and teshuvah (repentance) in the places to which they will be scattered. In this chapter, Moses highlights the commandment to worship only Adonai and to love God, prior to presenting the outlines of the mitzvot (commandments). This provides a model for later theology and law codes, such as the Mishneh Torah of Maimonides.

These laws make it possible for Israel to dwell in the land with security and compassion: "Observe them faithfully, for that will be proof of your wisdom and discernment to other peoples." The Torah then warns against idolatry, recalling the gift of the Ten Commandments at Mount Sinai, and calling on the Israelites to never give in to worshipping images of any corporeal being or astral body. Moses calls heaven and earth to witness against Israel, should the Jewish People transgress when he is no longer alive, and points out the penalty of exile should they sin. Yet he also assures his listeners that God will remain open to the possibility of teshuvah wherever they may be, "for Adonai your God is a compassionate God."

Moses then appeals to his listeners (and to us) to observe the commandments as a response to God's uniqueness and to God's kindnesses to our ancestors and to us. "Know therefore this day and keep in mind that Adonai alone is God in heaven above and on earth below; there is no other. Observe God's laws and commandments, that I enjoin upon you this day." Moses then establishes the three cities of asylum east of the Jordan.

The second address, the core of the biblical book, begins with a lengthy prologue in which Moses describes how God appointed him to lead the Israelites. He recapitulates the revelation at Mount Sinai, including the Ten Commandments and the people's selection of Moses as their intermediary with God.

Chapter 6 opens with the Shema, *the core affirmation of Israel's faith in God's uniqueness and special relationship with the people Israel. We are to tell our children about our miraculous liberation from slavery, and to remain distinct from the pagans in Canaan, faithful to our covenant with God, in the service of holiness and justice.*

◆≋◆

Parashat Va-Et'hanan/I Besought
Take 1
Do the Right Thing

When you think of the core teachings of Judaism, certain essentials quickly come to mind: the liberation from Egyptian slavery; the *Shema,* declaring the uniqueness of God; the Ten Commandments, affirming a moral and sacred order to human existence; and *mitzvot-halakhah,* Jewish law, which implements the love relationship between God and the Jewish People.

All of those insights are found in one remarkable *parashah,* the one we read this week. Here, in stirring eloquence, our greatest prophet and teacher reminds us that the central task of the Jew is to live in accord with the teachings of God—to conduct ourselves and our dealings with others in such a way that we cultivate the wisdom, compassion, and justice possible for all human societies.

At the very heart of Moses's speech is the belief that doing God's will and obeying the *mitzvot* are the sure path toward establishing a society of justice, of infusing every aspect of life with spirituality and allowing the fullest possible personal development and growth. *Halakhah* is the key—an authoritative network of sacred deeds which guides every step of our spiritual path, directing us what and how to eat, when and how to work, why and how to apply God's healing vision to human life.

These beliefs characterized Judaism from its earliest days, and all traditional forms of Judaism even today.

Particularly shocking, then, is one beautiful and yet seemingly extraneous verse in Moses's elegant and impassioned plea. After urging his followers to follow all of the *mitzvot,* he adds, "Do what is right and good in the sight of the Lord."

If God's will is expressed in *halakhah,* then why add, "do right and good"? And if we need to be told to do what is right and good, why bother with *halakhah*?

Ours is not the first generation to wrestle with the difficulty of knowing what, exactly, God wants from us. From the age of the prophets into our own, Jews have tried to discern the paths of righteousness. The command to "do what is right and good" may offer us a guidepost on our road.

Rashi suggests that this verse "implies a compromise, going beyond the letter of the law." In other words, there will be times when applying the law strictly will no longer embody doing what is right or good. In such moments, as obedient servants of God we are to have the courage to forge a compromise that may go beyond the current formulation of the tradition. The tradition itself provides for its own dynamic growth; *Halakhah* is a process, not an outcome.

The Ramban is even more explicit:

> Even in regard to those things where no specific command applies . . . it is impossible to record every detail of human behavior . . . . God included a general injunction to do what is good and right in every matter, accepting where necessary even a compromise in a legal dispute.

What both commentators recognize is that there are two ways to destroy a legal tradition: abandon its authority and relevance, on one hand, or reduce it to its rulings rather than its method, on the other. Both destroy the living tree of Judaism by undermining its jurisdiction or by denying its ability to respond to new insights and new phenomena.

The Talmud records the understanding of Rabbi Yohanan that Jerusalem was destroyed only because our ancestors acted in accordance with the letter of the Torah and did not go beyond it. In our age, as in times past, there are temptations to abandon the process initiated in the Torah, through excessive permissiveness or excessive rigidity. The command to do what is right and good is our summons to live our lives according to a *halakhah* that is dynamic, one the purpose of which is compassionate, and the details of which are just.

Our vitality and authenticity as Jews as well as individual growth and spirituality and, ultimately, God's love and sovereignty intersect at one place: in the continued flowering of a dynamic *halakhah,* one which seeks always to establish the right and the good.

✦

*Parashat Va-Et'hanan/*I Besought
Take 2

Doing Mitzvot and Loving God

In his farewell address to our people, Moses repeats the Ten Commandments, portrayed as the living words of God spoken before the entire people of Israel at Mount Sinai. He had first presented them in the Book of Exodus, offering an on-the-spot report of the revelation as it happened. For Moses that moment was so vital, he reiterates these commandments now, word for word.

In the midst of these stirring words, God promises to show "kindness to those who love Me and keep My *mitzvot* [commandments]."

Why should God distinguish between those "who love Me" and those who "keep My *mitzvot*"? After all, shouldn't a Jew who loves God also be a practitioner of *mitzvot*? And shouldn't someone who observes *mitzvot* also love God?

Sometimes it is difficult to realize that the questions that beset us today have troubled our forebears as well, that Jews of previous ages also wrestled with the challenge of faith in a world where God seems sometimes hidden or weak, and questioned the authority of Jewish tradition and the sacred nature of the Torah. But, of course, traditional Jewish writings, emerging from millennia of rabbis, philosophers, and sages, do cover the same concerns and ponder the same soul-searing questions as we ourselves do today.

Throughout Jewish history, as well as today, many Jews who love God did not observe the *mitzvot,* and many Jews zealous in their performance of *mitzvot* seemed not to grasp the implications of loving God.

For the former, love of God may devolve into a kind of self-worship, as if God is obligated to love each of us solely on our own terms. *Mitzvot* then may be performed because of their beauty, emotional power, or wisdom, with no sense at all that we perform *mitzvot* to please the Creator of the Universe, or to honor the sacred and commanding voice resonating throughout the mundane deeds of Jewish living.

For the latter, performance of the *mitzvot* may become a form of self-righteousness, in which piety in themselves and in others in measured by external punctiliousness. *Mitzvot* become a kind of cosmic scoreboard, in which the one who makes the most hoops, wins.

Both of these approaches present the danger of becoming forms of idolatry: One idolizes warm feelings and individual autonomy, the other idolizes sterile practice and unthinking obedience.

But a richly traditional and full Judaism, the kind portrayed in today's *parashah* and so lovingly developed throughout the millennia, insists on the observance of *mitzvot* as a method of cultivating a love of God and of responding to Divine command.

Through repeated deeds, we express our willingness to open ourselves to standards beyond those of our individual egos. By responding to a call which does not emerge from inside our own hearts, we learn to become sensitive to the needs of others, and, ultimately, of the One.

The *Mekhilta,* an ancient *midrash,* recognizes this same dynamic, explaining that "those who love Me" refers to Abraham and those who are like him. Abraham's spiritual greatness lay in his intimacy with God—an intimacy of loyalty, fidelity, and a readiness to disagree in love.

"Those who keep My *mitzvot,*" according to the *Mekhilta,* refers to the prophets and the elders; in other words, to Moses, the first prophet, and to the seventy elders who helped him implement the laws of the Torah, translating legal theory into living practice. The Judaism of the rabbis was and is rooted in both approaches, seeking to integrate a passion for God with a desire for godly living.

We are heirs of Abraham and of Moses, of a rich inner life coupled with, and cultivated by, a profound ritual practice. The challenge to contemporary Jewry is what it has always been: implementing the teachings of Judaism in order to reorient ourselves and our world to priorities that reveal and further a sacred vision.

By living *mitzvot* and by offering those holy deeds as acts of love, we demonstrate our fidelity to our people, our sages, and our God.

Parashat Va-Et'hanan/I Besought
Take 3
What We Do and Who We Are

No one is perfect. One of the inescapable realities of human life is that our shortcomings, preferences, or passions can interfere with our achievement of our own intended goals. Failure is the uninvited guest that accompanies us throughout our journeys.

We cannot banish failure and disappointment, but we *can* control how we respond to the latest evidence of our own errors. How can we best respond when told that we let someone down or failed to meet an important deadline?

One tempting response is to deny our failures, or to explain them away by turning against the person we have hurt. Or we can simply cover up our wrongdoing, trying to convince ourselves and others that it never really happened.

Quick to recognize this deception in others, we judge it as "defensive." In politicians, we consider such defensiveness cagey. But in our own cases, we are often so desperate to believe our own alibis, so eager to defy any flaw of our own making, that we buy into a whopper of a tale, only to appear deceitful to the rest of the world.

As in countless other instances, Moses, the greatest of the prophets and sages of ancient Israel, provides a role model. Confronting both his own magnificent accomplishments and his human failings, Moses realizes that hiding one's own errors only makes them appear worse.

In today's *parashah,* the Torah records his words "and I pleaded with the Lord at that time, saying . . ." The rabbis of the ancient *Midrash Sifre Devarim,* always attentive readers of every word, noticed that one word didn't add anything specific to this sentence. "Saying" seemed superfluous, and therefore available for a rabbinic interpretation.

What additional and unrecorded plea did Moses "say"? He asked, "*Ribbono Shel Olam,* Master of Space and Time, let any transgression that I have committed be recorded against me, so that people will not say, 'Moses seems to have falsified the Torah,' or 'Moses said something he was not commanded to say.'"

They compare this request—to list the particular sins for which he was prohibited from entering the Land of Israel—to that made by a woman aristocrat who gathered figs during the sabbatical year. Since such harvesting violates biblical law, the king ordered her to march through the center of town, so that the people would see her humiliation and would consequently avoid breaking the law themselves. As she began her march, she turned to the king and asked that her specific offense be publicly announced, so no one would accuse her of having committed a far more serious crime, such as murder or sexual immorality.

Similarly, Moses knew that later generations would wonder why he wasn't allowed to enter the Promised Land. If a specific reason wasn't given, we might assume that his transgression was far more severe than it actually was. In order to protect his own reputation, therefore, Moses insisted on complete revelation of his misdeed. Doubting God at the wilderness of Zin, and that alone, was the error that resulted in his punishment.

Unequaled among leaders of later generations, Moses's stern integrity remains a source of awe and marvel. Unswerving in his devotion to God and God's people, consistent in his pursuit of truth and justice, Moses was a true pinnacle of human candor and compassion. By admitting his own mistake publicly, he preempted his enemies from using it against him. He forestalled the possibility that others might accuse him of behavior far worse than anything he actually did. And he taught, through his own example, the importance of owning up to our mistakes.

If Moses erred, how can we not? But if he was not ashamed to admit his errors, then we need not be either. Mistakes are not weights that must be shouldered forever in silence. Guilt is healthy only if it provokes repentance, restitution, and renewal. By openly owning his own transgression, Moses took the essential first step toward transcending it.

Human identity is more than the sum total of our deeds. Those actions possess us only as long as we allow them to claim our core. By pronouncing their names in public, by dissociating ourselves from our actions, we banish those demons and liberate ourselves for the challenges and the growth yet to come.

EKEV/It Came to Pass
Deuteronomy 7:12–11:25

Parashat Ekev *opens with a reference to the blessings that will flow if the people live in harmony with God's rules. Moses reminds the Israelites that they do not have to worry about the Canaanites, despite their numbers or their power, since God is in their midst. Israel will thrive and prosper if it remains loyal to God and God's covenant, because "man does not live on bread alone, but on anything that* Adonai *decrees."*

God is giving Israel a rich and bounteous land. Gratitude is the optimal response to that graciousness, including thanking God after meals for the food and the land.

Moses then shifts tone, instructing against attitudes of self-righteousness that Israel's victories and conquest might engender. Instead, the Jews are to hold on to humility as a safeguard against arrogance and smugness. Toward that end, Moses reminds his listeners of the sin of the golden calf and of God's anger which was the result of that offense.

After that tragic incident, God renews the covenant with instructions to craft a second set of the Ten Commandments and the selection of the Levites for service in the Tabernacle (and later, the Temple).

Chapter 10:12–19 contains a summary of religious faith second to none, starting with God's sovereignty and uniqueness, moving through God's selection of Israel and its fidelity to God's commands, and ending with the need to bring justice to all peoples as the only proper fruit of faithfulness to God.

Chapter 11 exhorts Israel to love God and to observe God's commandments. Paragraphs from this chapter form the middle selections of the Kriyat Shema, *the daily recitation of the* Shema *in Talmudic and contemporary Judaism.* Ve-hayah Im Shamoa *speaks of the collective consequences of social greed and injustice, and of the need to teach and study these teachings repeatedly.*

Finally, the parashah *concludes with the assurance that faith and fidelity to God will secure the success of the conquest of* Eretz Yisrael.

Parashat Ekev/It Came to Pass
Take 1

Why We Give Thanks After Meals

"The unexamined life is not worth living," insisted the philosopher Socrates. For Sigmund Freud, the same thought became "where id is, let ego be." What both knew is that the great drive of human consciousness is toward understanding our place in the world, how and why we think what we think, and what and why we believe. Rather than exist only by our instincts, to live a fully human life is to act with understanding and volition.

To the extent that we transform rote behavior into conscious choice, we become more human. By exploring our motivations and our desires, we make our deeds meaningful, rather than simply functional.

Infusing behavior with meaning is the agenda of Judaism. For thousands of years, the structure of Judaism, embodied in *mitzvot,* infused routine behavior with the sacred. By transforming a deed into a *mitzvah,* we deepen its history, enrich its meaning, and connect ourselves with a community that spans the countries of the world. That kind of transformation is vividly exemplified in today's Torah portion.

After a meal, when "you have eaten your fill," says the Torah, "give thanks to the Lord your God for the good land which He has given you."

Why thank God *after* a meal? It makes a certain kind of sense to pray *before* a meal, when we have a need to be met. But afterward, we are already satisfied. And God surely does not need our prayers or gratitude. The prayer after eating, *birkat ha-mazon,* moreover, scarcely seems the appropriate time to make a request.

But there is more to prayer than simply focusing on our own needs. The act of praying has a larger purpose; it sensitizes us to the greatest marvel of all: that we exist, and that we are conscious of our existence.

Jewish prayer should shock us into an awareness that life itself is miraculous.

We did not ask to be born, and we did not create a world that could sustain human life. What a marvel, then, that we do exist, that we can sustain our bodies with food and drink! To eat as though eating is merely a humdrum event robs us of a chance for wonder, an occasion to recognize the magnificence of life. In the words of the Talmud, "benefiting from this world without saying a blessing is like stealing from God."

That food sustains us is miraculous. Each meal gives us an opportunity to encounter the unanticipated and unmerited bounty of the universe. Surely such an astounding match of inner need and outer response deserves our gratitude and our attention.

The Talmud records that our ancestor Abraham used to cause his guests to praise God. How did he do that? He would serve a lavish meal, at the end of which his guests would rise to praise him. Before they could utter a word, Abraham would say, "Did you eat what was mine? You ate what belongs to the God of the Universe. Praise and bless the One who spoke, causing the world to be."

We did not create the food that sustains us. We did not create the earth on which it grows, or the universe in which Earth itself floats. By summoning us to show gratitude for our food, Judaism reawakens our sense of marvel, restoring our ability to experience the extraordinary joy of truly living.

✦

Parashat Ekev/It Came to Pass
Take 2

What Are You Willing to Die For?

In the course of our daily routine, there are certain focal points—actions, comments, or individuals—which can ignite our passion like nothing else. While they may not receive a great deal of conscious thought or even much of our waking effort, their significance lies in how vital they are to our sense of identity, worth, and meaning.

Each of us may have our own reality for which we are willing to make sacrifices. Most parents would give up their lives for their children; some special individuals have given their lives for the children of others. On a very different level, many people get ulcers and heart attacks to serve their passion for wealth, prestige, or beauty.

How we live our lives is often shaped by what we value most. And that value can be identified simply by asking ourselves, What am I willing to die for? In the words of Rabbi Abraham Joshua Heschel,

> The most important decision a thinker makes is reflected in what he comes to consider the most important problem . . . there is only one really serious problem: And that is martyrdom. Is there anything worth dying for? We can only live the truth if we are willing to die for it.

Rabbi Heschel's point is that our lives derive their ultimate value and sense of purpose not necessarily by what receives most of our time, but what commands our deepest commitment.

Today's Torah portion relates to this issue in a specific context. This *parashah* speaks of "the Land which God swore to your ancestors," the Land of Israel. That land has been the focus of Jewish dreams and Jewish efforts throughout the millennia. The *mitzvah* of *Yishuv Ha-Aretz,* settling the land, became one of supreme importance.

There are many who are willing to sacrifice their own lives, and the lives of others, to acquire and to keep larger portions of that sacred soil.

In Israel today, and throughout world Jewry as a result, a vituperative debate rages between those who hold that *Eretz Yisrael* is the supreme value and others who insist that Jewish sovereignty and Jewish lives are the highest value. Because of that difference in perspective, some are willing to endanger Jewish lives to stake a claim to more of *Eretz Yisrael,* and some advocate abandoning some of the land in order to save Jewish lives, not to mention a sense of fairness for Palestinian nationalism as well.

Is the Land of Israel of ultimate value? Or is it a vehicle toward some more encompassing end?

The Torah portion we read this week is unambiguous on that score:

> Keep all the commandments which I command you this day, that you may be strong, and go in and possess the land, into which you go to possess it; and that you may prolong your days in the land.

The land is of importance, not as an end in itself, but as the *necessary backdrop for the fullest possible encounter with God.* Only within the Land of Israel is it possible to observe all the *mitzvot* commanded in the Torah and the Talmud, and only within the land are the rhythms of Jewish life and religion the basis of daily life.

Yet the significance of the land is not intrinsic to the land itself. The land is not the goal, but rather a sacred means to an even more sacred end. The ultimate goal is to observe all the commandments—including to "have one law for yourself and for the stranger," "seek peace and pursue peace," and "love the stranger."

The Land of Israel matters because it can lead to the creation of truly godly Jews. To the extent that we engage the promise of the land to become more compassionate, more loving, and more just—to that extent alone do we merit inhabiting the land. And only to that extent do we fulfill the purpose of our being there in the first place.

The ultimate goal of Judaism is to build godly Jews. The Land of Israel, as with every other aspect of Judaism, is a sacred rung on the ladder of holiness.

But the goal remains holiness, not the ladder itself.

✦

Parashat Ekev/It Came to Pass
Take 3

Serve the Coffee, Imitate God

Like many others, our culture enforces a rigorous hierarchy of authority. By watching how someone is dressed, the kind of work they do, how they are addressed, and how they address others, a member of American society can instantly determine a person's social standing. The boss is generally called by title ("Doctor") or by last name. The secretary isn't. The boss generally doesn't make the coffee, or water the plants; the secretary does. These nonverbal cues inform the participants and spectators of who's who in the pecking order at work and at home.

We tend to associate service tasks—cleaning, feeding, and watering—with a lower social status. The more powerful and important a person is, the less she is likely to sully her hands with these menial tasks.

Consider, for example, the path of a very motivated and intelligent teenage boy. For a first job, he might deliver papers or work in a fast-food restaurant clearing dishes. All who know him would admire his discipline, energy, and seriousness. But if he's still doing that ten years later, his parents will wring their hands in frustration at his lack of ambition. During his college years, he might volunteer to work in a politician's office, licking envelopes and answering the phone—again, a laudable demonstration of determination and drive. But if he's still doing that at the age of thirty, very few are going to see it as status enhancing. We expect a certain progression so that at some point, to retain our respect and admiration, this young man had better acquire an office of his own with his name on the door. And we don't expect him to answer his own phones, either. The fewer menial tasks he performs, the more we recognize his power and success.

Obviously, such a view of labor and service tends to encourage certain behaviors. If you are eager for prestige, don't be the one who brings drinks to your coworkers. We live with the subtle message to force others to care for you while you refuse to reciprocate on their behalf.

Not so Judaism.

In today's Torah portion, God compares the Land of Israel, which the tribes are about to enter, with the Land of Egypt. Praising *Eretz Yisrael,* God says, "There [Egypt] the grain you sowed had to be watered by your own labors . . . but the land you are about to cross into and possess . . . soaks up its water from the rains of heaven. It is a land which the Lord your God looks after."

The rabbis who compiled *Midrash Sifre Devarim* tell the story of a group of rabbis who were at a banquet held by the *Nasi,* the Jewish president, Rabban Gamaliel, in honor of his son. Rabban Gamaliel made a point of himself preparing and serving the wine, which one of the subordinate rabbis had refused to do, not wanting to appear to compromise the stature of the *Nasi.* His colleague, Rabbi Joshua, commented, "Let him serve. After all, Abraham, one of the great ones of the world, served the ministering angels when he thought they were pagans. . . . If Abraham, one of the great ones of the world, served those he thought were pagans, should not Gamaliel son of Rabbi serve us?"

Rabbi Zadok went even further in praise of serving others: "You have ignored God's honor in order to deal with the honor of flesh and blood. If the One-who-spoke-and-the-world-came-into-being causes winds to blow, brings up clouds, brings down rains, and raises vegetation, thus setting a table for everyone, should not Gamaliel son of Rabbi serve us?"

Rabbi Zadok and Rabbi Joshua understand that refusing to serve others does not enhance a person's dignity. Dignity is an inner quality—an ability to care about others and to embody responsibility and righteousness in one's deeds. Abraham serves as a biblical example of a prominent figure who saw his own dignity as enhanced by personally attending to the physical needs of others. And the ultimate role model of such meticulous care is God, who causes the rain to fall on *Eretz Yisrael* as a demonstration of love and support.

If *they* don't link status with a refusal to help others, why should we? Perhaps the foolish fear that one's dignity would be compromised by bringing someone a cup of coffee or by watering his plants is really an admission of insecurity, as if such trivial externalities really could diminish one's inner worth.

While executives, doctors, lawyers, and *machers* of all stripes eagerly avoid dirtying their hands to tidy up, perhaps it is their assistants and junior colleagues, rushing to care for the mundane needs of patients, colleagues, and clients, who are truly doing God's work in the world.

RE'EH/Behold!

Deuteronomy 11:26–16:17

Moses's preamble to the laws ends with the basic premise of the Torah: "See, this day I set before you blessing and curse." The choice, then as now, lies entirely in our own hands. Attention then shifts to the laws themselves, forming the longest section in Deuteronomy, and the royal road to a life rich in meaning, goodness, joy, and belonging. Rather than attempting to present a comprehensive code, complete with every detail, Deuteronomy lays out general principles, relying on an unwritten oral tradition to enumerate practice.

Moses begins with the sanctuary and maintaining religious consistency and purity. Idolatrous sites are to be destroyed, and God is to be worshipped only at a single site, the Temple in Jerusalem. "Together with your households, you shall feast there before Adonai your God, happy in all the undertakings in which Adonai your God has blessed you."

While sacrificial meat may only be offered in Jerusalem, provision is now made for the secular consumption of meat, through the laws of kashrut, *particularly removing the blood from any meat to be consumed.*

Eating in a way that is "good and right in the sight of God," the Jews are then told to shun religious syncretism (mixing alien forms of worship with Judaism). Toward that end, if someone, even a true prophet, seeks to get Jews to abandon the covenant, give up the mitzvot, *and to worship anyone other than Adonai, such a person is being sent to test their fidelity and courage. Jews are to resist that enticement and remove that prophet from their midst, "for he urged disloyalty to Adonai our God to make you stray from the path that Adonai your God commanded you to follow." This is the commanded response, for prophet, individual, or entire town seeking to separate Jews from Torah and Judaism.*

Laws of holiness follow, dealing with mourning and with dietary laws. Jews are prohibited from gashing ourselves in mourning, and are prohibited from eating any land animals except those with cloven hooves that chew their cud, sea animals with fins and scales, and particular birds. Again the Torah prohibits seething a kid in its mother's milk.

Finally, the Torah lays out recurrent obligations: tithes owed annually and every three years, the Sabbatical year remission of debts, freeing the eved Ivri (Hebrew servant) at the end of seven years (or arranging for permanent bondage if the servant chooses it), and the three annual pilgrimage festivals: Pesah (Passover), Shavuot (the Feast of Weeks), and Sukkot (the Feast of Booths).

✦

Parashat Re'eh/Behold!
Take 1

Smelling the Roses as Holy Act

We have enough reasons to let worry consume our lives. Parents don't meet our needs fully; children don't quite live up to our expectations. Spouses are all too human. Beyond these disappointments loom life's larger issues: aging, illness, fears of separation and mortality, the devastation of our environment, the threat of random violence, and so on, and so on.

In the midst of all these anxieties, how are we to live? Isn't unrelenting gloom a rational response? Many scholars and philosophers, struck by life's apparent pointlessness, have counseled emotional withdrawal from the passions of living for precisely that reason. Nothing will change, nothing will improve. We live and we die, without hope of any real breakthrough in human understanding or harmony. Is despair the most logical attitude to cultivate?

Perhaps it is. But people are never strictly rational, and life is far too variegated to fit any single response.

For the spiritually alive, life is a constant marvel. Without having asked to live, without doing anything to deserve the gifts of life, companionship, and joy, we are offered these gifts in an abundance that is staggering. Religion helps restore our thanks for everything we receive so effortlessly. Serving God implies the capacity to feel gratitude, a response of joy to the many wonders of living:

- For the miracle that parents and children can spend their lifetimes getting to know each other as people, growing to accept, appreciate, and love each other as independent human beings, not merely as objects to satisfy their own needs;

- For the miracle of being able to build and celebrate community—the joy of sharing in the struggles and rewards of other people's lives;
- For the miracle of being able to make this world a little better, a little more caring, a little more humane than it was when we entered it;
- For the miracle of being able to cultivate holiness in our daily lives, the miracle of *simhah shel mitzvah,* the joy of being a Jew and of observing the commandments;
- For the miracle—perhaps the greatest one of all—of simply *being*: having an opportunity to think, feel, experience, and wonder. Most of the time we take life for granted; we assume we deserve it, we have it coming to us. At the death of a loved one, that illusion is shattered. At rare moments in our lives—births, graduations, bar/bat mitzvahs, marriages—we see the marvel of life, and for brief spells are able to appreciate both the Giver and the gift.

Parashat Re'eh bids us "rejoice before the Lord of God." Judaism has consistently recognized *joy* as the most fitting response to God's abundant love. As the prophet Joel exclaimed, "Rejoice and be glad, for the Lord has done great things."

To look at the world and see those great deeds requires eyes trained to appreciate. Our tradition bids us to cultivate awareness, mindfulness, and beyond mindfulness, a thrill at being alive. Our traditions recognize that smelling the roses can be a religious act.

"One who has seen something pleasant and has not enjoyed it will be held responsible," Judaism teaches us. To reject a legitimate pleasure is to diminish the extent to which we truly live, to reject God's most fundamental gift. Enjoying life is a way to say "thank you."

And in the midst of enjoying the pleasures of living, Judaism bids us to remember those who cannot rejoice without our help.

In the words of the Rambam, "the Torah sensitizes us to assure the joy of the powerless, the poor, and the stranger." Reaching beyond the narrow boundaries of self and embracing our fellows as well, cultivating fellowship with our families, our communities, our people, and with God, we attain a true joy.

Parashat Re'eh/Behold!
Take 2

Commanded or Free?

The question of whether Jews are obligated by the practices and values of our religion is an issue that has divided our people into separate camps today.

On one hand, an intense and thriving religious coalition insists that the commandments come from God directly, and are therefore binding for all time, regardless of changing insight, circumstances, or preferences. Passionate about fidelity to the *mitzvot* of the Torah and the Talmud, these Jews hold *obedience* as the cardinal Jewish virtue. After all, we are told not to be "seduced by your heart or led astray by your eyes." Loyalty and obedience are the core of Jewish religion.

On the other hand, another large and thriving coalition of Jews is equally insistent that God's voice is unclear. While holding our traditional texts in great esteem as guides and as repositories of wisdom and historical experiences, these Jews nonetheless affirm that each individual must decide what is God's will for him or herself. We are urged not to "follow a majority to do evil." Autonomy, therefore, is the guiding, indeed preeminent, principle of Jewish faith.

Both of these perspectives offer a valuable insight for Jewish living and Jewish vitality.

It is unquestionable that Judaism has specific content. That content may be dynamic, but it has real contours and priorities that remain constant throughout the ages. Our religion's ability to construct a path to holiness and a relationship with God results from its wisdom and its viewpoint, both of which are distinctive and concrete. We cannot simply list our preferences and then call the emerging brew "Judaism."

It is also clear that the very basis of Judaism is the power of human beings to make choices, to be responsible for their own lives. In the words of the *Mishnah,* "All is foreseen, yet freedom of choice is given." In today's Torah portion, as well, God tells us, "See, this day I set before you blessing and curse."

The rabbis of the Talmud note that the Hebrew grammar of this phrase is surprising—it begins in the singular and ends in the plural! What lesson, they ask, is buried in that awkward construction?

According to our sages, we learn from the singular *re'eh*, see, that the *mitzvot* are given to the entire people—all Jews as a group. The contours of our religion are not the personal preference of each individual Jew.

Yet, at the same time, the phrase ends with *lif'neikhem*, before you (all), a plural construct, to remind us that each individual must decide whether to commit heart, mind, and soul to cultivating our *brit* with God. No one can force you to be obedient; no one can compel observance of the commandments. Each one of us has the power to choose to say yes or to say no.

In fact, the very notion of commandments implies the idea of free choice; otherwise, they mean nothing. Dogs don't need to be commanded to eat. When they see food, they eat out of an inner compulsion; there is no choice involved.

Jews do need to be commanded to keep kosher, love the stranger, visit the sick, and observe *Tishah b'Av*, because these actions don't come naturally to anybody. They require conscious choice, discipline, and desire.

For a *mitzvah*, a command, to have any ability to elevate and to make holy, we must retain the power to decline to act. Only then does our choice to be loyal to Torah, our efforts to serve God in all our ways, reflect a commitment of thoughtful acceptance, rather than an automaton's programming. Throughout history, Jews have had the power to choose.

But the power to choose doesn't mean that every choice is equally wise, equally sacred, or equally conducive to the transmission of Torah and Judaism.

We can choose to let the homeless remain on the streets. We have that power. We can choose to transform our eating into an act of holiness and solidarity with Jews throughout time. We have that power, too.

In ritual, as in ethics, we can choose. And we can choose incorrectly. God has given us the choice: "See, this day set before you blessing and curse: blessing, if you obey the commandments of the Lord your God . . . and curse, if you do not."

Choose wisely today.

Parashat Re'eh/Behold!

Take 3

Joy: Gratitude or Vanity?

Throughout the ages, we humans have struggled with integrating the reality of our own individual finitude with the vastness of human suffering and injustice. Is it moral to celebrate while others suffer? How much and what must I give up for the sake of the common good?

Assuming that there have always been paupers, outcasts, the vilified, and the deviant, to what extent must we give up our own joys and possessions to try to minimize their pain? Is it obscenity to feast in a world of hunger? Should we forgo a luxurious vacation because so many fellow citizens are homeless? Is there a moral justification to owning more than two suits or dresses when so many human beings on earth lack basic clothing or blankets?

There is no neat formula for balancing these two needs. Common sense urges some restraint; it is possible to be too lavish, too ostentatious. But it is no less possible to give up the legitimate joys of living without making any appreciable difference in the level of suffering in the world.

The Torah urges us to act with moderation, bidding us to reasonable celebration coupled with responsible *tzedakah* and restraint, in its approach to the most joyous days of the calendar year. In relaying God's commands for observing the festival of *Shavuot*, the Torah records, "You shall rejoice before the Lord your God with your son and daughter, your male and female slave, the Levite in your communities, and the stranger, the orphan, and the widow in your midst."

The first part of the instruction seems obvious: Anyone would include his or her children and household in a major celebration. What is less clear is why the celebrant must include the Levite, stranger, orphan, and widow.

Rashi provides a beautiful explanation. Noting the symmetry of numbers between the household of the celebrating Jew and the number of the needy, he puts the following into God's mouth: "Four of mine corresponding to four of yours: 'your son, your daughter, your male slave, and your female slave.' If you will gladden Mine, I will gladden yours."

The poor and the outcast have God's special concern and love. Just as our tradition informs us that God dwells in the broken heart, so here

Rashi is asserting that the poor lay special claim to God's love and therefore to our care. If we claim to serve God, there is no escaping the consequence of that relationship. Moving beyond inner spirituality, or political action, Judaism reflects the Divine imperative to personally nurture those abandoned by others and by society.

In fact, Rashi goes on to assert that the *mitzvah* of remembering that we were slaves in Egypt is the primary reason that God redeemed us in the first place.

An awareness of our own lowly origins and a memory of having suffered the hatred and scorn of Egyptian power can only lead us to adopt the weak and the despised as our own. Our holy days and festivals, then, become special occasions for demonstrating that we do remember what slavery feels like. Judaism seeks to enact God's command that every celebration must also become an opportunity for giving *tzedakah* and performing acts of *gemillut hasadim,* loving-kindness.

Caring for our own is a *mitzvah*. To refrain from celebrating is to diminish the joy and goodness of God's gift of life and community. Being alive is always an occasion for feasting and singing together; all the more so is the miraculous Jewish history of salvation and sanctification that stretches across the millennia. As heirs of that sacred past and messianic hope, our celebrations are properly an expression of gratitude and love.

But celebration that does not include *mattanot le-evyonim,* gifts to the poor, is the very opposite of gratitude. In fact, such celebration reveals mere vanity and self-absorption.

Reaffirming our membership in the larger family of humanity while still appreciating the pleasures that life offers, Jewish celebration builds community, sensitivity, and happiness. Such rejoicing is surely worth the effort.

SHOFTIM/Judges

Deuteronomy 16:18–21:9

Parashat Shoftim *deals with the primary arms of authority in biblical Israel: judges, monarchs, priests, and prophets. The Israelites are to appoint magistrates and judges in each settlement, and these are commanded to show impartiality toward all cases and petitioners, being scrupulous to avoid any bribes. "Justice, justice shall you pursue" was to guide their deliberations and their procedures.*

Three prohibited religious practices—setting up an asherah *(pagan wooden pillar), sacrificing an animal with a* mum *(blemish), allowing an apostate to remain—interrupt the discussion of judges, perhaps to indicate the importance of serving God properly as the cornerstone to true justice. The Torah provides a system of referral, from a local court to a high court, to handle cases that the local court cannot decide. This biblical grant of authority to "the magistrate in charge at the time" and the mandate to "observe scrupulously all their instructions to you" so that "you must not deviate from their verdict" forms the basis for rabbinic authority to this very day.*

The Israelites are permitted to establish a monarchy as they desire, but Moses places limits on the king's authority and power. The only responsibility that Deuteronomy explicitly assigns the king is to write and study a copy of the Torah. Clearly, this monarchy was to be under the authority of the law, and answerable to it. The king's wealth, stables, and harem were all limited so that "he will not act haughtily toward his fellows or deviate from the Torah." The section dealing with the clergy establishes that the kohanim *are to receive the offerings and sacrifices, from which they are to support themselves. The Torah then lists the specific portions they may rightfully claim. Finally, a Levite, no matter where in Israel he dwells, may claim the right to serve in the Temple. The prophet looms large in the Deuteronomic vision, and the book of Deuteronomy seeks to strengthen the authority and scope of the prophets. Alone of all biblical authorities, the prophet's basis is a quotation from God, rather than Moses's own words. The prophet is the heir to Moses himself. The* parashah *then restates the laws of the cities of asylum, establishes the law regarding intentional murder, and discusses the inviolability of boundaries and the law requiring not less than two witnesses. Chapter 20 establishes the laws of just warfare, limiting the extent to which the military can strike against civilians, who may be drafted, and the treatment of surrounding agriculture. Chapter 21 deals with a case of unsolved murder.*

✦

Parashat Shoftim/Judges
Take 1

The Divine Power of Shalom

Encamped on the borders of the Holy Land, preparing to conquer and inhabit *Eretz Yisrael,* the Jewish tribes hear a description of the laws of warfare for the first time. While we may take legal guidelines for combat for granted, the question of whether there should even be laws of war has been questioned in every age.

From its inception, Judaism has affirmed that war, being a human activity, is properly a subject for moral consideration and for legal limitation. An extensive "just war" tradition emerges out of the earliest layers of Jewish law, from the Torah, the *midrashim,* and the *Mishnah.* Jewish scholars have extended that tradition right into our own age, addressing issues of noncombatant immunity, siege warfare, and preemptive strikes from the perspective of the eternal values and structures of *halakhah.*

One of the first commandments about waging just war is found in *Parashat Shoftim.* In describing the procedures appropriate for the conquest of *Eretz Yisrael,* God mandates that "when you approach a town to attack it, you shall offer it terms of peace."

What a paradox! In responding to the most sacred war of Jewish tradition—the only war commanded explicitly by God, the one war which would allow Israel to live and thrive in its own land—even in that war the Jews are commanded to seek peace first.

Such is the greatness of peace.

In English, the primary meaning of the word *peace* is an absence of hostilities. Peace, itself, has no positive or inherent content; it is merely the lack of a negative condition.

In Hebrew, however, the connotation of *shalom* is one of fullness, completion, and wholeness. Peace is not simply a lack of violence; peace is the ultimate condition of fulfillment, the purpose of creation and of human creativity.

The rabbis of the Talmud and *midrashim* noted the centrality of the idea of *shalom* and enshrined it as the central value of rabbinic Judaism. Thus, they taught that "peace is the foundation and principle of the entire Torah, and the essential element in the creation of the world."

Those same rabbis took a relatively enigmatic biblical figure, Aaron the *Kohen Gadol* (high priest), and transformed him into a symbol of peace. As the great sage Hillel taught, "Strive to become a disciple of Aaron the kohen, one who loves peace and pursues peace." Tales were told of how Aaron would reconcile neighbors, friends, and even spouses—such was his passion in pursuing peace.

The Temple in Jerusalem was similarly transformed into a symbol of peace. Its altar restored peace between humanity and our Parent in Heaven; consequently, the use of any metal implement on its altar was prohibited. Why? Because "the altar was made to prolong life and iron is used to shorten it."

The same transformation elevated the Torah itself into a symbol of peace: "All her ways are pleasant, and all her paths are peace."

Shabbat, too, became the great day of peace throughout Jewish history, and, according to Kabbalistic legend, throughout the cosmos as well.

The central Jewish institutions—the Torah, *Shabbat,* the Temple—and the central religious figure, the *Kohen Gadol,* were transformed into living symbols of peace to demonstrate the centrality of that value at the core of Jewish teaching.

The rabbis went on to reinforce its centrality through the composition of Jewish prayer. Each major Jewish prayer—the *Kaddish,* the *Amidah,* and the *Birkat Kohanim* (priestly benediction)—concludes with a prayer for peace. In fact, the rabbis correctly understood that once humanity accepted peace as the essential goal of the universe, as a state of wholeness and completion, it would recognize a commitment to peace not as a sign of weakness, but rather as a commitment to a new and transforming kind of strength: "God will give strength to God's People; the Lord's People shall be blessed with peace."

You Can So Be Too Rich

We are justly proud of the ability of our economy to provide so many basics and so much comfort to our own people and to those around the world. The power of American enterprise, with its abundance and its energy, is remarkable by any standard. What used to be affordable only for nobility and the wealthy is now within reach of the average American.

We're all familiar with the popular adage, "You can never be too rich or too thin." Well, we've learned, of course, that indeed you *can* be too thin. We read of and perhaps ourselves know anorexics in our own society. As photographs of starving children flood our newspapers and television shows, we also see that for many of the world's people, being too thin is a dangerous part of the human condition.

But what about our wealth? Is it possible to be too wealthy? Imagine the wonderful activities and comforts you could buy with more money—a luxurious mansion, perhaps a *pied à terre* in some exotic part of the world, expensive art, magnificent jewelry—the possibilities are enticing and endless. Money may not be able to buy happiness, but it might well buy the things that buy happiness.

But today's Torah portion relates an example of too much wealth in ancient Israel: the king. The Torah says of the king,

> He shall not keep many horses or send people back to Egypt to add to his horses. . . . And he shall not have many wives, lest his heart go astray; nor shall he amass silver and gold to excess.

Apparently, it *is* possible to possess too much silver and gold. God's concern is that the king will become the captive of his wealth; that all those possessions will alter his perspective and determine his agenda.

In striking contrast to the rest of the world, ancient Israel was a notoriously democratic society. After leaving Egypt, the Israelite slaves did not establish a new state. Instead, they founded a system of laws that applied equally to every member of society. No nobility, no monarchy could alter the egalitarian nature of biblical Israel. In the eyes of God, all were equal. In the eyes of society, the only sovereign was God.

After two hundred years of this democracy, the people longed for a king to rule over them, so they could be "like all the nations." That repudiation of Jewish distinctiveness was the death knell for the sacred way that had sustained our people. The law in the Torah accurately summarized what happened with Israel's kings. Obsessed with adding more palaces, more slaves, more wives, and more wealth, they led the nation away from the moral rigor and passion for justice that characterizes the Torah. Instead of focusing on wealth, the Torah urges another form of responsibility for the king:

> When he is seated on his royal throne, he shall have a copy of this Teaching written for him on a scroll by the Levitical priests. Let it remain with him and let him read in it all his life, so that he may learn to revere the Lord his God, to observe faithfully every word of this Teaching as well as these laws. Thus he will not act haughtily toward his fellows, or deviate from the Instruction to the right or to the left.

Rather than focusing on his wealth, the king is commanded to focus on the Torah. By reading it repeatedly, he will retain a perspective about what is of eternal worth, and what is merely a tool for better living. When the ultimate focus in life is money and the things that money can buy, the feelings of other people are of little esteem, and the values of our tradition seem largely irrelevant.

Ironically, when wealth is the highest goal, no amount of money is enough. Insatiable demand can never be satisfied.

But if money and comfort are recognized for what they are, useful tools to allow us to focus on other things—character, compassion, justice, and spirit—then it becomes possible to experience contentment.

One can own enough, and enjoy sufficient income to be able to attend to the needs of others and one's own morality. More than that is too much.

"Who is rich?" the *Mishnah* asks. "One who is content with his portion."

This *Shabbat,* consider just how rich you already are . . . and how content.

Can't You Take a Joke?

Why is it that the first line of defense after hurting someone else is often an automatic, "Hey, can't you take a joke?"

How often have you heard a racist or anti-Semitic joke, only to have your discomfort met with, "It's only a joke!" People who humiliate gays or lesbians defend their hostility by insisting their remarks are meant as a joke, and that their victims are oversensitive. I've heard men joke about rape and then tell some offended woman that she has no sense of humor.

Jokes are serious business, the traditions of Judaism teach us, particularly when the apparent joke is really a thin veil for prejudice and hatred. For all behavior, the rabbis teach us, is interconnected, and moral standards are just as crucial for the seemingly trivial as for the more obviously significant.

These insights emerge from the rabbis' interpretation of a line from this week's Torah portion: the penalties exacted from a man who "hate[s] his neighbor, and lie[s] in wait for him, and rise[s] up against him."

The rabbis of *Midrash Sifrei Devarim* interpret that passage as elliptical: Some essential steps have been left out in the middle. According to their reconstruction, "If a person transgresses a minor commandment, he will eventually transgress a major commandment. If he transgresses 'you shall love your neighbor' he will eventually transgress 'you shall not bear a grudge' until he ends up shedding blood."

Commanded as we are to love one another, it is a small step to begin to hate another. Others may seem strange to us, different, unwilling to live the way we do. Rather than stretch ourselves to see the good that *they* embody, to understand their struggle to do the best *they* can, we cast them in the role of the enemy. Once we strip someone of her humanity, it is easy to create rationales for bearing a grudge against her. And after living with the grudge for long enough, it's not so tough to curdle that resentment into full-fledged hatred. Once the hatred is well established, justifying treating the object of one's hatred indecently—refusing to employ them, or to rent to them—or to serve them becomes very easy. Disgust shown passively melts easily into active disgust: curses shouted from a passing car escalate to brutal beatings.

The Torah, in shorthand, and the rabbis more explicitly, tell us that there is no such thing as a harmless joke. Any humor that stigmatizes and degrades people is directly linked to later acts of violence that erupt against those same people. Telling jokes against Jews, women, Poles, blacks, gays, or any other group of people is the first step down the slippery slope of abasement and abuse. Such comments create an atmosphere of acceptability for stripping a human being of humanity.

Hence, say the rabbis, the need for a commandment to love in the first place. Hence, they insist, the need to observe all the *mitzvot,* even those that seem paltry. In Rashi's summation: "Because he transgressed against 'you shall not hate' he will eventually come to shed blood."

Living with the consequences of this insight requires restructuring the way we speak of others, not only the way we act toward them. Our words become slings to wound, weaken, and create misery. These wounds are no less painful because they are not physical; what we *say* about other people can lead to physical violence we would abhor.

Someone else is a little too sensitive? Maybe the real problem is our *lack* of sensitivity.

Can't take a joke? Maybe because the joke resembles the tragedies of human hatred all too common in the world.

Don't have a sense of humor? Why should people laugh at their own degradation?

"Don't judge other people until you have stood in their shoes," instructs our *Mishnah.* And don't accuse them of lacking a sense of humor unless *you're* willing to laugh at being hated, too.

KI-TETZE/When You Go Forth
Deuteronomy 21:10–25:19

This lengthy parashah *contains the final collection of laws in Deuteronomy, a miscellany dealing with private concerns.* Here are laws *dealing with the individual and the family, communities, and neighbors, as opposed to matters of state or public authority.*

The parashah *begins with three family laws: laws limiting the prerogatives of a man who captures a woman in warfare, establishing the rights of a firstborn child in a polygamous family, and discussing the punishment of a* ben sorer u-moreh *(a stubborn and rebellious son).*

Given that *the body reflects the Divine image, the Torah mandates respectful treatment for the corpse of an executed criminal.*

Chapter 22 *presents a series of laws: on returning lost animals and lost property, assisting a fallen animal, maintaining gender distinction in dress, treatment of a mother bird and her eggs, and building a parapet on the roof. Laws follow prohibiting sowing mixed seeds in a single field, plowing with an ox and ass, and wearing clothing made of shaatnez (linen and wool). Four-cornered garments require tzitzit (tassels).*

A series of *laws about sexual misconduct deals with premarital sex, adultery, and rape. Chapter 23 continues the theme with a listing of forbidden relationships, then shifts to a discussion of who may or may not enter into God's assembly.*

The remaining laws *span a range of topics: the sanctity of the camp, asylum for escaped slaves, cultic prostitution. Lending on interest is prohibited, and the fulfillment of vows is mandated. One is allowed to eat in another person's vineyard.*

Chapter 24 *continues this eclectic listing, forbidding remarriage to an ex-spouse if she remarried in the interim. A man is allowed to postpone military service if newly married. There are laws on kidnapping, skin affliction, taking property to compel repayment of a defaulted loan, and prompt payment of wages.*

Passion for God *requires passion for justice, for "everyone who deals dishonestly is abhorrent to Adonai your God." The parashah ends with the ultimate symbol of dishonest, cruel treatment, that of Amalek, who "cut down the stragglers in your rear." Israel is commanded, therefore, to blot out Amalek's memory.*

✦✧✦

Parashat Ki-Tetze/When You Go Forth
Take 1
Making Waves

As we go about the routines of daily living, how often do we see someone who could use our help: a driver with a flat tire by the side of the road, someone burdened by too many packages, an elderly person afraid to cross a busy street?

How often do we silently sit through a joke that stereotypes and insults other people for their race, religion, gender, or sexual orientation? How often do we hear a bigoted remark or witness a racist act, and yet we still keep quiet?

How often have we passed a beggar and given nothing, or driven past someone asking for a job because he is homeless, and don't consider how we might help him?

We are tempted, in those situations and in countless others just like them, to do nothing. By our very nature, human beings simply do not like to rock the boat.

It may be human to be indifferent; it may be natural and it may be how we feel. But Jewish tradition, in this as in so many other arenas of human behavior, insists that we improve on nature, that we learn to override our feelings. The Torah commands us to make waves. When human suffering is at issue, we are not allowed to remain neutral or silent.

This week's Torah portion goads us beyond our usual complacency, and instructs us to involve ourselves in the struggles of our fellow human beings.

"If you see your fellow's ox or sheep gone astray, do not ignore it; you must take it back to your fellow." Not just your neighbor's animals, but also garments and any other property which belongs to someone else must be returned. All these obligations fit under the more general command "You must not remain indifferent."

This positive commandment obligates us all. It provokes us beyond our indifference, beyond our usual self-centered obsessions, and forces us to reorient our focus. Rather than allowing us to occupy our own total attention, the Torah shifts us to God and to God's perspective. While from our position, we may justify minding our own business, from God's perspective all life is a matter of spiritual concern. As God's agents on earth, we are charged with the care of every living thing.

Having articulated this perspective of responsibility and compassion in a positive commandment, the Torah also presents it through a negative example. The Torah tells us that no Moabite or Ammonite can ever be admitted into the congregation of the Lord, "because they did not meet you with food and water on your journey after you left Egypt."

Traditional commentators have understood this passage to mean that no Ammonite or Moabite can ever convert to Judaism, because they failed to demonstrate empathy and concern at that crucial moment.

An additional way to understand the verse is to recognize that the failure of the Ammonites and the Moabites to care and to act on their caring is itself evidence that they are not part of a holy congregation.

A person who claims to be religious, yet who cannot take an extra moment to respond to human need, demonstrates the shallowness of his or her own "faith." Such religiosity is still centered on selfish personal priorities. True spirituality, on the other hand, responds to God's needs.

※

Parashat Ki-Tetze/When You Go Forth
Take 2

You Are Unique, and So Is Your Donkey

Ours is a culture that maintains a paradoxical relationship to individuality. On the surface, America is a place that elevates the rugged individual above all others. It's you and me against the world, the popular song reminds us. By ourselves, we build our lives around initiative, energy, and a willingness to break from the past. American democracy is robust and passionate about personal liberty.

Our ideals may stress individualism, but our reality is starkly different. While praising the individual as the highest American ideal, we spend tremendous amounts of energy and money assuring ourselves that we don't differ too much from everyone else. We work hard to wear the same clothes, live in similar houses, pursue similar hobbies, and express remarkably similar opinions.

A person who acts too much like an individual is regarded as an eccentric if rich; a kook, if not; and, somehow, a threat to everybody else's convention and habit.

From the very first, we socialize our children into the rules and standards of the general culture. Standardization requires that they forsake the pleasures of simply being, the joy of aimless discovery. Instead, we foist a premature adulthood on our children, and then wonder at the immaturity that emerges from our adults.

Rather than permitting our children a period of undirected exploration, rather than teaching them to do something because of their own inner interests, we cultivate conformity in terms of achievement, awards, and, ultimately, careers.

Once the child enters adulthood, the preoccupation with compliance expands to include clothing styles, sexual expression, and even recreational activities. To a great degree, our frantic pursuit of leisure time reflects the monotony and stress of having to be like everybody else. It's simply too exhausting to have to keep up with the Joneses.

We forget the notion of age-appropriate behavior, the absence of a single standard for every single person, a child's need to live a child's life; we forget that each individual will express his or her personality in unique and changing ways. Just as human beings grow and evolve through every phase of life, so our expectations and our interests ought to shift and develop to incorporate new insight, new depth, and new contentment.

The Torah recognizes the need for standards to fit the personality of each individual. In today's reading, we are told "you shall not plow with an ox and a donkey together." Why not? Because the way an ox plows and the way a donkey plows are not the same. One animal would constantly feel pressured to adopt the standards of the other. In the process, the internal needs of that animal would be abandoned.

Each individual has needs and perceptions that change and evolve throughout his or her own life. No two people are in exactly the same place emotionally at the same time. Indeed, no one retains a static personality throughout time.

One aspect of the genius of Judaism is its ability to blend the changing and growing of each person with his or her continuing need for structure and belonging. Each different mood and thought adds to the sum of who we are. Each requires different times and modes of expression. In the words of *Kohelet,* "a season is set for everything, a time for every experience under heaven."

To be fully human means to seek out avenues to express responsibility and spontaneity, playfulness and seriousness, love and solitude. To focus only on one particular aspect of our personalities would be a diminution of our truest humanity.

Instead, by recalling the imperative not to link an ox and a donkey to the same plow, the Torah reminds us not to flatten our personalities into a homogeneous, unchanging mass.

Rather, by providing appropriate vehicles to express the range of human emotions and insight, Judaism assures a meaningful place for each individual within a caring and sacred community.

◆〰◆〰

Parashat Ki-Tetze/When You Go Forth
Take 3

Is Portnoy Responsible for His Mother? (And Is She, for Him?)

To what degree are children responsible for their parents' actions? And just how often must parents assume responsibility for the behavior of their children?

On the surface, most of us recoil from the notion that one person should share the blame for the actions of another. After all, if a parent acts recklessly, or accepts an ideology that is either foolish or dangerous, what does that have to do with the children? Perhaps they never found out what their parents believe. Or perhaps they know and protest inwardly, feeling bound to remain silent out of a sense of loyalty to their own family.

In a society founded on the notion of rugged individualism, it isn't hard to make the case that each of us is responsible only for our own actions. Consequently, we can easily agree with the instruction of this week's Torah portion, "You shall not execute the parent for the children, nor the children for the parents; each shall be executed only for their own sin."

Clearly, any moral or legal judgment about a person's deeds should not automatically include his family, religion, ethnicity, or nation. Only the individual is responsible for his own behavior.

But is that always true?

Elsewhere, the Torah describes God as One who "visits the iniquity of the parents on the children." That same description of God begins by affirming that God is "gracious and compassionate, patient, abounding in kindness and faithfulness." If all of those attributes describe God, perhaps it is possible to see some justice in holding children responsible for their parents, and holding parents responsible for their progeny.

The rabbis of antiquity wrestled with the fact that the same Torah contains both verses. Assuming that both verses cannot refer to the same issue, the *Sifrei*, a *midrash* on Deuteronomy, explains that today's portion deals with the question of testimony, establishing that "parents shall not be executed on the testimony of their own children, nor children on the testimony of their parents." In other words, immediate family members enjoy a right not to incriminate each other.

The Talmud offers a different way to understand the presence of the apparently contradictory passages. It explains that "one verse deals with children who continue in the same course as their parents, and the other verse with children who do not continue in the course of their parents." The distinction, according to this passage, is that children who allow the teachings and actions of their parents to dictate their own values and practices are responsible for their parents' deeds as well.

But that position raises yet another question: If we are responsible for our own actions, then whether we perpetuate the deeds of our parents is irrelevant. We will be punished, justly, for our own deeds, whether our parents initiated the practice or not. So why punish us for our parents' deeds even if we do continue them?

The Talmud offers us an insight into what it means to be a family. In our age, with so much emphasis placed on the individual identities of each family member, perhaps the Talmud's logic can serve as a useful reminder that being family means having your nose in each other's business. There is no way to separate intimacy and caring from involvement and intrusion. While it may be necessary to learn when to back off, it is also necessary to learn how to be *involved* in the lives of those we love.

In a sense, then, parents and children *do* shoulder a responsibility for the deeds of each other. As close relatives, we are responsible for sharing our insights and opinions with those we love. We are the only ones with the commitment to stay with a person throughout their errors and their folly. And that persistence carries with it the obligation to mediate reality for our parents and our children.

The two verses, then, both teach a necessary truth—that human law and human courts can only hold each individual accountable for her own deeds. And that God's perspective is one in which loving people act as guides, counselors, and occasionally as nudges, on behalf of their companions through life's journey.

KI-TAVO/When You Come In
Deuteronomy 26:1–29:8

Ki-Tavo *begins with the offer of prayers to be recited by farmers, one when bringing the first fruit offerings to the Temple and the other when giving the tithe to the poor every three years. These are the only examples of fixed liturgy addressing God the words of which are established by the Torah.*

All of the details of the laws are now enumerated, and Moses offers a conclusion to the lengthy series of rules and legislation completed. These are more than mere rules; they are the structure of a comprehensive relationship between the people Israel and God. In fulfilling these mitzvot, Israel "shall be, as God promised, a holy people to Adonai your God."

There are three ceremonies to be performed once Israel has entered the land:

1. *Erecting stone tablets with the text of the Torah, building an altar, and performing sacrifices at Mount Ebal.*
2. *The standing of the tribes on Mount Gerizim and Mount Ebal, there to proclaim the blessings and curses that the covenant can evoke.*
3. *The listing of the punishments by the Levites when people sin in ways difficult to try in human courts; the people are to affirm those punishments.*

The parashah *then proceeds with a lengthy description of the blessings awaiting Israel if it obeys God's law and lives by the terms of the covenant, and an even more extensive treatment of the punishments which will follow the violation of that covenant.*

This section concludes the second address: "These are the terms of the covenant which Adonai commanded Moses to conclude with the Israelites in the land of Moab, in addition to the covenant which God had made with them at Horeb."

Moses's third address urges ratification of the additional covenant: "Therefore observe faithfully all the terms of this covenant, that you may succeed in all that you undertake."

⁂

Parashat Ki-Tavo/When You Come In
Take 1

Normal Mystics and Wandering Arameans

From the first rays of the sun in the morning, through our meals, our chores, our friendships, our studies, and our work, we respond to a vast array of fragrances, sounds, visions, and thoughts each day. Whether we pay attention to all these sensations, whether they evoke a sense of joy and gratitude in us reveals more about our own attitudes than it does about these miracles of daily living.

For some of us, daily routine and a sense of entitlement blind us to the marvel of being alive. We notice how wonderful the faculty of sight is if we are threatened by its loss, and value good health only when we are ill. Living our lives retrospectively, the past seems ideal and the present, bland.

Yet the same events can be experienced as traces of something larger, Divine energy, symbols of God's desire to love and to be loved by human beings. Every day can ignite a response of wonder and awe.

Ki-Tavo, this week's Torah-reading, offers two prayers to be recited by each Israelite upon fulfilling a *mitzvah*. One prayer may be readily familiar, and the other more obscure, but both reveal the power of awe to inspire a sense of God's love and involvement in mundane ordinary activities.

Hebrew farmers recited the first prayer when they brought their first-fruit offerings, *bikkurim*, to the Temple in Jerusalem. Now found in the Passover *Haggadah*, it begins with the line "My father was a wandering Aramean." The prayer recounts the history of the Jewish People—our wanderings into Egypt and slavery, our miraculous liberation and settlement in the Land of Israel.

The second prayer was recited when a farmer set aside a tenth of his produce as a tithe, *Ma'aser Sheni*, for the poor, the Levite, or the non-Jew, three groups who would have needed special assistance in biblical

Israel. The farmer related what he had done, and then said: "I have obeyed the Lord my God. I have done just as You commanded me. Look down from Your holy abode, from heaven, and bless your people Israel."

Both prayers follow on the heels of fairly mundane activities. In the initial instance, the Jew has offered his first harvest. In the second, the farmer has provided food for the poor. Neither actions necessarily point beyond themselves; they happen all the time, and anyone can perform them. There is no need to see in them anything more than the generosity of a particular farmer and the fertility of one particular piece of land.

Jewish tradition, however, is not content with seeing the world as sufficient in itself. Instead, the Torah and rabbinic traditions repeatedly sensitize us to the role of diversity in our lives.

In reciting a prayer that summarizes Divine involvement, the farmer draws his own attention—and that of his listeners—beyond the limits of the event itself. Suddenly, on recital of a *berakhah,* a blessing, or the performance of a *mitzvah,* the Jew sees physical reality as embodying the transcendent.

Transforming an everyday practice into the occasion for a *mitzvah* infuses a dimension of holiness into an otherwise commonplace occurrence. *Normal mysticism* was the term that Rabbi Max Kadushin applied to Judaism's commitment to experience the presence of God in the mundane activities of daily living.

Awareness of the sacred awakens a new sensitivity to nature. "The Heavens declare the glory of God" only to the person open to looking for God's glory in the first place.

By involving us in a network of deeds, and by understanding those deeds as a response to the Divine, Judaism infuses our daily pattern of activities with a sense of wonder, with the possibility of mystical awakening at every turn.

A Still Small Voice

What Jew does not know the *Sh'ma,* the biblical declaration of God's unity, which the rabbis of the Talmud used as a pledge of allegiance? "Hear, O Israel, the Lord is our God, the Lord alone." This verse signified an acceptance of God's sovereignty over each individual Jew. To this day, observant Jews recite it during the *Shaharit* prayers of the morning, during *Ma'ariv* at night, and again in bed before falling asleep.

In *Parashat Ki-Tavo,* the Torah presents a second *Sh'ma,* one no less revolutionary in its insight. The Torah says, "Hear, O Israel, . . . the voice of the Lord your God and observe His *mitzvot* and His laws."

As it unfolds in the Torah and in rabbinic writings, Torah insists on the fusion of the ritual and the ethical. That blend of moral sensitivity and ritual profundity meets in the *mitzvah,* the commanded deed.

One would assume, therefore, that a Jew who observes the *mitzvot* is fulfilling all possible religious expectations. But if that is the case, why does this second *Sh'ma* need to add an additional category? "Observe His *mitzvot* and His laws" should suffice; why are we also told to "hear the voice of the Lord"?

The Torah alerts us to the central role of conscience within traditional Judaism. The requirement to go *mishurat lifnim ha-din,* beyond the limits of the law, springs from the perception that what is legal represents a moral minimum, a kind of popular consensus of the possible.

But law does not exhaust the full extent of morality. While establishing communal norms for minimal acceptable behavior, law is unable to cultivate the fullest and highest in human living.

Judaism recognizes the need for conscience to supplement the consensus of the law.

Thus, Abraham opposes God when God wants to destroy the city of Sodom and Gomorrah. Moses refuses to cooperate when God is enraged with the Jewish people in the wilderness. The prophet Jeremiah goes so far as to put God on trial!

Rabbi Moses ben Nahman, the Ramban, recognized the role of conscience when he spoke of a *naval birshut ha-Torah,* a scoundrel within the permissible limits of the Torah. Without the call of conscience, one can separate the letter of the law from its ultimate intention, to the detriment of both law and justice.

One can observe the *mitzvah* of *kashrut* and still be a glutton. One can pursue the *mitzvah* of *tikkun olam,* social justice, while still treating close associates as objects and neglecting the emotional needs of family members.

Observing the *mitzvot* is obligatory. The God of Israel calls us to a life of service, compassion, and sanctity.

But observing the *mitzvot* is not enough. We are also called to "hear God's voice," which the *Tanakh* portrays as "a still, small voice."

That voice corroborates a deeper truth within. It awakens us to a fuller understanding of ourselves and our obligations toward other human beings and to the planet as a nurturing home.

The *mitzvot* are necessary to provide a basic minimum. Just as with other legal systems, *halakhah* builds a communal consensus around the basic requirements of honesty, respecting the rights of others, and lawful living. Unique to Jewish law is its additional concern to make holiness a regular part of individual and communal behavior. But *halakhah* is not able to cope with the cement that holds civilization together: trust, decency, and goodness. These are matters of conscience, traces of the Divine within us.

The Holy One speaks to us through both.

Parashat Ki-Tavo/When You Come In
Take 3

Messengers Who Forgot the Message

In my family, different people possess different talents. My sister is a gifted artist; her etchings and sculptures add beauty to our lives. My wife, a brilliant attorney, is also a superb chanter of Torah. My brother is a budding actor, and his impersonations and drama enchant and compel.

Everyone has his or her own special blend of talent, interest, and skill. How we combine these gifts, and whether or not we choose to cultivate our strengths, can spell the difference between a contented life and one of frustration, between a useful contribution to society and a rather mediocre getting by.

What is true of individuals is true for a people as well. Each civilization has excelled in some areas, while being forced to rely on the achievements and insights of other peoples in other fields. Egyptian mathematics, Babylonian science, Greek sculpture and theater, Roman architecture, Indian philosophy, British literature, Chinese cooking, Dutch painting, and Arab grammar are all examples of a national culture reaching heights of excellence in a particular field.

The Jews, too, possess an area of special skill and interest in which we have shown distinction. We soar in the realm of the spirit, carrying much of the rest of humanity on the wings of our spiritual endeavors. Today's Torah portion addresses this unique religious genius. Moses relates,

> The Lord will establish you as His holy people, as He swore to you, if you keep the commandments of the Lord your God and walk in His ways. And all the peoples of the earth shall see that the Lord's name is proclaimed over you.

We are, in the words of Rabbi Abraham Joshua Heschel, messengers who have forgotten the message. We are a people with a purpose.

Unexceptional as an entity in so many other areas, the Jews are a rich and fertile source of spirituality and religion for all humanity and ourselves.

Throughout the millennia, our insights about the One God, creator of heaven and earth, source of morality and seeker of justice, have enlightened the lives and quiet moments of untold millions. The sacred writings of our teacher Moses, the stirring words of our prophets, reverberate wherever a commitment to human betterment, equality, and liberty remain.

Slaves seeking freedom quote Moses when they insist, "Let my people go!" Nations eager to guard their independence quote Leviticus when they demand, "Proclaim liberty throughout the land, and to all the inhabitants thereof!" And ethicists draw on the heritage of the Torah when they remind us of our obligation to love our neighbors as ourselves.

In a secular age, when people are valued for what they can do rather than for who they are, when esteem results from financial power rather than from character, it is difficult for Jews to remember our own national specialty, to remain true to our own unique skill. Our specialty is out of step with this age, as with every age.

The truths of the spirit involve a rejection of much that is prized by our neighbors.

The truths of the prophets demand an insistence on justice and compassion for all people.

The truths of the rabbis require an infusion of holiness even in the most mundane areas of human life and human discourses.

When we "walk in God's ways," when we "keep the commandments of the Lord," we reclaim our legacy of greatness, the one that projected the presence of Jews onto the stage of world history—a moderating, civilizing force for all humanity.

That legacy is ours to claim, even today. In the words of Isaiah, "Only let us be called by Your name."

NITZAVIM/You Are Gathered
Deuteronomy 29:9–30:20

Moses summons all of Israel—men, women, children, and strangers—to ratify the covenant. Indeed, this new covenant is so inclusive that it reaches beyond those present at the time: "I make this covenant, with its sanctions, not with you alone, but both with those who are standing here with us this day before Adonai our God and with those who are not with us here this day." He also points out the consequences of violating the covenant, and how dire those acts will be, but reminds his listeners that "concealed acts concern Adonai our God; but with overt acts, it is for us and our children ever to apply all the provisions of this Torah."

In the midst of enumerating the disasters that disobedience will elicit, Moses asserts the saving power of God's love and of teshuvah (repentance): "When you return to the Lord your God then the Lord your God will restore your fortunes and take you back in love." He asserts that these teachings are not too complex or too distant, but rather "the thing is very close to you, in your mouth and in your heart, to observe it."

And once again, Moses reminds us that this is about our own choices: "See, I set before you this day life and prosperity, death and adversity. For I command you this day, to love the Lord your God, to walk in God's ways, and to keep God's commandments. I call heaven and earth to witness against you this day: I have put before you life and death, blessing and curse. Choose life—if you and your offspring would live— by loving the Lord your God, heeding God's commands, and holding fast to God."

The Concealed and Revealed

Is it the good deed, or the right intention, which makes a person godly?

Moses tells the Jewish People, "That which is concealed is the Lord our God's; that which is revealed is ours and our children's forever, that we may fulfill all the words of this Instruction."

Traditionally, biblical commentators have understood both parts of this verse to apply to physical deeds. Tractate Sanhedrin, in the Babylonian Talmud, for example, explains that Moses is speaking about sins committed in private, which cannot be punished by a human court. The Talmud understands this verse to limit the power of our system of justice—people can be held accountable only for crimes committed in public. Only God can punish all other crimes.

According to this understanding, Moses is telling us that human beings should regard behavior as the stage on which to enact our humanity. In the words of Rabbi Israel Salanter, "Think about your fellow's body and your own soul, and not the reverse."

Our obligation as Jews and as human beings is to see that other people aren't starving, homeless, or lacking medical care. We should see that they are able to get an education, a job, and some security. The *nistarot,* that which is hidden, is properly God's concern, not ours.

There is great wisdom in that reading of the Torah, for it motivates us to concentrate on helping our fellow human beings in a very practical way.

It is also possible to interpret the words of Moses here very differently. External behavior is the limit of what human beings can see, measure, and judge. But that which underlies the behavior and is ultimately hidden from our view belongs to God.

A person can keep kosher and still treat others with cruelty. Someone can pray three times a day and still feel angry and bitter. Conversely, someone can never pray at all and focus all of his or her attention on good deeds, but perform those deeds to feed an insatiable ego.

The *meaning* of behavior is invisible to any outsider. And it is the *meaning* of the act—not just the act itself—that makes a "pleasing odor before the Lord."

The only one who can know whether our intentions are as sacred as our acts is God . . . and ourselves.

We know, in our hearts, whether we pray with sincerity or out of a sense of self-righteousness. We know whether our greeting another person is based on true concern for that person or motivated by wanting them to think well of us.

The hidden things are the Lord's. By seeking to align our concealed inner intentions with our revealed outer deeds, we can attain true godliness.

And that is our task.

Parashat Nitzavim/You Are Gathered
Take 2

On This Day, God Calls to You

Religion can transmit a sense of the majesty of the past. Traditions, because they come to us from a purer time, embody fragile vessels carrying remnants of a lost insight, the treasures of our ancestors' seeking and recording their relationship with God. The danger we face is idolizing the past, removing God from the theater of our own lives, trivializing the value of our own continuing journeys, ignoring the harvest of our own insight and response.

In this week's *parashah* Moses himself urges us against excessively venerating the past. "You stand *this day,* all of you, before the Lord your God . . . to enter into the covenant of the Lord your God, which the Lord your God is concluding with you *this day* . . . that He may establish you *this day* as His people and be your God."

Three times Moses stresses the phrase "this day." Rashi notices this repetition, and comments that the chorus of "this day" indicates that, "just as this day enlightens, so will God enlighten [the Jewish People] in the future."

God's relationship with humanity is a permanent expression of love, an ongoing reality no less than gravity or sunrise. Divine love is the source of the laws of nature, unifying human enterprise and the rhythms of nature.

To center one's faith in the past is to imprison God within a book or a set of books. To center one's faith in the living Source of life, the God of creation and of the revelation, is to liberate one's spirit to the continuous abundance of God's loving-kindness and grace.

Jewish tradition is sacred because it reflects our ancestors' intimacy with God and cultivates within us a responsiveness and an eagerness for that same intimacy, which means that Jewish tradition is only a vehicle in which to realize a love relationship with God.

For Jews, such a relationship may be attainable only through the practice of ritual acts and good deeds, through ongoing learning, and through prayer. At the same time, the Torah's emphasis on "this day" addressing "all of you" reminds us that the goal is not to perform *mitzvot*. The goal is God. *Mitzvot* are our special pathways leading to the splendor of the Holy One.

As with our ancestors, the Divine Creator beckons to each one of us. "Come, My beloved, come away."

Today, this day, God calls to you, and to your neighbor, and to me. Today, even now, the Holy One of Israel awaits our response.

Parashat Nitzavim/You Are Gathered
Take 3

Not in Heaven

We Americans are justly proud of our heritage of religious freedom, whereby a person is judged not by denominational affiliation, but on merit. At the same time, the spirit of tolerance is often expressed in public discourse as deriving from a "Judeo-Christian" heritage, reflected in "three religious traditions": Protestant, Catholic, and Jewish.

But Judaism isn't only a religion. If Judaism were just a religion, someone who stopped believing in Judaism would no longer be Jewish. Yet every Jew can tell you that a nonreligious Jew is . . . a Jew!

Judaism certainly includes many elements of a religion. Jewish civilization has always been passionate about God, holiness, and morality. We celebrate religious holidays, and have holy books, religious leaders, and religious symbols. But being a Jew also involves identifying with a specific people and with their history, culture, and identity. Particularly in the modern age, Jewish religion and Jewish culture are often in opposing positions on specific issues.

The Talmud tells of a giant who owned a bed. When a guest was too tall for the bed, he would cut off the guest's arms and legs to make the fit exact. Defining Judaism solely as a religion is that same kind of amputation. We do it so that Jewish reality can fit into a Gentile category of thought, but we know that the definition excludes a great deal of what being Jewish is all about.

One of the most famous passages in the entire Torah addresses the nature of the Torah itself. "It is not in the heavens, that you should say, 'Who among us can go up to the heavens and get it for us and impart it to us, that we may observe it,'" God tells us. Angels may be in heaven. Demons, possibly. But the Torah, the path joining the Jewish People and the Divine, is a very earthly book. Its concerns, its logic, and its language are the stuff of human life and human need.

The *Midrash Devarim Rabbah* explains that this verse means "the Torah is not to be found among astrologers, whose work is to gaze at the heavens."

In the weeks that have passed, we have taken a look at the Torah's attention: how to live in harmony with the land, how to establish standards of justice for the stranger and the citizen alike, how to establish seasons and festivals of holiness, how to live in the presence of God, how to educate ourselves and our children to the responsibilities and the grandeur of being a Jew.

Much of the Torah tells us how to build the Tabernacle, an earthly dwelling for God. Not only is the Torah not in heaven, but we even bring God from remote distances to become an intimate partner in human life and society.

Judaism believes in paradise, but insists that the Torah is not in heaven because we know that our task as children of God is to redeem Creation, to use the considerable resources of prayer, contemplation, study, and piety in order to establish the paradise of God's sovereignty here and now.

A Torah in heaven would be helpful in heaven. Our lives, our destiny, and our challenge is right here on our planet. By building communities of justice and compassion, by giving families the tools they need to raise good and honest Jews, we make our Torah a living force.

Right here on earth.

VA-YELEKH/He Went
Deuteronomy 31:1–31:30

With Parashat Va-Yelekh, Moses begins the epilogue, concluding the great series of addresses that are the Book of Deuteronomy. He begins by announcing his own impending retirement, and the transfer of leadership to Joshua. It will be Joshua who will lead the Israelites in the conquest of the land, and Moses exhorts them to "be strong and resolute, be not in fear or in dread of them; for Adonai your God marches with you: God will not fail you or forsake you." Moses then transfers the mantle of leadership to Joshua by repeating his charge to Joshua in the presence of the entire people.

Moses writes down the Torah and puts it into the care of the priests and elders, who are charged with its interpretation and its regular public recital every Shemittah (Sabbatical Year). Strikingly, the public reading is for men, women, children, and the strangers who are now part of the confederation Israel.

God calls Moses and Joshua, to prepare the transfer of leadership by directly appointing Joshua. Then God informs Moses that the Israelites are bound to disobey in the future, and he instructs Moses to compose a poem-song that will warn the Israelites and serve as to witness to them about the punishment their disloyalty will incur. Only then does God actually install Joshua, using similar language to that of Moses.

Moses then follows up with the Levites, informing them about the care of the Torah, and convenes the Israelites to hear the chanting of the song of witness.

Parashat Va-Yelekh/He Went
Take 1

If Not Now, When?

One of the most painful rabbinic duties is to try to offer comfort after a doctor has informed someone that he has a terminal illness. What is there to say in the face of the unfairness of life, of the horror of the decree, and of the despotic way that illness ignores our most carefully conceived plans for the future?

Recently, I was called to the hospital to attend to a man who had just been informed of an advanced cancer that would probably take his life in the near future. Neither he nor his wife had any prior inkling that he was sick. A physical examination, prompted by a recurrent pain in his side, culminated in this awful prognosis.

I sat with the man and his wife for several hours, listening to their anger, sorrow, and pain. Toward the end of my visit, his wife became especially angry, telling me that they had saved their money for years, denied themselves meals out and new clothes, postponed trips and vacations, all in anticipation of a "golden years" retirement. Now, they would never have the years or the health to enjoy their savings, never be able to luxuriate in some idyllic future. "This cancer is cheating us of our retirement!" she stormed.

Her complaint fits far too many of us. How often do we postpone a legitimate pleasure—time with our loved ones, an afternoon walk by the beach, a weekend vacation—anticipating some time in the future when we will have the leisure we deprive ourselves of today.

In today's Torah portion, the rabbis of *Midrash Devarim Rabbah* comment on God's abrupt announcement to Moses, "Behold, your days approach that you must die." They relate a tragic tale of a father at his son's circumcision. The father takes some special wine that is being served at the *simhah,* and puts it away to be used at the boy's wedding, unaware that the child will die thirty days hence. Later that same evening, Rabbi Shimon ben Halafta meets death on the road, and notices that death looks strange. He inquires about the unusual experience, and death responds that the strange look is "on account of the talk of human beings who say 'This-and-that we will do,' while none of them know when they will be summoned to die."

None of us knows the hour of our death, nor the condition of our health in the future. Rabbi Shimon wisely observes that death is no respecter of personal status or wealth: "No one, when about to die, can say, 'I will send my slave in my stead.' No one has the power to say to death, 'wait for me until I have settled my accounts,' or 'until I have set my house in order.'"

Without knowing our own future, lacking any ability to avoid death, we act as if we have all the time in the world. The truth is, however, that only the present is real. All our pleasure, hope, love, and purpose is wrapped into this moment, this time. We may cherish our memories, but we possess only today. Even a man as great as Moses had to die, and so do we all. In the meantime, however, we can choose life—by making sure that we make time in the present for what is truly important and truly gratifying, even should tomorrow never come.

Obviously, some planning, some saving, some denial is essential. The likelihood is great that tomorrow *will* come, and we must prepare for it today. But it is also possible to overemphasize the importance of deferring pleasure. Moses, when told he would die, had no way to postpone the inevitable, nor do we.

Rather than putting off that vacation until retirement, take it now. Rather than working extra hours now in the hopes of spending time with our children a few years hence, luxuriate in their youth, already too fleeting. Rather than postponing the chance to grow spiritually, the time for us to act is now.

Hillel, a great sage of the *Mishnah,* taught us "Do not say 'when I have leisure, I will study,' for you may never have leisure." That wise advice applies to all areas of our lives. Don't put off letting your husband, wife, or sweetheart know that you care—he or she may not wait around for you to show you love. Don't postpone calling a dear friend, or writing a letter to a beloved relative with whom you haven't communicated in years. Neither they nor you will be around forever.

Perhaps the best balance is to live each day as if it were our last, while at the same time preparing for tomorrow in a way that will leave our loved ones, our faith, and our world a little stronger, a little better, and a little more capable of facing the future, whether or not we are there to share it.

Parashat Va-Yelekh/He Went
Take 2

The People of the Book

"Read this Teaching aloud in the presence of all Israel," Moses instructs the *kohanim,* the priests. "Gather the people—men, women, children, and the strangers in your communities—that they may hear and so learn to revere the Lord your God and to observe faithfully every word of this Teaching."

It's easy to be an impressive leader when you are the only one with any information. To gain the respect of a group of people who don't have the knowledge or the sources to challenge a ruling takes little real leadership. But from the beginning, Moses made it impossible for the Jewish community to be burdened with that kind of leadership by default. He taught the *kohanim* so they could teach the people—women as well as men, Gentiles as well as Jews.

No rabbi, educator, cantor, or teacher can hide the sources of his or her own learning. All Jews have access to the *Tanakh,* the Talmud, the *midrashim,* Jewish philosophy, and Jewish history.

What a liberation the Torah initiated! Suddenly, religion was elevated beyond the realm of mystery and clergy, and was transformed into the possession of anyone willing to set aside a little time for learning.

In learning, a Jew hears the voice of God. In study, a Jew joins a dialogue that has been in progress for three thousand years—a dialogue of love between God and the Jewish People.

Rabbis Louis Finkelstein, former chancellor of the Jewish Theological Seminary, said, "When I pray, I speak to God. When I study, God speaks to me."

We are, all of us, invited to a venerable interaction. The God of Israel doesn't glory in secrets, mysteries, or magic. Our God wants mature, thinking, feeling partners in the ongoing work of Creation, men and women willing to use their hearts and their minds in the service of spirituality, which means that thinking, no less than feeling, is a religious act.

Thinking, the *mitzvah* of Talmud Torah, is one of Judaism's greatest gifts to its children. In the process of thinking in response to ancient, medieval, and modern Jewish writings, we have an opportunity to remake ourselves in their image, to realign ourselves with their values, and to reread them in the light of our own insights and needs.

We are still, after all, the People of the Book.

✦◗◗◆◗✦

Parashat Va-Yelekh/He Went
Take 3

Our Children

When I was growing up, my childhood synagogue had a "don't ask, don't tell" policy about kids. We were expected to remain silent and invisible, so that the service could retain the decorum and majesty necessary for the adults to feel uplifted. One result of that policy was that the worship was indeed beautiful and focused. Another result was that no one brought children to pray. An additional result was that few young adults (the people who had the little children to begin with) participated in the worship service, since they were responsible for handling their own children, and the children weren't welcome.

Today, a few decades later, the pendulum has shifted, and many synagogues now go to great lengths to welcome young children. Using my own congregation as an example of a general phenomenon, we now run three parallel services for children: a tot *Shabbat* for the very young, a kid's service for the preschool age, and a Junior Congregation for the postkindergarten years. On *Shabbat* evening, the children ascend the *bimah* to hold little cups of wine during the recitation of *Kiddush,* and on *Shabbat* morning, the children march around the sanctuary for both Torah processions, often carrying their own stuffed Torah toys. One result of this policy is that the worship is chaotic and occasionally disrupted. Another is that there are periodic complaints when a parent isn't sufficiently attentive or a child is exceptionally rambunctious. Yet another result is that lots of children and young parents fill our worship services each *Shabbat* morning.

Is this progress? Or have we simply returned to the errors of an earlier time? When Jews first came to America in large numbers, they and their leadership resolved to establish services that were dignified and decorous precisely because they did not like the chaos of their hometown *shuls*. We, having grown up with these more staid and fastidious services, are returning to the chaos they abandoned. Are we making a mistake? Of course, the hope is that children who feel at home in the synagogue will mature to become adults who feel at home in the synagogue. But this gamble comes at a price: Kids, after all, are distracting and noisy. A *shul* filled with kids is hardly an island of repose, an oasis of tranquility. Is the venture worth the sacrifice?

We aren't the first to ask that questions. Indeed, today's Torah portion raises this very issue. Moses ordains the establishment of the *Hakhel,* a gathering of the entire Jewish People in *Sukkot* every seven years. During the *Hakhel,* the entire Torah was read anew, and discussed among the entire population. As Rabbi Aaron ha-Levi, fourteenth-century author of the *Sefer Ha-Hinnukh,* observes: "The ensuing discussion will lead to an appreciation of our Torah, its greatness and supreme value, which in turn will arouse great longing for it. With this attitude they will study and attain a more intimate knowledge of God. Thus they will merit good life and God will rejoice in their works."

The *Hakhel* was the chance for all community members to discuss the Torah and to renew their passion for it. So the Torah mandates: "Gather the people—men, women, children, and strangers." This commandment seemed strange to at least one Talmudic rabbi. Rabbi Eleazar ben Azariah asked, "If the men came to learn and the women to hear, why do the little ones come?" Won't their presence disrupt the very purpose of the *Hakhel,* making discussion and listening more difficult?

His answer is that we bring the children "in order to grant reward to those that bring them." Bringing the children entails a sacrifice indeed, but one that earns a great reward. The truth is that little children disturb the adults so that they are not able to pay attention and hear well, thus the question: Why do the children come? Why all the care and trouble about the children if they just disturb the adults? Isn't it more worthwhile to leave them at home where they won't disturb the worship? The answer comes: "In order to grant reward to those that bring them." There is a great reward in bringing children, and the reward is greater than the loss. Children are emotional, and the holy atmosphere makes a deep impression on the hearts of children, and draws them near to the worship of God. There is a reward and a benefit in this, even though there is an element of neglect of Torah study.

For the sake of educating children in Torah and good deeds, it is worthwhile to impair one's personal well-being. That is the wisdom of the ages, and the hope of this age, too. Always trying to balance the needs of every congregant, we still must make room for our littlest—and sometimes our noisiest—members: our children.

HA'AZINU/Give Ear!

Deuteronomy 32:1–32:52

Ha'azinu *is an extended poem, warning the Israelites of their future betrayal of God's covenant, and the disastrous consequences that this disloyalty will entail. It begins with an invocation of heaven and earth as witnesses against Israel when the poet is no longer alive.*

Then it moves through the history of God's relationship with the people Israel, and of Israel's consistent lack of gratitude and loyalty in the face of God's saving acts. The poet declares that God will, indeed, punish Israel for its rebelliousness, but will limit the severity of that punishment, and will ultimately turn Divine anger against Israel's enemies, the tools of God's temporary anger against Israel.

Ultimately, God will deliver a repentant Israel, and Israel will sing in celebration of that eventual redemption and salvation.

Moses concludes, after the end of the poem, that the people must remain devoted to Torah, since "this is not a trifling thing for you; it is your very life."

✦

Parashat Ha'azinu/Give Ear!
Take 1

Outer Garments and Inner Truth

Today's Torah-reading offers us one of the most exquisite poems ever written. At its outset, the poet invokes the faithful reliability of nature to witness God's faithfulness to the Jewish People:

Give ear, O heavens, let me speak;
Let the earth hear the words I utter!
May my discourse come down as the rain,
My speech distill as the dew.

In powerful words, Moses recites the history of Jewish enslavement in Egypt and of God's bountiful love in liberating the people and leading them to their own land. The poem then continues by warning the Jews to remember God's love and to remain faithful to their covenant with their Creator and Liberator.

How striking that the summation of the entire narrative of the Torah should be cast as a poem! That when God looks for a style intense enough to communicate passion and urgency, only poetry will suffice! Indeed, looking at God's instruction to Moses to "write down this poem and teach it to the people of Israel," the Talmud records the view that the poem in question is not simply this song of Moses, but actually the entire Torah.

What does it mean to claim that the whole Torah is poetry?

At its simplest level, this assertion recognizes the meticulous care that went into every word, every sentence of the Torah. A tremendous amount of attention resulted in a text of vivid beauty, in which each sentence contains precisely the right words, in exactly the right form. There is nothing haphazard or unintentional in the way the Torah is written.

On a deeper level, poetry is writing refined to its essence. Poetry can communicate in brief what it takes prose many pages to convey.

In this way, too, the Torah is poetry. A relatively short book, it has nonetheless been the mother of libraries. In commenting on the Torah, in considering the consequences of its instructions, men and women of all generations and of many religions have written millions of words, expanding on its insights. An ever-fresh fountain, the water of Torah fertilizes and energizes whatever it touches. Its brevity is a veil; its face is of infinite wisdom, love, and piety.

Finally, poetry is striking in that its most essential message is not its most overt. When Robert Burns wrote, "O my Love's like a red, red rose" he was conveying a truth of a higher order. On the level of literal truth, his statement was simply false—it is unlikely that his lover was green and prickly from the neck down, pungent and red from the neck up! A botanist would not agree that his lover shared the characteristic of a rose.

But a lover would intuitively understand that the kind of truth Robert Burns was communicating was not the sort that can be weighed, tested, or measured. Only paltry truths—the truths of things and objects— submit to that standard. The truth of meaning and value—truths of love, of exaltation, of good, and of right—such truths cannot be pinched, bartered, or measured.

And they cannot be conveyed in prose. Only poetry contains sufficient respect for the intangible and the overwhelming to make such truth audible to the human ear, remaining faithful to the heart.

The Torah's truths are true in that sense. And in that sense, all of the Torah, from the narratives of Creation to the lists of laws to the summary speech of Moses at the end, all of it is poetry. Its artfulness, its concise language, and its profound insight bear the hallmark of poetry.

In the words of the Zohar, the classic mystical commentary to the Bible:

> If one looks upon the Torah as merely a book presenting narratives and everyday matters, alas! Such a teaching . . . we too could compile. But the Torah, in all its worlds, holds supernal truths and sublime secrets. . . . Just as wine must be in a jar to keep, so the Torah must be contained in an outer garment. The garment is made up of the tales and stories, but we, we are bound to penetrate beyond!

May this year have been for you one of penetration to the very core of Torah's meanings, and may your further explorations bring with them joy, solace for sorrow, and redemption.

♦≈♦

Parashat Ha'azinu/Give Ear!
Take 2

Religion for a Secular Age

It is commonplace for religious leaders to mourn the weakening religion has suffered in modern times. In the "good old days," people took religion seriously. Now, however, science, psychology, and secularism dominate the way people think about issues and the way they live their lives.

Today's religion is, at best, occasional. Once a week, Americans sit in their houses of worship for a few hours of quiet contemplation and song. Then, having paid off their debt to God, they can return to their normal lives, with busy social schedules, leisure time, and career demands.

We separate religion from life. Issues of personal identity and meaning, questions about human frailty or aggression, political conflicts and how to resolve them—these become questions for "experts." All we ask of religion is to make us feel good and to provide our children with moral values.

Today's Torah-reading stands in opposition to the creeping trivialization of religion. The Torah says of religion that "it is no emptiness for you; it is your life."

Religion that is less than our very lives is not religion at all. It is a convenience for the comfortable. A tool for appeasing guilt and enforcing conformity, religion becomes—in such cases, one more aspect of social respectability.

The religion of the Torah and the rabbis, on the contrary, embraces every aspect of Jewish communal and individual life. What people eat (and how we prepare it); how we conduct our business affairs; how we treat our spouses, parents, and children; the structure of our homes; the fabric of our clothing; the institutions in the community and the extent to which the community cares for the poor and the weak—all these are understood to be religious issues which require a religious response.

Judaism is that response. It beckons us beyond ourselves. It seeks to implement that earliest agenda—to recognize the divine image in every human being, to confirm God's prophecy that Creation is very good.

Judaism is the vehicle for reflecting those values in our deeds, our relationships, and our society.

Such a religion has nothing to fear from science. In fact, science can be a useful tool, a source of information and of healing. Such a religion can use the perceptions of psychology to illuminate its own timeless insights into the human psyche. Such a religion can even benefit from a secularism that prods it beyond complacency and smug self-satisfaction.

The only threat to religion is from those who would limit it to being nice, comfortable, and occasional. That constricted faith may work for a while, but when the jagged edges of life's tragedies require a response, or when the joy of a *simhah* is reduced to simply a party, then modern, tailored, rational religion is unable to provide profundity, meaning, or comfort.

Life is not rational, nice, or comfortable. It is all encompassing, overwhelming, and mysterious. To be able to bring comfort to the afflicted and justice to the suffering, religion must also retain elements of mystery and aspects of discomfort.

As a full-time way of living, Judaism is without peer. It "is not emptiness for you; it is your life."

✦✦✦

Parashat Ha'azinu/Give Ear!
Take 3

The Spark of Eternal Life

For many Jews, the assertion that life extends beyond the grave sounds thoroughly Christian. Television preachers and evangelists may insist on eternal life, but surely Judaism doesn't coddle that kind of prescientific superstition!

Or does it?

The notions of life after death, the resurrection of the dead, and an eternal paradise for the righteous of *all* nations were recognized as essential elements within Jewish tradition until very recently. It is only with the modern infusion of panscientism—the insistence that only what can be measured, tested, or weighed is real—that some Jews began to ignore or deny Judaism's assurance of life eternal.

In fact, Judaism recognized the eternity of each human being from its earliest stages. In the Bible, human souls went to a place called *She'ol,* where they existed forever. The Judge Samuel is even summoned from *She'ol* to speak to the overcurious King Saul!

Such a belief is explicit in the Book of Samuel, where Hannah praises God as "the Lord [who] deals death and gives life, casts down into *She'ol* and raises up," and in the Book of Daniel, where the prophet reveals that "many of those that sleep in the dust of the earth will awake."

In our Torah-reading as well, the rabbis of the Talmud recognize a reference to human transcendence of death. God exclaims, "I deal death and give life; I wounded and I will heal." Just as a person is first wounded and later healed, so one first dies and is later given life. Just as healing will happen in the future, so God will give life in the future as well. Such a belief may be a cornerstone of Judaism, but we must still ask, is a belief in human immortality reasonable?

An afterlife is no more astounding than life itself. After all, it is highly unlikely that a collection of five organic elements (carbon, hydrogen, nitrogen, oxygen, and potassium) would be able to write or read an article on the Torah. Yet we do precisely that. We are able to care, learn, relate, and build together. That there is life at all is a miracle. Is it any more or less miraculous to expect that the power that could make us live once would allow us to live again?

A *midrash* tells a tale of two fetuses inside their mother's womb, immediately preceding birth. As their mother's contractions begin, one fetus turns to the other and announces, "I know that out there is no more umbilical cord, so we cannot eat. There is no surrounding sack of liquid, so we cannot survive. This is the end, there is nothing beyond the womb."

The second fetus responds, "Although I cannot prove it, since I've never been out there, I believe that everything we've been going through for the past nine months has been preparing us for something beyond. All our experiences and growth are for a reason. Maybe we don't *need* an umbilical cord or to be surrounded by liquid in our next form of existence." Judaism asserts that the God who created life can sustain life, that the source of our existence pervades and girds the cosmos, that being made in God's image, all human beings contain a spark of eternity. That we are eternal is God's gift of love to us. How we use that sacred spark is in our hands, a gift of love we offer back to the One who will redeem us from death itself.

VE-ZOT HA-BERAKHAH/
This Is the Blessing
Deuteronomy 33:1–12

The final parashah of the Torah ends on a joyous note; it is appropriately called "This Is the Blessing." Moses's final words to Israel are of benediction. Throughout his long leadership, Moses showed the people his authority as lawgiver, and his moral rigor as chastiser. Only now does he reveal to them what he has already shown God: his deep love for and loyalty toward the Jewish People.

He begins with praise of God's power, and God's devotion to Israel: "Lover, indeed, of the people, Their hallowed are all in Your hand." God's sovereignty is placed in the hands of the Jewish People.

Moses then goes through each tribe, offering a vision of its future, its character, and its challenges. After reviewing each tribe, he again praises God's love of the entire people: "O Jeshurun (Upright one), there is none like God, Riding through the heavens to help you . . . O happy Israel! Who is like you, a people delivered by Adonai."

After concluding his final blessing to his beloved people, Moses ascends Mount Nebo. Before dying, he gazes on the vista of the land that Israel will enter, and in which it will shape the history of all humanity. Then he dies, at the age of 120 years, "his eyes . . . undimmed and his vigor unabated."

The Torah pauses in its narrative to praise this "nursing father" of a prophet: "Never again did there arise in Israel a prophet like Moses—whom Adonai singled out face to face—for the various signs and portents that Adonai sent him to display in the land of Egypt, against Pharaoh and all his courtiers and his whole country, and for all the great might and awesome power that Moses displayed before all Israel."

Some of the Commentators
and the Commentaries
Influencing The Bedside Torah

Ancient

Avot de-Rabbi Natan—a *midrash* on *Pirkei Avot*

Mekhilta—a Halakhic *midrash* on the Book of Exodus; first- and second-century Israel

Midrash Rabbah—a collection of *midrashim* on each of the five books of the Torah: *B'raisheet Rabbah, Sh'mot Rabbah, Va-Yikra Rabbah, Ba-Midbar Rabbah,* and *Devarim Rabbah*; Israel, fifth through twelfth centuries

Mishnah—the authoritative compilation of rabbinic law and tradition by Rabbi Judah ha-Nasi; second-century Israel

Philo—philosopher whose comments on the Torah often were allegorical; first-century Egypt

Pirkei de-Rabbi Eliezer—aggadic *midrash*; eighth-century Israel

Pesikta de-Rav Kahana—sermons on the synagogue reading cycle; fifth-century Israel

Sifra—*midrash* to the Book of Leviticus; fourth-century Israel

Sifrei—Halakhic *midrash* to the Book of Numbers and Deuteronomy; fourth-century Israel

Talmud—extensive collection of rabbinic law, tradition, and narrative. The Jerusalem Talmud dates from the early fifth century; the Babylonian Talmud dates from the early seventh century.

Torat Kohanim—another name for the *Sifra*.

Medieval

Aaron Ha-Levi—thirteenth-century Spain; *Sefer Ha-Hinnukh*

Abravanel, Isaac ben Judah—fifteenth-century Portugal and Spain

Bahya ben Asher—thirteenth-century Spain

Bekhor Shor, Joseph ben Isaac—twelfth-century France

Levi ben Gershom (Gersonides or Ralbag)—fourteenth-century France

Hizkuni, Hezekiah ben Rabbi Manoah—thirteenth-century France

ibn Ezra, Abraham—twelfth-century Spain

Kimhi, David ben Joseph (the Radak)—twelfth-century France

Moses ben Maimon (Maimonides or the Rambam)—twelfth-century Spain and Egypt

Moses ben Nahman (Nachmanides or the Ramban)—thirteenth-century Spain and Israel

Rashi (Rabbi Shlomo ben Isaac)—eleventh-century France

Saadia ben Joseph (Saadia Gaon)—ninth-century Babylonia

Samuel ben Meir (the Rashbam)—twelfth-century France

Sforno, Ovadiah ben Jacob—sixteenth-century Italy

Modern

Alter, Robert—*The Art of Biblical Narrative, The Art of Biblical Poetry*

Douglas, Mary—*Purity and Danger*

Eliade, Mircea—*The Sacred and the Profane, Myth and Reality, The Myth of the Eternal Return, The Quest*

Epstein, Barukh Ha-Levi—*Torah Temimah*

Fox, Everett—*In the Beginning, And These Are the Names*

Freud, Sigmund—*Character and Culture, Totem and Taboo, The Interpretation of Dreams*

Fromm, Erich—*Escape from Freedom, You Shall be as Gods, Man for Himself*

Gillman, Neil—*Sacred Fragments*

Ginzberg, Louis—*Legends of the Jews*

Gottwald, Norman—*The Hebrew Bible: A Socio-Literary Introduction*

Greenberg, Moshe—*Understanding Exodus*

Greenberg, Simon—*A Jewish Philosophy and Pattern of Life*

Greenstein, Edward—*Understanding the Sinai Revelation*

Heschel, Abraham Joshua—*God in Search of Man, The Sabbath, The Insecurity of Freedom, What Is Man?*

Hirsch, Samson Raphael—*Horeb*

Kadushin, Max—*The Rabbinic Mind, Worship and Ethics*

Leibowitz, Nehama—*Studies in Genesis, Studies in Exodus, Studies in Leviticus, Studies in Numbers, Studies in Deuteronomy*

Levenson, Jon—*Sinai and Zion, Creation and the Persistence of Evil*

Levine, Baruch—*The JPS Torah Commentary: Leviticus*

Milgrom, Jacob—*The JPS Torah Commentary: Numbers*

Miller, Allan—*Towards a Philosophy of Conservative Judaism, Transference to Religion and Religious Personnel*

Neusner, Jacob—*The Enchantments of Judaism*

Plaut, Gunther—*The Torah: A Modern Commentary*

Rosenberg, Yaakov—Vice-Chancellor of the Jewish Theological Seminary

Rosenzweig, Franz—*The Star of Redemption, On Jewish Learning*

Rubenstein, Richard—*After Auschwitz, The Religious Imagination*

Sarna, Nahum—*The JPS Torah Commentary: Genesis, Understanding Genesis, Exploring Exodus*

Wyschograd, Michael—*The Body of Faith*

Index

community
  defining, 27
  dietary laws and, 185
  support of, 62, 93–94
compassion, 262–63
  elderly and, 105
  honesty and, 24
  leadership with, 250–51
  Seven Laws of Noah and, 14,
    132–33
competition, and money, 76
compromise, politicians and, 110–11
conflict resolution, dreams and, 73
conformity, 323–24
conscience, 330–31
conservation of environment, 7–8
contentment, wealth and, 316–17
corrupt behavior, 129–30, 132
courage, 251, 252
Creation story, 7–8
  equal rights for men and women
    and, 5–6
  ways of interpreting, 4–5
creativity, 47
crises, deepened perception and,
  28–32
culture, Jewish, 337

daily living
  enjoying pleasures of, 307–8
  experiencing holiness in activities
    of, 307–8, 329
  Jewish laws of, 131
  Judaism as way of, 349–50
death. See also loss; mortality
  commitment and, 118–20
  coping with reality of, 203
  facing terror of, 168–69, 203
  life after, 350–51
  and living in present, 340–41
  plans for future and, 340–41
  putting off, 104
  red cow purification and, 259
  taking life for granted and, 308

dependency on others, 94
  child's, 126–27
despair, resistance to, 84–85
dietary laws. *See kashrut*
dignity, 304–5
disabled persons, 206–8
  as catalysts, 208
  dehumanization of, 206–7
disconnectedness, feeling of, 160
discrimination, response to, 269–71
diversity, 7, 236–37, 248–49, 274,
  286–87, 329
dreams, 50–51
  conflict resolution and, 73
  interpretation of, 71–73
  Jacob's, 47–48
  Joseph and, 61–62, 68, 72
dust of the earth, Jews compared to,
  48–50

eating, prayer after, 300–301, 310
ecological awareness, 211
education, Jewish, supporting, 149–51
elderly, 104–6, 111, 213
empathy, 188, 272, 322
environment, 112
  conservation of, 7–8
  heredity versus, 11, 191–92
  of Israel, renewal of, 211
envy, 70
equality, 6, 95–96, 248, 249
  of men and women, 5–6, 111
  in sight of God, 290–91
  of young and old, 111
eternal life, 350–51
ethics
  rituals and, 198–200, 330
  situational, 228, 229
  spirituality and, 147
evil deeds
  individual responsibility for,
    252–53
  Jewish reaction to, 270–71
  silence in face of, 244–46, 277–78

as lifelong process, 238
leavening, 166–67
legacy, 40–41, 86–87. *See also* heritage
   spirituality as, 332–33
   traditions, 336–37
liberation, 101–3
   partial, 108–10
liberty. *See* freedom
life
   eternal, 350–51
   reverence for, 185, 195–96, 307–8
light(s) eternal, 144–45
   of menorah, 135–36, 234–35
living each day as if last, 340–41
loneliness, love and, 80
loss, growth of soul and, 80
love, 71
   for God, 143–44, 336–37
   God's, 143, 336–37
   of humanity, 222
   importance of, 30–31
   meaning of, 79–80
   power of, 37–38
   revelation and, 157

marriage, 228–29
martyrdom, 301–2
meekness, 33–35
men
   Creation myth and, 5–6
   moral development, 228–29
   and women, differences, 191–92
menorah, 135–36, 234
mindfulness, 307–8
miracles, 84, 117
mission of Judaism, 62, 63
mitzvot, 48, 132–33, 233, 235, 293,
   300, 310
   conscience and, 330, 331
   cultivating practice of, 116,
     118–20, 123, 131
   health considerations, 195–96
   holy light and, 145
   Jewish identification and, 116

Jewish study as, 239, 342–43
   loving God and, 295–96
   normal mysticism and, 329
   as pathways to God, 337
   prayer following, 328–29
morality, 64–65, 83, 129–30
   conscience and, 330–31
   human relationships and, 228–29
   Seven Laws of Noah and, 14
   situational, 228, 229
mortality, insights from awareness of,
   28–32
murder, 129–30, 278–79
mysticism, normal, 329

names, lists of, 92–94
Nazirites, 230–31
negotiation, 250
number seventy, significance of, 236

obedience, 309–10

parents
   behavior toward, 126
   honoring, 126–27
   responsibilities for children's
     deeds, 324–26
passive resistance, 269–71
Passover, 166–67
peace
   commitment to work toward,
     12–13
   honesty and, 23–24
   meaning of, 314–15
   rainbow as symbol of, 12–13
   symbols of, 315
perception
   power of, 243–44
   reality versus, 82
perspective
   human versus divine, 82–83
   of the "seeking Jew," 113
planning for future, 340–41
pleasures of life, enjoying, 307–8